CARDIAC POSITRON EMISSION TOMOGRAPHY
Viability, Perfusion, Receptors and Cardiomyopathy

Developments in Cardiovascular Medicine

VOLUME 166

The titles published in this series are listed at the end of this volume.

CARDIAC POSITRON EMISSION TOMOGRAPHY

Viability, Perfusion, Receptors and Cardiomyopathy

edited by

E. E. VAN DER WALL

Department of Cardiology,
University Hospital Leiden,
Leiden, The Netherlands

P. K. BLANKSMA

Department of Cardiology,
University Hospital Groningen,
Groningen, The Netherlands

M. G. NIEMEYER

Department of Cardiology,
Martini Hospital,
Groningen, The Netherlands

and

A. M. J. PAANS

PET Centre,
University Hospital Groningen,
Groningen, The Netherlands

This publication has been made possible with an educational grant from
Lorex Synthélabo, Maarssen, The Netherlands

LOREX
SYNTHÉLABO

SPRINGER-SCIENCE+BUSINESS MEDIA, B.V.

A C.I.P. Catalogue record for this book is available from the Library of Congress.

ISBN 978-94-010-4014-3   ISBN 978-94-011-0023-6 (eBook)
DOI 10.1007/978-94-011-0023-6

Printed on acid-free paper

TABLE OF CONTENTS

PART FOUR: *Myocardial perfusion*

In 1991 the National PET (Positron Emission Tomography) Research Center in Groningen, The Netherlands, has started its research activities. Besides brain research and oncology, cardiology has been one of the main areas of research of the Groningen PET center. A joint effort of the PET Center and the Department of Cardiology has lead to a comprehensive study program, in which a number of important issues are covered. A total of over 500 patients, volunteers, and animal cardiac studies have until now been accomplished using five different PET tracers: nitrogen-13 (^{13}N)-ammonia for myocardial perfusion, fluorine-18-fluorodeoxyglucose (^{18}FDG) for myocardial viability, carbon-11 (^{11}C)-CGP-12177 and ^{18}F-fluorocarazolol for myocardial β-receptor density, and ^{11}C-acetate for myocardial oxidative metabolism.

The fields of study closely correlate with the issues dealt with in this book, and include the following:

1. Myocardial viability is usually studied with the combination of ^{13}N-ammonia myocardial perfusion at rest and during a dipyridamole stress test, and ^{18}FDG after glucose loading or during a euglycemic glucose clamp. A new method of quantification with parametric polar maps was developed and described in the literature. A close cooperation European level is pursued in the EEC concerted action on PET investigations of cellular regeneration and degeneration in cardiology, and at the national level within the Interuniversity Cardiology Institute of the Netherlands (ICIN), comparing PET with other methodologies (^{18}FDG SPECT, ^{201}Tl and ^{99m}Tc SPECT, dobutamine stress echocardiography, MR imaging and ^{31}P MR spectroscopy).

2. Myocardial perfusion heterogeneity has been studied in normal volunteers (smokers and non-smokers), patients with syndrome X, patients with idiopathic ventricular fibrillation, and patients with hypertrophic cardiomyopathy. The findings have been compared with other cardiological techniques. The cold pressor test has been found to be a feasible non-invasive alternative to intracoronary acetylcholine for testing coronary endothelial function in a number of patient categories.

3. Myocardial oxidative metabolism is now studied with ^{11}C-acetate at rest and during dobutamine stress testing. This method is used to improve the accuracy of viability

studies, to investigate the working mechanisms of newly developed anti-ischemic drugs, and to increase the insight in fundamental mechanisms of myocardial hibernation.

4. Adrenergic beta-receptor density can very well be studied using PET imaging. The emphasis in Groningen has been placed on improving the existing compartment modelling, originally described by the group in Orsay, and by developing new ligands with other metabolic and affinity characteristics and improved applicability in several organs (heart, lung, brain).

Positron emission tomography has great potential. However, PET research and clinical application is rather complex. Therefore, a successful further development of PET, also in cardiology, heavily depends on a close interdisciplinary cooperation, also on an international basis.

We hope that this book, which reflects the Cardiac PET Conference in June 1995 in Groningen, contributes to a mutual international cooperation of all disciplines working in the field of PET.

Kong I. Lie
Willem Vaalburg

Clinical cardiology has made significant contributions to the understanding of cardiac perfusion and metabolism primarily through positron emission tomography (PET). Currently, PET plays a dominant role in defining regional myocardial viability and identifying patients with ischemic left ventricular dysfunction who might benefit from coronary revascularization. Based on simultaneous assessment of perfusion and metabolism, PET may be decisive for further patient management. Apart from the value of PET in patients with coronary artery disease, PET has been shown to provide unique information in patients with cardiac muscle disease, such as hypertrophic cardiomyopathy, and in patients with syndrome X. In addition, PET allows neuronal control assessment of the heart by receptor imaging.

To understand the present and future role of PET, one should be thoroughly acquainted with its main advantages and limitations. The advantages of PET are 1) its noninvasive character, 2) the availability of a virtually unlimited number of radiotracers, 3) its excellent temporal and spatial resolution, and 4) the ability to quantify myocardial perfusion and metabolism in absolute terms using physiologically appropriate mathematical models. Major limitations of PET are 1) the price of a PET scanner (up to 3 million US$), 2) the start-up and operational costs, and 3) the technical and logistic complexities, all resulting in a limited availability of PET facilities.

At present almost 200 PET facilities have been installed world-wide (the January 1995 figures for the USA were 76, Japan 36, and Western Europe 44). In order to compete favorably with the more conventionally applied techniques in clinical cardiology, such as echocardiography or single photon emission computed tomography (SPECT), the inherent weaknesses and strengths of PET should be weighed against the advantages and limitations of echocardiography and SPECT imaging. In particular in the era of cost-containment, health care departments require the development of adequate diagnostic and therapeutic strategies with the emphasis on cost/effectiveness for the different imaging modalities. Regarding the patient in whom the question of viability is predominant, one might consider starting a PET study rather than using PET as a last resort (*'ultimum refugium'* policy) following echocardiography, SPECT, and coronary

xi

arteriography. The algorithm of using PET as an initial test, which seems highly justified by its superior diagnostic accuracy over the other techniques, would shorten the diagnostic procedure and thereby reduce costs. To diminish the start-up and operational costs of PET imaging itself, one may think of stand alone cameras supported by generator produced radiotracers or by local PET radionuclide distribution centers. These options mandate a lot of patient studies per day or the use of radionuclides with a suitable half-life of several hours or more. Of course, expenses of all PET issues will go down as soon as the cardiology community is fully aware of its potential in daily clinical practice; increasing demands will lead to increasing patient studies per day, increasing use of radionuclides, a wider dissemination of PET facilities, all of which may ultimately reduce health care costs. To summarize, PET has currently provided clinicians with a unique powerful approach to evaluate myocardial perfusion, metabolism, and neuronal function. Whether future applications will continue to flourish depends largely on a better understanding of the clinical potential of PET in cardiology, its role in the decision-making process for specific patient groups, and reduction of 'hardware' costs; all these factors are pivotal in gaining cardiac PET a prosperous future.

Cardiac Positron Emission Tomography is a bibliographical reflection of a Symposium, held on June 8 and 9, 1995, Groningen, The Netherlands. At this Symposium all major issues dealing with cardiac PET were discussed from myocardial perfusion to viability, and from receptor imaging to cardiac muscle disease. A cost-benefit analysis of PET has been presented, which is -in view of the above-mentioned aspects of PET- of eminent importance for the future development of PET facilities. In addition, other competing imaging modalities such as echocardiography, SPECT imaging, and magnetic resonance imaging were broadly discussed.

Herewith we like to acknowledge all individuals, societies and institutions who have had a substantial contribution to our Symposium and, hence, to the appearance of *Cardiac Positron Emission Tomography*. First of all, we thank all authors and co-authors for making great efforts in preparing their superb up-to-date chapters. They are all excellent investigators in the field of cardiac PET or related imaging techniques, and they have stimulated both basic and clinical research with the aim of improving patient care. We are very proud to have included the *Wenckebach Lecture* presented by Dr. Paolo Camici, one of the foremost pioneers in cardiac PET imaging. We like to acknowledge our sponsors i.e. the Netherlands Society of Cardiology (NVVC), the Working Group on Nuclear Cardiology and MRI of the NVVC, the Interuniversity Cardiology Institute of the Netherlands (ICIN), the Netherlands Society of Nuclear Medicine (NVNG), the European Society of Cardiology (ESC), and the European Association of Nuclear Medicine (EANM), all of whom tremendously contributed to the success of our Symposium. We are very grateful for the indispensable assistance offered by the Board of Directors of the University Hospital Groningen, who laid the basis for the Symposium. We want to thank Prof.dr. K.I. Lie (Head Department of Cardiology, Groningen) and Prof.dr. W. Vaalburg (Head PET Center, Groningen) for their invaluable driving force behind the Symposium.

The appearance of our book would not have been possible without a generous educational grant from Lorex Synthélabo (Maarssen, The Netherlands), being the Founding Father of the Working Group on Nuclear Cardiology and MRI of the NVVC.

We are most grateful for the support by Nettie Dekker (Kluwer Academic Publishers, Dordrecht), Annelies Kwant-Joppe (Secretary Department of Cardiology, Groningen), and Jan Schoones (Leiden Medical Library). Lastly, we are very much indebted to Anneke van der Meij (Secretary Department of Cardiology, Leiden) who put a lot of effort in the preparation and completion of *Cardiac Positron Emission Tomography*.

We hope that this book will assist the clinical cardiologist, the nuclear medicine physician, the fellows in cardiology and nuclear medicine, the radiochemist, the physiologist, the basic research fellow, and the technician in understanding the most recent attainments in cardiac PET.

The Editors

Ernst E. van der Wall
Paul K. Blanksma
Menco G. Niemeyer
Anne M.J. Paans

LIST OF CONTRIBUTORS

Rutger L. Anthonio, National PET Research Center, University Hospital Groningen, Oostersingel 59, P.O. Box 30.001, 9700 RB GRONINGEN, The Netherlands
Co-authors: Aren van Waarde, Antoon R.M. Willemsen, Jan Pruim, Wiek H. van Gilst, Paul K. Blanksma, Willem Vaalburg and Kong I. Lie

Jeroen J. Bax, Department of Cardiology, Free University Hospital, De Boelelaan 1117, 1081 HV AMSTERDAM, The Netherlands
Co-authors: Jan H. Cornel, Frans C. Visser, Paolo M. Fioretti, Arthur van Lingen, Johannes M. Huitink, Otto Kamp, Gerrit J.J. Teule and Cees A. Visser

Paul K. Blanksma, Department of Cardiology, University Hospital Groningen, Oostersingel 59, P.O. Box 30.001, 9700 RB GRONINGEN, The Netherlands
Co-authors: Jan L. Posma, Richard M. de Jong, Jan Pruim, Antoon T.M. Willemsen, Rutger L. Anthonio, Evert van der Wall, Willem Vaalburg and Kong I. Lie

Otto-Erich Brodde, Institute of Pharmacology and Toxicology, Martin-Luther University Halle-Wittenberg, Medical Faculty, Magdeburger Strasse 4, D-06097 HALLE (Saale), Germany

Paolo G. Camici, MRC Cyclotron Unit, Hammersmith Hospital, Du Cane Road, LONDON W12 0NN, U.K.

Jan H. Cornel, Thoraxcenter, Room Ba 350, University Hospital Rotterdam, P.O. Box 1738, 3000 ROTTERDAM, The Netherlands
Co-author: Paolo M. Fioretti

Willem Flameng, Department of Cardiology, University Hospital Gasthuisberg, Herestraat 49, B-3000 LEUVEN, Belgium
Co-authors: Bharati Shivalkar and Marcel Borgers

Raymond W.M. Hautvast, Department of Cardiology, University Hospital Groningen, Oostersingel 59, P.O. Box 30.001, 9700 RB GRONINGEN, The Netherlands

Maria G.M. Hunink, Department of Health Sciences, University Groningen, Office for MTA, Ant. Deusinglaan 1, 9713 AV GRONINGEN, The Netherlands

Lukas Kappenberger, Department of Internal Medicine, Division of Cardiology, Centre Hospitalier Universitaire Vaudois, CH-1011 LAUSANNE, Switzerland
Co-authors: Xavier Jeanrenaud and Nicole Aebischer

Joan G. Meeder, Department of Cardiology, University Hospital Groningen, Oostersingel 59, P.O. Box 30.001, 9700 RB GRONINGEN, The Netherlands

Menco G. Niemeyer, Department of Cardiology, Martini Hospital, P.O. Box 30.033, 9700 RM GRONINGEN, The Netherlands
Co-authors: Joan G. Meeder, Aaf F.M. Kuiper, Paul K. Blanksma and Ernst E. van der Wall

Anne M.J. Paans, National PET Research Center, University Hospital Groningen, Oostersingel 59, P.O. Box 30.001, 9700 RB GRONINGEN, The Netherlands

Jan L. Posma, Thoraxcenter, University Hospital Groningen, Oostersingel 59, P.O. Box 30.001, 9700 RB GRONINGEN, The Netherlands
Co-authors: Paul K. Blanksma and Kong I. Lie

Christian A. Schneider, III Clinic for Internal Medicine, University Hospital Cologne, Joseph Stelzmannstrasse 9, D-50924 COLOGNE, Germany
Co-authors: Frank Baer, Eberhard Voth, Peter Theissen and Udo Sechtem

Markus Schwaiger, Clinic & Policlinic of Nuclear Medicine, Technical University Munich, Klinikum rechts der Isar, Ismaniger Strasse 22, D-81675 MUNICH, Germany
Co-authors: Götz Münch, Ngoc Nguyen and Don Wieland

Eng-Shiong Tan, Department of Cardiology, University Hospital Groningen, Oostersingel 59, P.O. Box 30.001, 9700 RB GRONINGEN, The Netherlands

Ernst E. van der Wall, Department of Cardiology, Building 1, C5-P25, University Hospital Leiden, Rijnsburgerweg 10, 2333 AA LEIDEN, The Netherlands

Aren van Waarde, PET Centrum, University Hospital Groningen, Oostersingel 59, P.O. Box 30.001, 9700 RB GRONINGEN, The Netherlands
Co-authors: Philip H. Elsinga, Rutger L. Anthonio, Ton J. Visser, Paul K. Blanksma, Gerben M. Visser, Anne M.J. Paans and Willem Vaalburg

William Wijns, Cardiovascular Centre, O.L.V. Hospital, Moorselbaan 164, B-9300 AALST, Belgium
Co-authors: Anne Bol and Jacques A. Melin

Antoon T.M. Willemsen, PET Center, University Hospital Groningen, Oostersingel 59, P.O. Box 30.001, 9700 RB GRONINGEN, The Netherlands
Co-authors: Paul K. Blanksma and Anne M.J. Paans

STATE OF THE ART IN CARDIAC POSITRON EMISSION TOMOGRAPHY
Wenckebach Lecture

Paolo G. Camici

Introduction

The great potential of positron emission tomography (PET) to elucidate tissue function is reflected in the increasing number of centers being established. Not only does the technique offer greater accuracy in the measurement of regional radioactivity concentration but it also enables the use of true biological tracers. PET is still seen as an expensive tool, principally because of the need of a cyclotron to produce the short-lived isotopes. However, much development has been carried out in recent years into compact, self-shielding cyclotrons which do not need a team of engineers for their maintenance. In addition, automated kits for the production of commonly used tracers are now available. In some cases, central cyclotron facilities are being installed to distribute tracers [principally fluorine-18 (^{18}F)-labeled compounds] to nearby centers. Parallel innovations in tomographic scanner design continue to blossom. These are providing greater efficiency of photon detection and improved image resolution. New detector and electronic designs are bringing with them greater reliability.

There has been much discussion about the dual roles of 'research' and 'clinical' PET.[1] A number of centers, particularly in the United States, have installed PET systems purely for clinical diagnosis, mainly in the determination of myocardial viability but also for applications in oncology and neurology. Diagnostic testing of this kind is clearly derived from original work carried out at research establishments. The terms 'research' and 'clinical' should therefore be regarded as complementary. PET centers devoted to medical research will, by their very nature, not become widespread. They rely on close connection with clinical research institutes and the collaboration between clinicians, radiochemists, tracer modellers, physicists and radiographers. Naturally, this will be an expensive undertaking, but the survival of such centers and, just as importantly, collaboration between them, is vital for the survival of PET in general.

1

E. E. van der Wall et al. (eds.), Cardiac Positron Emission Tomography, 1–14.
© 1995 *Kluwer Academic Publishers.*

Applications of PET in cardiology

Current applications of PET imaging in cardiology can be divided into three main categories: studies of regional myocardial blood flow, metabolism and pharmacology.

Myocardial blood flow

Radionuclide imaging techniques, e.g. thallium-201 (^{201}Tl), have enabled the assessment of nutritive tissue perfusion as opposed to measurements of epicardial coronary flow as measured by either thermodilution[2] or Doppler catheter techniques.[3,4] Prior to the advent of PET imaging technology, only directional changes of regional myocardial blood flow could be assessed using either planar gamma scintigraphy or single photon emission computed tomography with different single photon emitters.[5] Quantification of myocardial blood flow using these techniques was rendered impossible due to the physical limitations of the imaging systems and the tracers available. PET overcomes the physical limitations of previously available imaging systems mainly by providing the means for accurate attenuation correction, thus enabling absolute quantification of the concentration of radiolabeled tracer in the organ of interest.[6] As PET technology has advanced and rapid dynamic imaging has become possible, quantification of myocardial blood flow has been achieved following the development of suitable tracer kinetic models.

A number of tracers have been used for measurement of myocardial blood flow using PET, in particular, oxygen-15 labeled water ($H_2{}^{15}O$),[7-10] nitrogen-13 labeled ammonia ($^{13}NH_3$),[11-14] the cationic potassium analogue rubidium-82 (^{82}Rb)[15] and carbon-11 and gallium-68 labeled albumin microspheres.[16,17] Early PET studies used $^{13}NH_3$ and ^{82}Rb to provide qualitative assessments of myocardial blood flow.[11,18] Although kinetic models have been proposed for quantification of myocardial blood flow using ^{82}Rb,[19] these are limited by the dependence of the myocardial extraction of this tracer on the prevailing flow rate and myocardial metabolic state.[20] Therefore, quantitation of myocardial blood flow either under hyperemic conditions or in metabolically impaired myocardium is inaccurate. Furthermore, the high positron energy of this radionuclide results in relatively poor image quality and in a reduced spatial resolution due to the relatively long positron track of ^{82}Rb.[20] Although positron-labeled albumin microspheres can provide accurate estimates of myocardial blood flow, they require intraventricular injection which renders their use impractical. Currently, $H_2{}^{15}O$ and $^{13}NH_3$ are the most widely used tracers for the quantitation of regional myocardial blood flow with PET. Tracer kinetic models for quantification of myocardial blood flow have been successfully validated in animals against the radiolabeled microsphere method over a wide flow range for both $H_2{}^{15}O$[7-10] and $^{13}NH_3$.[13,14,21] The values of myocardial blood flow determined in normal human volunteers at rest or during pharmacologically-induced coronary vasodilatation are similar.[7,14] $H_2{}^{15}O$ is theoretically superior to $^{13}NH_3$ in that $H_2{}^{15}O$ is a metabolically inert and freely diffusible tracer[22] which has a virtually complete myocardial extraction which is independent of both flow rate[23] and myocardial metabolic state.[8] This makes $H_2{}^{15}O$ a particularly suitable tracer for measurements of absolute perfusion also under circumstances where metabolic abnormalities, which could affect myocardial trapping of $^{13}NH_3$,[24] may be present. On the other hand, the quality of myocardial $^{13}NH_3$ images is superior to that of $H_2{}^{15}O$ images. Both $H_2{}^{15}O$ and $^{13}NH_3$ have short physical half-lives (2 and 10 minutes respectively) which allow repeat measurements of myocardial blood flow in the same session.

Prior to the advent of PET technology, investigations of regional coronary blood flow in man were restricted to the level of the epicardial coronary artery. However, it is well established that the major regulatory site of tissue perfusion is at the level of the arterioles which are not amenable to catheterization. With the development of quantitative myocardial blood flow measurement using PET, it is becoming possible to challenge the function of the coronary microvasculature by measuring the coronary vasodilator reserve which is generally calculated as the ratio of the maximal flow following pharmacological challenge to the resting flow level. This definition of coronary vasodilator reserve is however dependent on the coronary perfusion pressure and also assumes that maximal vasodilatation has been achieved.[25] PET studies in healthy human volunteers have established that the normal coronary vasodilator reserve in response to a standard intravenous dose of dipyridamole (0.56 mg/kg over 4 minutes) is approximately 3.5 to 4.0.[24] This data is similar to those reported using the Doppler catheter technique for measuring epicardial coronary flow velocity.[26] The measurement of coronary vasodilator reserve is useful for the assessment of the functional significance of coronary stenoses in patients with coronary artery disease.[27] In addition, PET is particularly helpful in those circumstances where the coronary vasodilator reserve is diffusely (and not regionally) blunted, e.g. in patients with hypertrophic cardiomyopathy,[28] due to a widespread abnormality of the coronary microcirculation.

Myocardial metabolism

PET imaging has been used to probe a variety of cardiac biochemical pathways. Studies have been performed using labeled amino acids to measure amino acid metabolism and protein turnover rates.[29] However, the majority of PET metabolic studies have focused upon investigation of the pathways involved in energy metabolism and the alterations which occur in disease.

Oxidative metabolism
The normoxic heart relies mainly upon aerobic metabolism of free fatty acid (FFA) by ß-oxidation as its main source of high energy phosphates. In order to measure the flux through this pathway during normoxic and ischemic conditions, PET imaging has been performed after intravenous administration of the natural free fatty acid palmitate labeled with carbon-11 (^{11}C). These studies indicated that the clearance of ^{11}C-palmitate from the myocardium was related to the degree of oxidative metabolism, though absolute quantification of utilization rates was not possible due to the over-complexity of the model required to explain the behaviour of ^{11}C-palmitate in tissue.[29] Interpretation of myocardial uptake and clearance of ^{11}C-palmitate is further complicated by the dependence of these two parameters on the prevailing blood flow and dietary state. In ischemic tissue the clearance rates were found to be reduced, suggesting reduced free fatty acid utilization in these regions.[30] A few additional

studies have been performed using synthetic FFA analogues to assess oxidative metabolism,[29] but currently only a few PET studies with labeled free fatty acids are being performed. In this respect, studies with radionuclide free fatty acids appear more promising (Chapter van der Wall).

Carbon-11 labeled acetate (^{11}C-acetate) has been advocated as a tracer of tricarboxylic acid cycle activity[31] and has been used as an indirect marker of myocardial oxygen consumption (MVO$_2$) by PET in both experimental animals[31-34] and humans.[35] A number of studies have shown that the rate constant describing the clearance of ^{11}C-acetate from the myocardium correlates well with catheter measurements of oxygen extraction fraction from analysis of arteriovenous differences of blood oxygen content using the Fick Principle.[32-34] Clinical studies using ^{11}C-acetate have demonstrated a decreased clearance rate from infarcted myocardium.[36] More recently, ^{11}C-acetate clearance in reperfused myocardium has been found to be reduced to a similar extent to the reduction in myocardial perfusion.[37] However, the lack of appropriate models which accurately describe the complex tissue kinetics of ^{11}C-acetate have prevented absolute quantification of MVO$_2$ using this tracer. Furthermore, measurements of MVO$_2$ using this tracer will be subject to blood flow and dietary constraints similar to those encountered during measurements made using labeled FFA's. Therefore, it has been suggested that standardization of metabolic status is important to make meaningful assessments of MVO$_2$ using this tracer.[38]

A new method to quantify MVO$_2$ by inhalation of oxygen-15 labeled molecular oxygen gas ([15]O$_2$) has been developed recently.[39] The accuracy of this approach to quantify oxygen ejection fraction and MVO$_2$ has been successfully validated over a wide range of values in experimental animal studies.[40] Studies in human subjects yielded mean oxygen ejection fraction and MVO$_2$ values of 61 ± 8 % and 9.4 ± 1.8 ml/min/100g, respectively,[39] which are consistent with those values previously reported for man obtained from invasive catheterization studies. This technique promises to be of great use in the measurement of aerobic metabolism in human cardiac disease.

Glucose metabolism
Studies of glucose metabolism have been performed using PET, principally using fluorine-18-fluorodeoxyglucose ([18]FDG) as a tracer. This tracer is transported into the myocyte on the same trans-sarcolemmal carrier as glucose and is then phosphorylated to [18]FDG-6-phosphate by the enzyme hexokinase. This is essentially a unidirectional reaction, as no glucose-6-phosphatase has yet been identified in cardiac muscle,[41] and results in [18]FDG-6-phosphate accumulation within the myocardium. Thus, although measurement of the myocardial uptake of [18]FDG is proportional to the overall rate of trans-sarcolemmal transport and hexokinase-phosphorylation of circulating glucose by heart muscle, no information about the further intracellular disposal of glucose can be derived from measurements of [18]FDG uptake. A number of kinetic modelling approaches have been used for the quantification of glucose utilization rates using [18]FDG.[42] The major limitation of these approaches is that quantification of glucose metabolism requires the knowledge of the lumped constant, a factor which relates the kinetic behaviour of the [18]FDG to naturally occurring glucose in terms of the relative affinity of each molecule for the trans-sarcolemmal transporter and for hexokinase. Unfortunately, the value of the lumped constant in humans under different physiological and pathophysiological conditions is not known, thus making true *in vivo*

quantification of myocardial metabolic rates of glucose very difficult.

PET studies with [18]FDG and [82]Rb for assessment of myocardial glucose metabolism and perfusion respectively, were performed in fasting patients with chronic stable angina pectoris and angiographically proven coronary artery disease following supine exercise on a bicycle ergometer.[43] In the regions which demonstrated perfusion defects during exercise, an increased [18]FDG uptake was observed. This would be consistent with an increased glycolytic metabolism in the ischemic zone. Furthermore, the augmented glucose uptake in the ischemic territory was sustained well after the reversal of the perfusion defects and it was demonstrated that the glucose was probably being used to replenish glycogen stores which were depleted during the ischemic episode.

Additional [18]FDG studies were performed at rest in healthy volunteers, patients with chronic stable angina and patients with unstable angina under fasting conditions.[44] It was demonstrated that [18]FDG uptake was significantly higher in the unstable angina patients off therapy than in the normal subjects and patients with stable angina. The resting glucose utilization in the latter two subject groups were similar. This data indicates the presence of resting ischemia in these patients which could be alleviated by intravenous infusion of nitrates, as evidenced by a decrease in resting myocardial [18]FDG uptake.[44] Of interest was the finding that in patients with unstable angina, increased resting [18]FDG uptake could be observed in myocardial territories subtended by epicardial coronary arteries with non-critical stenoses.

Assessment of myocardial viability

With the advent of coronary revascularization and thrombolysis, it has become apparent that restoration of blood flow to asynergic myocardial segments may result in improved regional and global ventricular function. This is particularly important as left ventricular function is the most important factor for assessing prognosis in patients with coronary artery disease.[45,46] In addition, the greatest clinical benefit from revascularization is seen in those patients with the most severe forms of left ventricular dysfunction.[47] Therefore, the clinically important task is to be able to detect, pre-operatively, those dysfunctional segments which contain viable myocardium and thus, select those patients who may benefit from revascularization. Initial studies indicated that myocardial ischemia and infarction could be distinguished by analysis of PET images of the perfusion tracer [13]NH$_3$ and the glucose analogue [18]FDG, acquired after an oral glucose load.[48] Regions which showed a concordant reduction in both myocardial blood flow and [18]FDG uptake ('flow-metabolism match') were hypothesized to be infarcted and irreversibly injured, whereas regions in which [18]FDG uptake was relatively preserved or increased despite having a perfusion defect ('flow-metabolism mismatch') were considered ischemic and viable.[48] This hypothesis was tested by Tillisch et al.[49] who performed pre-operative PET scans in 17 patients undergoing coronary artery by-pass grafting. Regional wall motion increased after surgery in 35/41 segments displaying 'flow-metabolism mismatch' and remained depressed in 24/26 segments demonstrating 'flow-metabolism match'. This method has identified the presence of viable myocardium in regions that were considered necrotic, and thus non-viable, on the basis of conventional investigations, in particular:

1) Q waves on the electrocardiogram;[50] and 2) fixed defects on standard[51] and late redistribution[52] [201]Tl perfusion imaging. More recent studies have shown that a significant proportion of myocardial regions which have reduced end-diastolic wall thickness and no systolic wall thickening, as defined by spin-echo gated magnetic resonance imaging, have residual [18]FDG uptake on PET imaging.[53] Recent data from 82 patients with advanced coronary disease and severe left ventricular dysfunction suggest that the 'flow-metabolism mismatch' pattern identifies a subgroup of patients who are at an increased risk of sudden death and adverse cardiac events (i.e. myocardial infarction, cardiac arrest, late revascularization) and who may thus benefit most from revascularization.[54]

Other groups have proposed that [18]FDG images should be acquired alternatively, in either the fasting state[55] or using the euglycemic hyperinsulinemic clamp technique.[56,57] With the former, variable [18]FDG uptake in the heart has been demonstrated in normal subjects[58] and image quality is poor. Variability in regional [18]FDG uptake in normal volunteers has also been demonstrated after oral glucose loading,[56] and it is possible to observe 'flow-metabolism mismatch' in normal subjects.[59] This is a potentially confounding factor in the interpretation of images acquired from patients. With recent suggestions that semi-quantitative[60,61] and quantitative analyses of [18]FDG uptake may enhance detection of viable myocardium using PET, there is an urgent need to fix rigorously the study conditions, as the uptake of [18]FDG by the heart is dependent on many factors. In addition, many patients with coronary artery disease are insulin resistant (i.e. the amount of endogenous insulin released after feeding will not induce maximal stimulation due to partial resistance to the action of the hormone). This will results in poor [18]FDG image quality after an oral glucose load in many cases. To circumvent the problem of insulin resistance, an alternative protocol has been recently applied to the PET viability studies. This protocol is now accepted by most European PET centers that take part in an E.E.C. sponsored multicenter study. This protocol is based on the use of the hyperinsulinemic euglycemic clamp which basically consists in the simultaneous infusion of insulin and glucose that acts on the tissue as a metabolic stressor stimulating maximal [18]FDG uptake. The use of the euglycemic hyperinsulinemic glucose clamp provides excellent image quality, demonstrates uniform tracer uptake throughout the heart, and enables PET studies to be performed under standardized metabolic conditions.[56,57] This will allow a comparison of the absolute values of the metabolic rate of glucose (μmol/g/min) amongst different subjects. This approach is particularly useful in studying patients with coronary disease, many of whom have some degree of insulin resistance, as well as enabling more meaningful comparisons of data from different patient populations and study centers.

It has recently been suggested that the degree of myocardial viability may be overestimated when using radiolabeled deoxyglucose.[62,63] In particular, animal studies have demonstrated that the accumulation of ^{14}C-deoxyglucose overestimated the amount of viable tissue assessed according to histological criteria.[64,65] Several possible explanations may account for this observation. First, the presence of inflammatory cells in the necrotic zone which take up radiolabeled deoxyglucose may account for the elevated uptake of deoxyglucose in the infarct zone. Secondly, the elevated deoxyglucose signal may be accounted for by the presence of an admixture of necrotic and ischemic but viable tissue within the infarcted region. The enhanced uptake of deoxyglucose due to a reliance on glycolytic metabolism in the latter tissue type may result in an elevated estimation of the mean deoxyglucose uptake in the functionally compromised region as a whole.

Myocardial pharmacology

PET studies of myocardial pharmacology have principally concerned the sympathetic nervous system and tracers have been developed to probe the integrity of both pre- and post-synaptic sites. Alterations of this system have been implicated in the pathophysiology of a number of cardiac disorders, in particular, heart failure,[66] ventricular arrhythmogenesis,[67] coronary artery disease,[68] idiopathic dilated[69] and hypertrophic cardiomyopathy.[70,71] With the development of suitable tracers using PET, it may be possible to identify a more precise role for sympathetic nervous system dysfunction in the development of the above conditions.

Several ß-blocker drugs have been labeled with ^{11}C for imaging by PET.[72] The most promising of these is CGP 12177. This is a non-selective ß-adrenoceptor antagonist which is particularly suited for PET studies due to its high affinity and low lipophilicity, thus enabling the functional receptor pool on the cell surface to be studied.[73] Initially, racemic (R,S)-CGP 12177 was successfully labeled with ^{11}C and used to produce images in dogs.[72] However, it became clear that better quality data could be obtained by using the pure active enantiomer, (S)-CGP 12177, labeled with carbon-11. Studies in animals[74] demonstrated significantly improved myocardial uptake using the labeled (S)-enantiomer compared to the racemic compound. Analysis of plasma samples by high performance liquid chromatography taken up to one hour after intravenous injection of both (RS)- and (S)-CGP 12177 labeled with ^{11}C indicated the presence of 30% radiolabeled metabolites in rats and virtually none in greyhounds.[75]

A graphical method for quantification of ß-adrenoceptor density (B_{max}, pmol.ml^{-1}) from the PET data has been developed.[76] This approach requires two injections of ^{11}C-(S)-CGP 12177, one at a high specific activity followed by a second at a lower specific activity. Studies in our institution in a group of young healthy subjects have yielded B_{max} values of 10.4 ± 1.7 pmol.ml^{-1}, using a modified version of the above graphical analysis. ß-Adrenoceptor density was uniformly distributed throughout the different regions of the left ventricular myocardium. These data are consistent with literature values of B_{max} for ß-adrenoceptors in human ventricular myocardium determined *in vitro*.[66] Data indicate that ß-adrenoceptor density is decreased in patients with hypertrophic cardiomyopathy by approximately 25-30% relative to values in normal subjects.[77] The decrease in receptor density occurs in both hypertrophied and non-hypertrophied portions of the left ventricle. This data is consistent with the hypothesis that sympathetic overdrive might be involved in the phenotypic expression of hypertrophic cardiomyopathy. It is noteworthy that the density of ß-adrenoceptor is correlated with the systolic and diastolic function of the left ventricle. Reductions in the myocardial ß-adrenoceptor density of approximately 50% have been reported in patients with heart failure of different causes,[77,78] using in vitro ligand binding to homogenized myocardial biopsy samples. In a recent study, Merlet et al.[79] using S-^{11}C-CGP 12177 and PET reported a 53% decrease in myocardial ß-adrenoceptor density in patients with dilated cardiomyopathy compared to normal controls. Attempts have been made to study alpha-1 adrenoceptors *in vivo* using ^{11}C-labeled prazosin and PET,[72] but to date clinical studies have not been performed. Investigations of the alpha adrenergic system would be of interest as their levels have been found to alter as a result of myocardial ischemia[80] and they have also been implicated in arrhythmogenesis.[81]

In addition to post-synaptic receptor studies, PET has also been used to investigate the integrity of pre-synaptic sympathetic innervation of the heart. Three tracers have been used for this purpose: [18]F labeled fluorometaraminol,[82] ^{18}F-labeled fluorodopamine,[83] and ^{11}C labeled hydroxyephedrine.[84] These tracers compete with endogenous noradrenaline for the transport into the pre-synaptic nerve terminal via the neuronal uptake-1 transport system. Once within the neurone these compounds are metabolized and trapped and hence serve as markers of sympathetic innervation. Recent studies have demonstrated decreased retention of ^{11}C labeled hydroxyephedrine in patients after cardiac transplant which is consistent with the heart being denervated.[85] However, with time, some sympathetic re-innervation occurred particularly in the anteroseptal regions of the heart. This has recently been correlated with the recovery of sensation of angina pectoris in these patients.[86]

Furthermore, PET studies using ^{11}C labeled MQNB have been used to quantify the density of myocardial muscarinic cholinergic receptors in both experimental animals[87] and man.[88] These studies should be extended to patient groups given the possible pathophysiological role of muscarinic receptors in arrhythmogenesis and control of sympathetic nerve function. Investigations of peripheral type benzodiazepine receptors have also been reported using ^{11}C labeled PK11195 as a ligand.[89] Clinical studies using this tracer have not been performed, though are indicated by virtue of the linkage between these binding sites and dihydropyridine calcium channels.[90]

References

1. Coleman RE, Robbins MS, Siegel BA. The future of PET in clinical medicine and the impact of drug regulation. Semin Nucl Med 1992;12:193.
2. Ganz W, Tamura K, Marcus HS, Donoso R, Yoshida S, Swan HJC. Measurement of coronary sinus blood flow by continuous thermodilution in man. Circulation 1971;44:181.
3. Hartley CJ, Cole JS. An ultrasonic pulsed Doppler system for measuring blood flow in small vessels. J Appl Physiol 1974;37:626.
4. Cole JS, Hartley CJ. The pulsed Doppler coronary artery catheter. Preliminary report of a new technique for measuring rapid changes in coronary artery flow velocity in man. Circulation 1977;56:1.
5. Van der Wall EE. Nuclear cardiology and cardiac magnetic resonance. The Netherlands, Hans Soto Productions, 1992.
6. Hoffman EJ, Phelps ME. Positron emission tomography: principles and quantitation. In: Phelps ME, Mazziotta JC, Schelbert, editors: Positron emission tomography and autoradiography: principles and applications for the brain and the heart. New York: Raven Press, 1986:113-48.
7. Araujo LI, Lammertsma AA, Rhodes CG et al. Non-invasive quantification of regional myocardial blood flow in normal volunteers and patients with coronary artery disease using oxygen-15 labeled carbon dioxide inhalation and positron emission tomography. Circulation 1991;83:875-85.
8. Iida H, Kanno I, Takahashi A et al. Measurement of absolute myocardial blood flow with $H_2^{15}O$ and dynamic positron emission tomography: strategy for quantification in relation to the partial-volume effect. Circulation 1989;78:104-15.
9. Bergmann SR, Fox KAA, Rand AL et al. Quantification of regional myocardial blood flow in vivo with $H_2^{15}O$. Circulation 1984;70:724-33.
10. Bergmann SR, Herrero P, Markham J, Weinheimer CJ, Walsh MN. Noninvasive quantification of myocardial blood flow in human subjects with O-15 labeled water and positron emission tomography. J Am Coll Cardiol 1989;14:639-52.
11. Schelbert HR, Phelps ME, Hoffman EJ, Huang SC, Selin CE, Kuhl DE. Regional myocardial perfusion assessed by N-13 labeled ammonia and positron computerized axial tomography. Am J Cardiol 1979;43:209-18.
12. Krivokapich J, Smith GT, Huang SC et al. Nitrogen-13 ammonia myocardial imaging at rest and with exercise in normal volunteers: quantification of coronary flow with positron emission tomography. Circulation 1989;80:1328-37.
13. Bellina CR, Parodi O, Camici P et al. Simultaneous in vitro and in vivo validation of nitrogen-13 ammonia for the assessment of regional myocardial blood flow. J Nucl Med 1990;31:1335-43.
14. Hutchins GD, Schwaiger M, Rosenspire KC, Krivokapich J, Schelbert H, Kuhl DE. Noninvasive quantification of regional blood flow in the human heart using N-13 ammonia and dynamic positron emission tomographic imaging. J Am Coll Cardiol 1990;15:1032-42.
15. Herrero P, Markham J, Shelton ME, Weinheimer CJ, Bergmann SR. Noninvasive quantification of regional myocardial perfusion with rubidium-82 and positron emission tomography. Exploration of a mathematical model. Circulation 1990;82:1377-86.
16. Beller GA, Alten WJ, Cochavi S, Hnatowich D, Brownell GL. Assessment of regional myocardial perfusion by positron emission tomography after intracoronary administration of Ga-68 labeled albumin microspheres. J Comput Assist Tomogr 1979;3:447-52.
17. Wilson RA, Shea MJ, De Landsheere CH et al. Validation of quantification of regional myocardial blood flow in vivo with 11C-labeled human albumin microspheres and positron

emission tomography. Circulation 1984;70:717-23.

18. Selwyn AP, Allan RM, L'Abbate A et al. Relation between regional myocardial uptake of rubidium-82 and perfusion: Absolute reduction of cation uptake in ischemia. Am J Cardiol 1982;50:112-21.

19. Huang SC, Williams BA, Krivokapich J, Araujo LI, Phelps ME, Schelbert HR. Rabbit myocardial ^{82}Rb kinetics and a compartmental model for blood flow estimation. Am J Physiol 1989;256:H1156-H64.

20. Araujo LI, Schelbert HR. Rubidium-82: Dynamic positron emission tomography in ischaemic heart disease. Am J Cardiac Imag 1984;1:117-24.

21. Shah A, Schelbert HR, Schwaiger M, Hansen H, Selin C. Measurement of regional myocardial blood flow with N-13 ammonia and positron emission tomography in intact dogs. J Am Coll Cardiol 1985;5:92-100.

22. Johnson JA, Cavert HM, Lifson N. Kinetics concerned with distribution of isotopic water in isolated dog heart and skeletal muscle. Am J Physiol 1952;171:687-93.

23. Yipintsoi T, Bassingthwaite JB. Circulatory transport of iodoantipyrine and water in the isolated dog heart. Circ Res 1970;27:461-7.

24. Bergmann SR, Hack S, Tewson T, Welch MJ, Sobel BE. The dependence of accumulation of ^{13}NH$_3$ by myocardium on metabolic factors and its implications for the quantitative assessment of perfusion. Circulation 1980;61:34-43.

25. De Silva R, Camici PG. Role of positron emission tomography in the investigation of human coronary circulation. Cardiovasc Res 1994;28:1595-612.

26. Rossen JD, Simonetti I, Marcus ML, Winniford MD. Coronary dilatation with standard dose dipyridamole and dipyridamole combined with handgrip. Circulation 1989;79:556-72.

27. Uren NG, Melin JA, De Bruyne B, Wijns W, Baudhuin T, Camici PG. Relation between myocardial blood flow and the severity of coronary artery stenosis. N Engl J Med 1994;330:1782-8.

28. Camici PG, Chiriatti G, Lorenzoni R et al. Coronary vasodilation is impaired in both hypertrophied and nonhypertrophied myocardium of patients with hypertrophic cardiomyopathy: a study with nitrogen-13 ammonia and positron emission tomography. J Am Coll Cardiol 1991;17:879-86.

29. Schelbert HR, Schwaiger M. PET studies of the heart. In: Phelps ME, Mazziotta JC, Schelbert HR, editors. Positron Emission Tomography and Autoradiography. Principles and Applications for the Brain and the Heart. New York: Raven Press, 1986:581-662.

30. Schelbert HR, Henze E, Schon HR et al. C-11 Palmitic acid for the noninvasive evaluation of regional myocardial fatty acid metabolism with positron computed tomography. IV. In vivo demonstration of impaired fatty acid oxidation in acute myocardial ischemia. Am Heart J 1983;106:736-50.

31. Buxton DB, Schwaiger M, Nguyen A, Phelps ME, Schelbert HR. Radiolabeled acetate as a tracer of myocardial tricarboxylic acid cycle flux. Circ Res 1988;63:628-34.

32. Armbrecht JJ, Buxton DB, Schelbert HR. Validation of [1-^{11}C]acetate as a tracer for noninvasive assessment of oxidative metabolism with positron emission tomography in normal, ischemic, postischemic, and hyperemic canine myocardium. Circulation 1990;81:1594-605.

33. Brown MA, Myears DW, Bergmann SR. Noninvasive assessment of canine myocardial oxidative metabolism with carbon-11 acetate and positron emission tomography. J Am Coll Cardiol 1988;12:1054-63.

34. Buxton DB, Nienaber CA, Luxen A et al. Noninvasive quantitation of regional myocardial oxygen consumption in vivo with [1-^{11}C]acetate and dynamic positron emission tomography. Circulation 1989;79:134-42.

35. Armbrecht JJ, Buxton DB, Brunken RC, Phelps ME, Schelbert HR. Regional myocardial

oxygen consumption determined noninvasively in humans with [1-^{11}C] acetate and dynamic positron tomography. Circulation 1989;80:863-72.

36. Walsh MN, Geltman EM, Brown MA et al. Noninvasive estimation of regional myocardial oxygen consumption by positron emission tomography with carbon-11 acetate in patients with myocardial infarction. J Nucl Med 1989;30:1798-808.

37. Vanoverschelde JLJ, Melin JA, Bol A et al. Regional oxidative metabolism in patients after recovery from reperfused anterior myocardial infarction. Relation to regional blood flow and glucose uptake. Circulation 1992;85:9-21.

38. Hicks RJ, Herman WH, Kalff V et al. Quantitative evaluation of regional substrate metabolism in the human heart by positron emission tomography. J Am Coll Cardiol 1991;18:101-11.

39. Iida H, Rhodes CG, Yamamoto Y et al. Quantitative measurement of myocardial metabolic rate of oxygen (MMRO$_2$) in man using positron emission tomography. Circulation 1990;82:III-614 (Abstract).

40. De Silva R, Yamamoto Y, Rhodes CG, Iida H, Maseri A, Jones T. Non-invasive quantification of regional myocardial oxygen consumption in anaesthetized greyhounds. J Physiol 1992;446:219P (Abstract).

41. Gallagher BM, Fowler JS, Gutterson NI, MacGregor RR, Wan C-N, Wolf AP. Metabolic trapping as a principle of radiopharmaceutical design: Some factors responsible for the biodistribution of [^{18}F] 2-deoxy-2-fluoro-D-glucose. J Nucl Med 1978;19:1154-61.

42. Huang SC, Phelps ME. Principles of tracer kinetic modeling in positron emission tomography and autoradiography. In: Phelps ME, Mazziotta JC, Schelbert HR, editors. Positron emission tomography and autoradiography. Principles and applications for the brain and heart. New York: Raven Press, 1986:287-346.

43. Camici P, Araujo LI, Spinks T et al. Increased uptake of ^{18}F-fluorodeoxyglucose in postischemic myocardium of patients with exercise-induced angina. Circulation 1986;74:81-8.

44. Araujo LI, Camici P, Spinks T, Jones T, Maseri A. Beneficial effects of nitrates on myocardial glucose utilization in unstable angina pectoris. Am J Cardiol 1987;60:26H-30H.

45. Mock M, Ringvist I, Fisher LD et al. Survival of medically treated patients in the Coronary Artery Surgery Study (CASS) Registry. Circulation 1982;66:562-8.

46. The Multicenter Postinfarction Research Group. Risk stratification and survival after myocardial infarction. N Engl J Med 1983;309:331-6.

47. Califf RM, Harrel FE, Lee KL et al. Changing efficacy of coronary revascularization. Implications for patient selection. Circulation 1988;78(Suppl I):I-185-I-91.

48. Marshall RC, Tillisch JH, Phelps ME et al. Identification and differentiation of resting myocardial ischemia and infarction in man with positron computed tomography, ^{18}F-labeled fluorodeoxyglucose and ^{13}N ammonia. Circulation 1981;64:766-78.

49. Tillisch J, Brunken R, Marshall R et al. Reversibility of cardiac wall motion abnormalities predicted by positron tomography. N Engl J Med 1986;314:884-8.

50. Brunken R, Tillisch J, Schwaiger M et al. Regional perfusion, glucose metabolism, and wall motion in patients with chronic electrocardiographic Q wave infarctions: evidence for persistence of viable tissue in some infarct regions by positron emission tomography. Circulation 1986;73:951-63.

51. Brunken R, Schwaiger M, Grover-McKay M, Phelps ME, Tillisch J, Schelbert HR. Positron emission tomography detects tissue metabolic activity in myocardial segments with persistent thallium perfusion defects. J Am Coll Cardiol 1987;10:557-67.

52. Brunken RC, Mody FV, Hawkins RA, Nienanber CA, Phelps ME, Schelbert HR. Positron emission tomography detects metabolic viability in myocardium with persistent 24-hour

single-photon emission computed tomography ^{201}Tl defects. Circulation 1992;86:1357-69.
53. Perrone-Filardi P, Bacharach SL, Dilsizian V et al. Metabolic evidence of viable myocardium in regions with reduced wall thickness and absent wall thickening in patients with chronic ischemic left ventricular dysfunction. J Am Coll Cardiol 1992;20:161-8.
54. Eitzman D, Al-Aouar Z, Kanter HL et al. Clinical outcome of patients with advanced coronary artery disease after viability studies with positron emission tomography. J Am Coll Cardiol 1992;20:559-65.
55. Tamaki N, Yonekura Y, Yamashita K et al. Positron emission tomography using fluorine-18 deoxyglucose in evaluation of coronary artery bypass grafting. Am J Cardiol 1989;64:860-5.
56. Hicks RJ, Herman WH, Kalff V et al. Quantitative evaluation of regional substrate metabolism in the human heart by positron emission tomography. J Am Coll Cardiol 1991;18:101-11.
57. Knuuti MJ, Nuutila P, Ruotsalainen U et al. Euglycemic hyperinsulinemic clamp and oral glucose load in stimulating myocardial glucose utilization during positron emission tomography. J Nucl Med 1992;33:1255-62.
58. Gropler RJ, Siegal BA, Lee KJ et al. Nonuniformity in myocardial accumulation of ^{18}F fluorodeoxyglucose in normal fasted humans. J Nucl Med 1990;31:1749-56.
59. Berry JJ, Pieper S, Hanson MW, Hoffman JM, Coleman RE. The effect of metabolic milieu on cardiac PET imaging with fluorine-18 deoxyglucose and nitrogen-13 ammonia in normal volunteers. J Nucl Med 1991;32:1518-25.
60. Bonow RO, Dilsizian V, Cuocolo A, Bacharach SL. Identification of viable myocardium in patients with chronic coronary artery disease and left ventricular dysfunction. Comparison of thallium scintigraphy with reinjection and PET imaging with ^{18}F-fluorodeoxyglucose. Circulation 1991;83:26-37.
61. Perrone-Filardi P, Bacharach SL, Dilsizian V, Maurea S, Frank JA, Bonow RO. Regional left ventricular wall thickening. Relation to regional uptake of ^{18}F-fluorodeoxyglucose and ^{201}Tl in patients with chronic coronary artery disease and left ventricular dysfunction. Circulation 1992;86:1125-37.
62. Bonow RO, Berman DS, Gibbons RJ et al. Cardiac positron emission tomography. A report for health professionals from the committee on advanced cardiac imaging and technology of the council on clinical cardiology, American Heart Association. Circulation 1991;84:447-54.
63. Kalff V, Schwaiger M, Nguyen N, McClanahan TB, Gallagher KP. The relationship between myocardial blood flow and glucose uptake in ischemic canine myocardium determined with fluorine-18-deoxyglucose. J Nucl Med 1992;33:1346-53.
64. Sebree L, Bianco JA, Subramanian R et al. Discordance between ^{14}C deoxyglucose and ^{201}Tl in reperfused myocardium. J Mol Cell Cardiol 1991;23:603-16.
65. Depre C, Melin JA, Essamri B, Grandin C, Wijns W, Borgers M. Ultrastructural correlates of metabolism-flow mismatch pattern on positron emission tomography. Circulation 1991;84:(Suppl. II):II-90 (Abstract).
66. Brodde OE. β_1 and β_2-adrenoceptors in the human heart: Properties, function, and alterations in chronic heart failure. Pharmacol Rev 1991;43:203-42.
67. Haverkamp W, Gülker H, Hindricks G, Breithardt G. Effects of b-blockade on the incidence of ventricular tachyarrhythmias during acute myocardial ischemia: experimental findings and clinical implications. In: Heusch G, Ross Jr. J, editors. Adrenergic mechanisms in myocardial ischemia. New York: Springer-Verlag, 1991:293-303.
68. Hjalmarson A. Heart rate and b-adrenergic mechanisms in acute myocardial infarction. In: Heusch G, Ross Jr. J, editors. Adrenergic mechanisms in myocardial ischemia. New York: Springer-Verlag, 1991;325-33.

69. Merlet P, Dubois-Randé J-L, Adnot S et al. Myocardial b-adrenergic desensitization and neuronal norepinephrine uptake in idiopathic dilated cardiomyopathy. J Cardiovasc Pharmacol 1992;19:10-6.
70. Maron BJ, Bonow RO, Cannon RO, Leon MB, Epstein SE. Hypertrophic cardiomyopathy: Interrelations of clinical manifestations, pathophysiology, and therapy (Part I). N Engl J Med 1987;316:780-9.
71. Maron BJ, Bonow RO, Cannon RO, Leon MB, Epstein SE. Hypertrophic cardiomyopathy: Interrelations of clinical manifestations, pathophysiology and therapy (Part II). N Engl J Med 1987;316:844-52.
72. Syrota A. Positron emission tomography: Evaluation of cardiac receptors. In: Marcus ML, Schelbert HR, Skorton DJ, Wolf GL, editors. Cardiac imaging. A companion to Braunwald's HEART DISEASE. Philadelphia: WB Saunders Company, 1991;1256-70.
73. Staehelin M, Hertel C. [^{3}H]CGP12177: a b-adrenergic ligand suitable for measuring cell surface receptors. J Recept Res 1983;3:35-43.
74. Araujo LI, Rhodes CG, Hughes JMB et al. Assessment of myocardial ß-receptors in vivo using C-11 (S) CGP12177 and positron emission tomography (PET). J Nucl Med 1991;32:S927 (Abstract).
75. Jones HA, Rhodes CG, Law MP et al. Rapid analysis for metabolites of ^{11}C-labeled drugs: fate of [^{11}C]-S-4-(tert.-butylamino-2-hydroxypropoxy)-benzimidaz ol-2- one in the dog. J Chromatography 1991;570:361-70.
76. Delforge J, Syrota A, Lançon J-L et al. Cardiac ß-adrenergic receptor density measured in vivo using PET, CGP12177, and a new graphical method. J Nucl Med 1991;32:739-48
77. Lefroy DC, De Silva R, Choudhury L et al. Diffuse reduction of myocardial ß-adrenoceptors in hypertrophic cardiomyopathy. J Am Coll Cardiol 1993;22(6):1653-60.
78. Bristow MR, Ginsburg R, Minobe W et al. Decreased catecholamine sensitivity and ß-adrenergic receptor density in failing human hearts. N Engl J Med 1982;307:205-11.
79. Bristow MR. Pathophysiologic and pharmacologic rationales for clinical management of chronic heart failure with ß-blocking agents. Am J Cardiol 1993;71:12C-22C.
80. Merlet P, Delforge J, Syrota A et al. Positron emission tomography with 11C CGP-12177 to assess ß-adrenergic receptor concentration in idiopathic dilated cardiomyopathy. Circulation 1993;87:1169-78.
81. Corr PB, Crafford WA. Enhanced alpha-adrenergic responsiveness in ischemic myocardium: role of alpha-adrenergic blockade. Am Heart J 1981;102:605-12.
82. Sheridan DJ, Penkoske PA, Sobel BE, Corr PB. Alpha-adrenergic contributions to dysrhythmias during myocardial ischemia and reperfusion in cats. J Clin Invest 1980;65:161-71.
83. Wieland D, Rosenspire K, Hutchins G et al. Neuronal mapping of the heart with 6-[F-18]-Fluorometaraminol. J Med Chem 1990;33:956-64.
84. Goldstein DS, Chang PC, Eisenhofer G et al. Positron emission tomographic imaging of cardiac sympathetic innervation and function. Circulation 1990;81:1606-21.
85. Schwaiger M, Kaliff V, Rosenspire K et al. Noninvasive evaluation of the sympathetic nervous system in the human heart by PET. Circulation 1990;82:457-64.
86. Schwaiger M, Hutchins GD, Kalff V et al. Evidence for regional catecholamine uptake and storage sites in the transplanted human heart by positron emission tomography. J Clin Invest 1991;87:1681-90.
87. Stark RP, McGinn AL, Wilson RF. Chest pain in cardiac-transplant recipients. Evidence for sensory reinnervation after cardiac transplantation. N Engl J Med 1991;324:1791-4.
88. Delforge J, Janier M, Syrota A et al. Noninvasive quantification of muscarinic receptors in vivo with positron emission tomography in the dog heart. Circulation 1990;82:1494-504.

89. Delforge J, Le Guludec D, Syrota A, Crouzel C, Merlet P. In vivo quantification of myocardial muscarinic receptors in humans with PET. Circulation 1991;84(Suppl II):II-423 (Abstract).
90. Charbonneau P, Syrota A, Crouzel C, Vallios JM, Prenant C, Crouzel M. Peripheral-type benzodiazepine receptors in the living human heart characterized by positron emission tomography. Circulation 1986;73:476-83.

MYOCARDIAL VIABILITY:
STUNNING AND HIBERNATION

Willem Flameng, Bharati Shivalkar,
and Marcel Borgers

Myocardial stunning

DEFINITION

Myocardial stunning is defined as a transient postischemic myocardial dysfunction, occurring during full reperfusion after a short episode of non-lethal ischemia. This phenomenon was first recognized by Heyndrickx et al.[1] and termed "myocardial stunning" by Braunwald and Kloner.[2] The initial description of stunning i.e. a total coronary occlusion of only 5 to 15 minutes that was not associated with detectable myocardial necrosis, resulted in impairment of ventricular systolic function that lasted for several hours following reperfusion. Since then, myocardial stunning has been demonstrated experimentally under a variety of conditions and in many different animal species. Several of these conditions become extremely important for a better understanding of the clinical relevance of myocardial stunning. At first there is the problem of "peri-infarction stunning". It has been well established that during prolonged coronary artery occlusion only a variable fraction of the area at risk will become necrotic.[3] A "border zone" of myocardial tissue, adjacent to necrotic myocardium will survive mainly due to collateral flow, and myocardial stunning can be demonstrated in this border zone after delayed reperfusion of the blocked vessel.[4] Therefore, the akinetic area related to infarction can easy be overestimated in the early reperfusion phase: at this stage differentiation between viable and necrotic tissue cannot be made on the basis of regional function studies alone. Second, not only regional ischemia will result in stunning upon reperfusion but also global ischemia or anoxia. This finding has important implications because it explains why hearts of patients undergoing cardiac surgery are very often dysfunctional in the early period of reperfusion after cross clamping of the aorta despite cardioplegic protection. A third important circumstance under which stunning can be demonstrated is that stunning also occurs in the presence of partial coronary stenosis instead of complete occlusion

15

E. E. van der Wall et al. (eds.), Cardiac Positron Emission Tomography, 15–24.
© 1995 Kluwer Academic Publishers.

followed by reperfusion.[5] Obviously relative ischemia due to imbalance between oxygen supply and demand can induce stunning as well as a complete occlusion of the coronary vessel. This observation is important because it explains why transient coronary spasm may result in regional myocardial dysfunction.

Stunning and myocardial viability

By detailed assessment of subcellular myocardial structure during progression of ischemia, a clear sequence of morphological changes can be described. After a few minutes of ischemia, the first subtle morphological alterations are found in the mitochondria: the small osmiophilic granules embedded in the mitochondrial matrix disappear. When ischemia proceeds, more pronounced alterations occur in the mitochondria: clearing of the mitochondrial matrix, swollen and disrupted cristae, and rupture of inner and outer mitochondrial membrane. These lesions can be used to create a scoring system for the semi-quantitative grading of ischemic injury. However, when ischemia passes the "point of no return" in terms of cell viability, a clear morphological picture is found: disruption of the sarcolemma, inclusion of typical amorphous dense bodies in the mitochondria, intracellular edema, and chromatin clumping and margination in the nucleus. It is remarkable that under all these conditions, the contractile system (sarcomeres and myofibrils) remain structurally intact as far as can be detected with the electron microscope. Only at a late stage after the onset of irreversible damage, does the contractile system disintegrate.

It is obvious that irreversibly damaged myocytes are, and remain, non-functional. There is, however, no direct correlation between the amount of myocardial necrosis and the extent of myocardial dysfunction in a given perfusion area of the blocked and reperfused coronary vessel. Indeed, viable postischemic tissue will be non-contractile as well for hours to days while ultrastructure reveals only very minor abnormalities. In a previous experimental study,[6] we showed that upon reperfusion after 90 minutes of coronary occlusion in dogs, salvage of 68 % of the perfusion area of the occluded artery was obtained. Viability of the myocardium in this area was demonstrated by electron microscopy. However, postischemic regional function was completely lost in the first 24 hours, despite this considerable amount of viable time. Nevertheless, regional function recovered after 1 week of reperfusion, which suggests the presence of stunned myocardium in the early postischemic phase.

These observations imply that indirect noninvasive assessment of viability (i.e. differentiation between ischemia, necrosis and stunning) cannot be based only upon the lack of regional function in the presence of flow i.e. reperfusion. Indeed, in a previous study,[7] we could demonstrate that necrotic tissue is transiently hyperperfused in the initial reperfusion phase before the "no reflow phenomenon" develops while the viable, stunned borderzone transiently looses its maximal dilatory capacity.

Mechanisms of stunning

The basic mechanisms responsible for this transient reduction of postischemic contractility (up to 7 days before complete recovery) are not fully elucidated.

At first glance, a loss of high energy phosphates via a washout of nucleotide precursors (mainly adenosine and inosine) upon reperfusion is the most plausible cause of stunning. Indeed, the de novo synthesis of adenosine triphosphate (ATP) takes at least 72 hours.

In recent experiments, however, we have shown that, under conditions of short periods of ischemia (up to 10 minutes), myocardial ATP is catabolized to adenosine diphosphate (ADP) and adenosine monophosphate (AMP) without significant accumulation of adenosine and inosine. Reperfusion resulted in a rephosphorylation of nucleotides to ATP at near normal levels. Postischemic dysfunction, however, remained unaltered. Additional possible mechanisms of myocardial stunning may include defects in processes of energy production, transport, or utilization.

Energy producing processes
Such a defect would consist of decreased oxidative phosphorylation in the mitochondria of the postischemic myocardium. In a recent experimental study we have demonstrated that in cases of stunning the energy state of the heart is intact in terms of high energy phosphate content and mitochondrial function.[8]

Energy transport processes
ATP cannot diffuse freely from its site of production (mitochondria) to its site of utilization (myofibrils). Energy is transferred via the creatine phosphate shuttle from production to utilization sites via two separate isoenzyme systems, the mitochondrial and the myofibrillar creatine kinase isoenzyme. Hypothetically, the loss or inactivation of, for example, the myofibrillar bound creatine kinase (CK) isoenzyme can be responsible for stunning and can even explain the "overshoot" of postischemic tissue levels of creatine phosphate. Experimental evidence for this kind of mechanism was given recently.[9]

Energy utilizing processes
Recent studies of Schaper et al.[10] on ATP turnover and on the relation between energy metabolism and function after repeated short periods of ischemia provided evidence that ATP utilization in reperfused myocardium is reduced in the presence of a sufficient ATP supply. Moreover, postischemic contractile dysfunction can be reversed by inotropic stimulation indicating that, even in the presence of reduced tissue levels, ATP turnover can be increased. The mechanism for reduced ATP splitting by the sarcomeres is unclear: it may reside in the sarcomeres themselves or in disturbances of the electromechanical coupling.

Ito et al.[11] reported that an intracoronary infusion of calcium increased regional contractile function in stunned myocardium and suggested a defect at the level of the excitation-contraction coupling, probably involving calcium fluxes.

Bolli[12] focused on the role of oxygen radicals, the amplification of damage by calcium overload and the resulting excitation-contraction uncoupling. The subcellular seat of the defect which is probably caused by free radicals is however nuclear. Our results do not support hypotheses that pinpoint the defect to the sarcoplasmic reticulum.[13,14]

Kusuoka et al.[15] suggested that the crucial lesion in stunning occurs at the level of the contractile proteins, rather than more proximally, and that the sensitivity to calcium of the contractile proteins is altered.

Clinical relevance of myocardial stunning

a) Stunning in the surgical setting:

In routine cardiac surgery, myocardial stunning is probably the most frequent cause of postoperative myocardial dysfunction and low cardiac output syndrome. Even in uncomplicated operations, a transient depression of left ventricular stroke work index is observed. In several studies we could show that such a depression of function during the reperfusion phase is associated with an almost normal ultrastructural aspect of the myocardium.[16] Under these conditions, the hearts typically respond to intravenous application of calcium.

As mentioned before, most pharmacological interventions that increase intracellular calcium improve function of the stunned myocardium. When these interventions however cannot reverse the low output syndrome, prolonged reperfusion can be achieved by the use of left ventricular assist devices.

In cases of regional acute ischemia and evolving infarction, early reperfusion by emergency coronary artery bypass surgery can salvage a considerable amount of myocardial tissue. During the immediate postoperative phase, the reperfused viable portion of the area at risk remains akinetic as can be demonstrated by transoesophageal echocardiography. Late postoperative technetium-99m studies however, revealed a significant improvement of contractility in these "stunned" areas.[17]

b) Stunning in the cardiological setting:

Studies in patients with stable angina pectoris suggest that exercise-induced myocardial ischemia may result in prolonged contractile and metabolic abnormalities in the absence of evidence of persisting ischemia. Either two-dimensional echocardiography[18] or positron emission tomography[19] were used in these studies. The time course of such abnormalities remains to be defined, as these studies have been limited to the first 60 minutes after exercise. Also in patients suffering from unstable angina, the myocardium may be reversibly depressed because improvement in regional wall motion is observed in this syndrome after coronary angioplasty.[20]

Myocardial hibernation

DEFINITION

In 1984, Rahimtoola proposed the concept of hibernating myocardium to describe "a state of persistently impaired myocardial and left ventricular function at rest due to reduced coronary blood flow that can be partially or completely restored to normal if the myocardial oxygen supply/demand relationship is favorably altered, either by improving blood flow and/or by reducing demand".[21] This theory was based on clinical observations and the concept was not universally accepted when first proposed.[22]

Even much earlier, we made the observation that between patients suffering from coronary artery disease, a subpopulation exists having severely depressed contractile function in the presence of severe coronary artery stenosis but without evidence of myocardial infarction.[23] We studied postrevascularization recovery of myocardial function in these patients and could demonstrate that these areas functionally improve after coronary artery bypass surgery.[24] We studied also myocardial viability in these hypocontractile regions and found that these "hibernating" areas are not only perfectly viable but show some specific subcellular alterations.

Viability of the hibernating myocardium

Severe, long lasting coronary artery stenosis is associated with a 30% reduction in myocardial nucleotide content and regional wall motion abnormality.[25] This observation of reduced adenylate pool parallelling the reduction in local contractility, does not necessarily imply that the depression of local function is caused by this reduction in adenylate pool. Indeed, the ADP/ATP ratio, the energy charge and the creatine phosphate levels are in the normal range and this is very suggestive for an intact mitochondrial function, that is, a normal energy production. Such a situation resembles well that of the "stunned myocardium", but now induced by chronic intermittent ischemia. However, recurrent episodes of ischemia may not only induce stunning and purine loss, but also may activate proteolytic systems responsible for myofibrillar lysis. It is also possible that chronic or intermittent ischemia alters sarcoplasmic reticulum function and interrupts excitation contraction coupling. When this process prevents the myocardium to contract for a longer period of time without inducing necrosis, the critical balance between protein synthesis and breakdown may be disturbed and, in analogy with atrophy, a kind of dedifferentiation of the myocytes will be induced, resulting in a reduced volume fraction of contractile proteins. We observed this phenomenon when we studied the relationship between structural alterations and left ventricular contraction abnormalities in patients with coronary artery disease.[26] Transmural biopsies of the left ventricular anterior free wall were taken during aortocoronary bypass surgery. When preoperatively anterior wall motion was reduced, significant myocardial cell "dedifferentiation" was found in patients without previous anterior infarction. A typical example of these ultrastructural findings is presented in Figure 1.

Myofibrillar lysis is a typical finding in myocardial cells from chronically hypokinetic or akinetic areas. Most interesting is the finding that such a myocardial "dedifferentiation" without fibrosis is related to chronic ischemia.[23,24] In segments with severely reduced contractile function but without significant fibrosis, that is, in segments without remote infarction, loss of contractile material is massive mainly in the subendocardium. The most striking subcellular alteration is the loss of contractile material which is replaced by large amounts of glycogen, sarcoplasmic reticulum and mitochondria. In many cells only a small rim of sarcomeres arranged marginally is preserved. It is clear that contractile function of these myocardial cells must be severely reduced. On the other hand, other vital cellular components (nucleus, mitochondria cell membranes, etc.) although altered, remained viable. Therefore this phenomenon is referred to as hibernating myocardium.

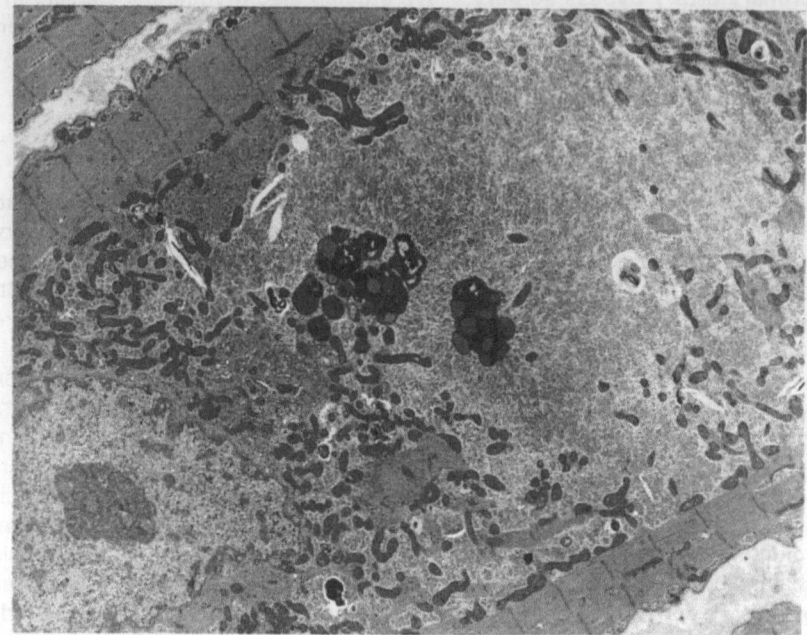

Figure 1. Electron micrograph of a myocardial cell (x 11180) originating from hibernating myocardium. The cell is viable but the volume fraction of sarcomeres is severely reduced, leaving some rims of myofibers. The cytoplasm contains an increased amount of glycogen and small, irregularly shaped mitochondria.

Myocardial hibernation: a clinical entity

In patients with chronic coronary artery disease without acute, evolving infarction multivariate analysis of angiographic, histologic and electrocardiographic data revealed three definite groups of patients.[23]

A first group comprised patients with normal histologic findings associated with severe coronary stenosis without abnormal wall motion. Electrocardiographic abnormalities were limited to ST-segment changes. The second group of patients had important myocardial cell abnormalities with severe fibrosis associated with severe coronary stenosis and severely depressed wall motion. In this group there was a high incidence of infarction apparent on the electrocardiogram. The third subpopulation of patients comprised patients with severe myocardial alterations with only modest fibrosis, associated with severe coronary stenosis and severely impaired wall motion. The incidence of infarction on the electrocardiogram was low. In this subgroup of "hibernating" myocardium the myocytes were viable but the volume fraction of contractile proteins was severely reduced and replaced by glycogen and small mitochondria.

Late postrevascularization studies showed that contractile function is partially restored in these segments indicating that reversal of early myocytolytic changes or "redifferentiation" may occur when chronic ischemia is reversed in time.

Myocardial hibernation: own results

The recognition that myocardial tissue can hibernate under ischemic conditions and can show recovery after revascularization, has had important therapeutic and investigational implications. Initially, it was thought that a severe degree of coronary stenosis was responsible for the reduced contractility and that there was immediate recovery of the hibernating myocardium after revascularization. In a recent study[27] we studied 36 coronary artery bypass surgery (CABG) candidates, who had pre- and three months post-operatively positron emission tomography and equilibrium nuclear angiography. An intraoperative transmural needle biopsy of the anterior wall was also taken and processed for histological analysis.

The individual preoperative data ranged from very low to very high values ; regional ejection fraction from 9 to 95% (46±23%, mean ± SD), flow from 41 to 100% (70±17%), and metabolism from 38 to 118% (79±22%).

The preoperative data including the regional ejection fraction, metabolism, flow and histology were displayed as a biplot using principle component analysis. A biplot is a two-dimensional graphical display of multivariate data. A multivariate cluster analysis further separated the patients in nonoverlapping subgroups as follows:

The *first* cluster had normal regional ejection fraction, flow, metabolism (76±13%, 91±10%, and 92±11% respectively), low degree of transmural fibrosis (8±4%) as determined by morphometry and viable myocytes (n = 9). These patients did not show a significant change in regional ejection fraction, flow and metabolism three months postoperatively.

The *second* subgroup (n = 19) had low regional ejection fraction and low flow, but normal metabolism (39±11%, 67±10% and 94±16% respectively). There was a low degree of fibrosis (14±9%), and 23±10% of myocytes (as determined by planimetry analysis) showed a variable loss of myofibrils. Three months after CABG these patients showed a significant recovery of the regional ejection fraction at 50±13% (p<0.05), and a better flow (78±8%, p<0.05), denoting successful revascularization.

The *third* cluster of patients (n = 5) had low regional ejection fraction, reduced flow and diminished metabolism (20±8%, 50±13% and 51±9% respectively), with a high degree of fibrosis (62±16%). Furthermore, a substantial number of myocytes showed a variable loss of myofibrils (23±15%). Post CABG there was no significant recovery in the regional ejection fraction (REF), flow or metabolism (14±9%, 51±4%, 51±5% respectively, p>0.05).

The *fourth* cluster of patients (n = 3) also showed reduced regional ejection fraction, flow and metabolism (49±11%, 69±10%, 69±11% respectively), a substantial degree of fibrosis (29±10%), and a large number of myocytes showing variable loss of myofibrils (57±23%). There was a high degree of glycogen accumulation (26±5%), as shown by the use of a special staining (periodic acid Schiff), determined planimetrically as the volume fraction of glycogen per cell, and calculated further as the average volume percent per biopsy. There was no significant improvement in the regional ejection fraction, and the flow and metabolism showed a non-significant improvement, probably due to the small number of patients.

A stepwise logistic regression analysis showed that a combination of low preoperative regional ejection fraction and maintained metabolism (high [18]FDG uptake) was the best predictor of functional recovery (p < 0.008). Furthermore, there was a negative correlation between regional ejection fraction, flow and metabolism versus the fibrosis, with metabolism having the best correlation with fibrosis (p < 0.0001). Postoperatively, there was an improvement in these correlations (p < 0.0001). This indicates that fibrosis plays an important role in determining the postoperative regional outcome in terms of function, flow and metabolism.

References

1. Heyndrickx GR, Millard RW, Mc Ritchie RJ et al. Regional myocardial functional and electrophysiological alterations after brief coronary artery occlusion in conscious dogs. J Clin Invest 1975;56:978-85.
2. Braunwald E, Kloner RA. The stunned myocardium: Prolonged, postischemic ventricular dysfunction. Circulation 1982;66:1146-9.
3. Flameng W, Lesaffre E, Vanhaecke J. Determinants of infarct size in non-human primates. Basic Res Cardiol 1990;85:392-403.
4. Ellis SG, Henschke CI, Sandor T et al. Time course of functional and biochemical recovery of myocardium salvaged by reperfusion. J Am Coll Cardiol 1983;1:1047-55.
5. Thaulow E, Guth BD, Heusch G et al. Characteristics of regional myocardial stunning after exercise in dogs with chronic coronary stenosis. Am J Physiol 1989;257:H113-9.
6. Flameng W, Vanhaecke J, Borgers M. Histology of the postischaemic myocardium and its relation to left ventricular function. Br J Anaesth 1988;60:145-225.
7. Vanhaecke J, Flameng W, Borgers M, Jang IK, VandeWerf F, Degeest H. Evidence for decreased coronary flow reserve in viable postischemic myocardium. Circ Res 1990;67:1201-11.
8. Flameng W, Andres J, Ferdinande P, Mattheussen M, Van Belle H. Mitochondrial function in myocardial stunning. J Mol Cell Cardiol 1991;23:1-11.
9. Greenfield RA, Swain JL. Disruption of myofibrillar energy use: mechanisms that may contribute to postischemic dysfunction in stunned myocardium. Circulation 1985;72(Suppl 3):68.
10. Schaper W, Buchwald A, Hoffmeister HM, Ito BR. "Stunned myocardium" is a problem of energy utilization and not of energy supply. Circulation 1985;72(Suppl 3):119.
11. Ito BR, Tate H, Schaper W. Calcium induced increases in regional contractile function before and after transient coronary occlusion in dog. Circulation 1985;72(Suppl 3):68.
12. Bolli R. Mechanism of myocardial "Stunning". Circulation 1990;82:723-38.
13. Kaplan P, Hendrikx M, Mattheussen M, Mubagwa K, Flameng W. Effect of ischemia and reperfusion on sarcoplasmic reticulum calcium uptake. Circ Res 1992;71:1123-30.
14. Mattheussen M, Mubagwa K, Rusy BF, Van Aken H, Flameng W. Potentiated state contractions in isolated hearts: effects of ischemia and reperfusion. Am J Physiol 1993;264:H1663-73.
15. Kusuoka H, Koretsune Y, Chacko VP, Weisfeldt ML, Marban E. Excitation-contraction coupling in postischemic myocardium: Does failure of activator Ca^{2+} transients underlie "Stunning"? Circ Res 1990;66:1268-76.
16. Flameng W, Van der Vusse J, Borgers M. Methods for assessing preservation techniques-Invasive techniques. In: Engelman R, Levitsky L, editors. Handbook of clinical cardioplegia. Mount Kisco, New York: Futura Publishing Company, 1982:63-80.
17. Flameng W, Sergeant P, Vanhaecke J, Suy R. Emergency coronary bypass grafting for evolving myocardial infarction: effects on infarct size and left ventricular function. J Thorac Cardiovasc Surg 1987;94:124-31.
18. Robertson WS, Feigenbaum H, Armstrong WF, Dillon JC, O'Donnell J, McHenry PW. Exercise echocardiography: a clinical practical addition in the evaluation of coronary artery disease. J Am Coll Cardiol 1983;6:1085-9.
19. Camici P, Araiyo LI, Spinks T et al. Increased uptake of ^{18}F-fluorodeoxyglucose in postischemic myocardium of patients with exercise-induced angina. Circulation 1986;74:81-8.
20. Renkin J, Wyns W, Ladha Z, Col J. Reversal of segmental hypkinesis by coronary angioplasty in patients with unstable angina, persistent T wave inversion, and left anterior

descending coronary artery stenosis. Additional evidence for myocardial stunning in humans. Circulation 1990;82:913-21.

21. Rahimtoola SH. A perspective on three large multicenter randomized clinical trials of coronary bypass surgery for chronic stable angina. Circulation 1985;72(Suppl V):123-5.

22. Rahimtoola SH. The hibernating myocardium. Am Heart J 1989;117:211-21.

23. Flameng W, Wouters L, Sergeant P et al. Multivariate analysis of angiographic, histologic and electrocardiographic data in patients with coronary heart disease. Circulation 1984;70:7-17.

24. Flameng W, Suy R, Schwarz F et al. Ultrastructural correlates of left ventricular contraction abnormalities in patients with chronic ischemic heart disease: determinants of reversible segmental asynergy. Am Heart J 1981;102:846-57.

25. Flameng W, Vanhaecke J, Van Belle H, Borgers M, De Beer L, Minten J. Relation between coronary artery stenosis and myocardial purine metabolism, histology and regional functions in humans. J Am Coll Cardiol 1987;9:1235-42.

26. Borgers M, Thone F, Wouters L, Ausma J, Shivalkar B, Flameng W. Structural correlates of regional myocardial dysfunction in patients with critical coronary artery stenosis: Chronic Hibernation? Cardiovasc Pathol 1993;2:237-45.

27. Shivalkar B, Borgers M, Maes A, Mortelmans L, Flameng W. Low regional function associated with high metabolism predicts functional recovery after coronary bypass surgery. Circulation 1994;90,4:I-251.

2   POSITRON EMISSION TOMOGRAPHY ASSESSMENT OF MYOCARDIAL VIABILITY

Eng-Shiong Tan

Introduction

The concept of "hibernating myocardium",[1] defined as impaired regional myocardial contractility with preserved viability, bears important clinical implications. Revascularization of patients with hibernating myocardium brings about a clear and convincing reduction of mortality and morbidity. Revascularization of necrotic / infarcted tissue does not show any effect.[2] Therefore, it is foreseeable that accurate diagnostic methods to differentiate hibernating from necrotic myocardium will help in reaching a decision to revascularize. Although the magnitude of the problem of differentiating viable from necrotic tissue in areas of diminished contractility, is estimated to be only 10% of all patients eligible for revascularization,[3] the high cost of revascularization and ensuing cardiac morbidity and the major impact on quality of life justify the cost and effort of a diagnostic intervention to avert these problems by far.

"Stunned myocardium", defined as prolonged depressed myocardial function after an episode of ischemia when perfusion is fully restored,[4] is another situation where viability may come into question. In the case of pure stunning, viability is preserved and the myocardium will recover spontaneously, albeit after quite some time. If the episode of ischemia has damaged the myocardium irreversibly, no recovery of contractility will follow. This situation is encountered, for instance, in the setting of thrombolytic therapy after an acute myocardial infarction.

Both stunning and hibernation represent clinical entities whereby myocardial viability comes into question. The seriously affected myocardial function could both be caused by necrotic as well as by temporarily dysfunctional, viable myocardial tissue with the ability to recover.

Several diagnostic methods for the detection of viability have been proposed. Stress echocardiography with dobutamine (DSE), single photon emission computed tomography (SPECT) with thallium-201 (^{201}Tl) as isotope or technetium-99m-Sestamibi (^{99m}Tc-MIBI), and fluorine-18-deoxyglucose (^{18}FDG) as tracer and positron

25

E. E. van der Wall et al. (eds.), Cardiac Positron Emission Tomography, 25–35.
© 1995 Kluwer Academic Publishers.

emission tomography (PET) with measurement of perfusion and metabolic imaging have emerged as the most practical and promising tools. It is already sufficiently demonstrated that PET represents the most powerful diagnostic method,[5] but until now there are no conclusive data to support the notion that the more accurate diagnosis gained by PET at a higher cost, will translate in a cost effective way to guide the decision to revascularize a patient with impaired myocardial contractility. The diagnostic modalities other than PET will be reviewed elsewhere in this book. The methodology of assigning a value of cost effectiveness to a diagnostic method will be reviewed in a separate chapter of this book dedicated to medical decision making. This chapter will focus on PET as a method to delineate viable myocardium. Only perfusion measurement pertinent to the question of viability will be mentioned here. The chapter written by Bol and Wijns will deal in detail with the perfusion measurement per se.

Basic concepts

Myocardial perfusion, contractility, and metabolism are all closely interrelated. A reduction in regional perfusion will be followed by a proportional reduction in contractility concomitant with a change in substrate use. This is shown in animal studies during total coronary occlusion.[6,7] Beside the perfusion and oxygen content of the arterial blood, other factors, like the availability of substrates and neurohumoral activity, also determine the substrate use of the myocardial cell. Normally fatty acids are metabolized for up to 80% to satisfy the energy demands. During of ischemia, that is when perfusion is low, the myocardial cell will shift its substrate to glucose.[8]

The induction of longstanding serious ischemia not resulting in necrosis has been extremely difficult to realize in the animal model. Until now, a model of chronically low perfused myocardium with preserved viability for longer than a few hours is still lacking. It is however assumed that the shifts in substrate use from free fatty acids to glucose, seen in the more acute phase of ischemia, will become permanent in the chronic phase.

Both the decrease in contractility as the use of glucose instead of free fatty acids as substrate will result in diminished oxygen use for the same amount of energy produced and therefore could be seen as a means of the myocardial cell to reduce oxygen expenditure. Although the complete experimental evidence is missing, considering the overwhelming amount of clinical clues, a state of hibernation of the myocardial cell in which the diminished supply of nutrients is met by a decreased function, does seem to be possible. It is not clear though, for how long the cell can maintain its integrity and ability to return to normal function. There seems to be a time dependent factor. The longer the ischemia, the less likely the tissue will remain viable. The degree of ischemia may be another factor. The more serious the ischemia, the shorter the cell is able to stay in the state of hibernation. A cause for hibernation other than stable and longstanding serious ischemia, may be repetitive short bouts of serious ischemia, inducing "longstanding stunning". Indications for such a mechanism is found in PET studies in man. Here, very remarkably, perfusion measurements in rest only show slightly reduced to normal perfusion in hibernating segments, i.e. segments with reduced contractility and signs of preserved viability. There is however a markedly reduced perfusion reserve. So, possibly in the recent past, these segments may have suffered repetitive episodes of ischemia caused by episodes of increased demand which cannot be met by the reduced perfusion reserve, for instance during physical exercise, producing the dysfunction.[9] If this holds true, it may be possible that a low perfusion state, causing serious dysfunction, simply cannot be endured for a long time, being the reason that an experimental set up with longstanding low perfusion and maintained viability till now could not be realized.

Instead of induction of ischemia by reduction of supply, an increase of demand through an increase of heart rate for instance during atrial fibrillation is suggested to induce the same adaptive cellular mechanisms in the atrial cells. The first experiments using this model have yielded promising results.[10] Early research in dogs also has used rapid pacing of the ventricles as a means to induce chronic ischemia by increasing the demand of blood. The prospects to explore further along this avenue are very exciting and will most certainly contribute to a better understanding of hibernating myocardium in the future.

Positron emission tomography

PET uses positron emitting isotopes. During the radioactive decay of these isotopes, positively charged electrons are emitted, so-called positrons. These particles will annihilate with a negatively charged electron in the surrounding environment, yielding energy in the form of two photons, each 511 keV, radiating in two opposite directions of 180 degrees. The photons are registered by detectors grouped in rings around the patient. Through electronic linkage of opposite detectors, the location of each annihilation is detected and in due time backprojected in a tomographic representation. As the two photons will travel through the whole space between the two opposite detectors, it is possible to perform a transmission scan, in order to correct for the attenuation of all the tissue and other material between the two detectors. This is one of the major advantages of PET compared to SPECT, beside the higher resolution, enabling us to quantify the measurements. Due to the detection of only one photon in single photon techniques, on theoretical grounds, reliable attenuation correction and quantification of the data cannot be realized with SPECT.

The tracers currently used for PET studies are labeled with the following positron emitting radionuclides: oxygen-15 (^{15}O) (half life 2.4 minutes), nitrogen-13 (^{13}N) (half life 10 minutes) carbon-11 (^{11}C) (half life 20.4 minutes), and fluorine-18 (^{18}F) (half life 110 minutes). Although the short physical half live is beneficial to the patient because of the low burden of radiation, except for ^{18}F, they also necessitate an on site accelerator, raising the cost of PET studies considerably. The tracers, like ^{11}C labeled acetate and ^{15}O labeled water, are naturally occurring physiologic substrates or analogues of these normal chemical molecules. Some radiopharmaceuticals can be made using generators. These radiopharmaceuticals are limited to studies of perfusion and blood pool imaging and they do not constitute of naturally occurring biological molecules.

The amount of data collected in one patient compels us to use certain representation modes to summarize the data as much as possible without reducing the data in the process. We therefore developed the paramap tool as described in the chapter "Parametric imaging of myocardial perfusion and metabolism".[12] In short, the transversal tomographic slices of the heart is reoriented along the long axis of the heart. The short axis slices, obtained by reslicing the heart perpendicular to the reoriented long axis, is represented in a so called bull's eye view, the apical short axis slice in the middle, the basal (near the valves) slice at the perimeter. Ten short axis slices are reconstructed and each slice is divided in forty eight segments, forming a total of 480 segments. With color coding of each segment, a value for perfusion, glucose metabolism rate, or combinations of these values per segment can be visualized. The "paramap" is now able to exhibit a complete view of the left ventricle and provides at the same time a sufficiently detailed segmental distribution of any studied function or derived parameter of the myocardium at a glance (Figure 1).

Perfusion

A minimum level of myocardial perfusion is necessary for survival of myocardial tissue. Several investigators have tried to determine a threshold level of perfusion under which myocardial viability is not possible and above which viability is likely. This has not been overtly successful. One reason may be that a segment of necrosis induced by a relative shortlived episode of ischemia, for instance a thrombus superimposed on a non-significant coronary stenosis lysed after more than 6 hours, still can enjoy a relatively high perfusion after this episode of ischemia, without really consisting of vital myocardium anymore. At the other end of the flow spectrum, low levels of flow may be a result of down-regulation induced by hibernating but viable myocardium. This may result in a considerable overlap of flow values around this hypothetic threshold, making measurement of only perfusion for assessment of viability either with PET or SPECT, a somewhat precarious enterprise.

Lately, it appeared possible to use a perfusable tissue index using PET with $H_2^{15}O$ as tracer.[13] The perfusion tissue index probably represents the part of the myocardium still capable of exchanging water rapidly and therefore vital. If proven reliable, it will add a fast and easy alternative approach to delineate viable myocardium. There has been some criticism however from other groups suggesting that heterogeneity of perfusion may be the origin of difference in perfusable tissue index.

Metabolism

^{18}FDG

The change in substrate use from free fatty acids to glucose both in aerobic as anaerobic metabolism during and after ischemia lies at the root of the assessment of viability with imaging of glucose metabolism. ^{18}FDG, a glucose analogue, traces

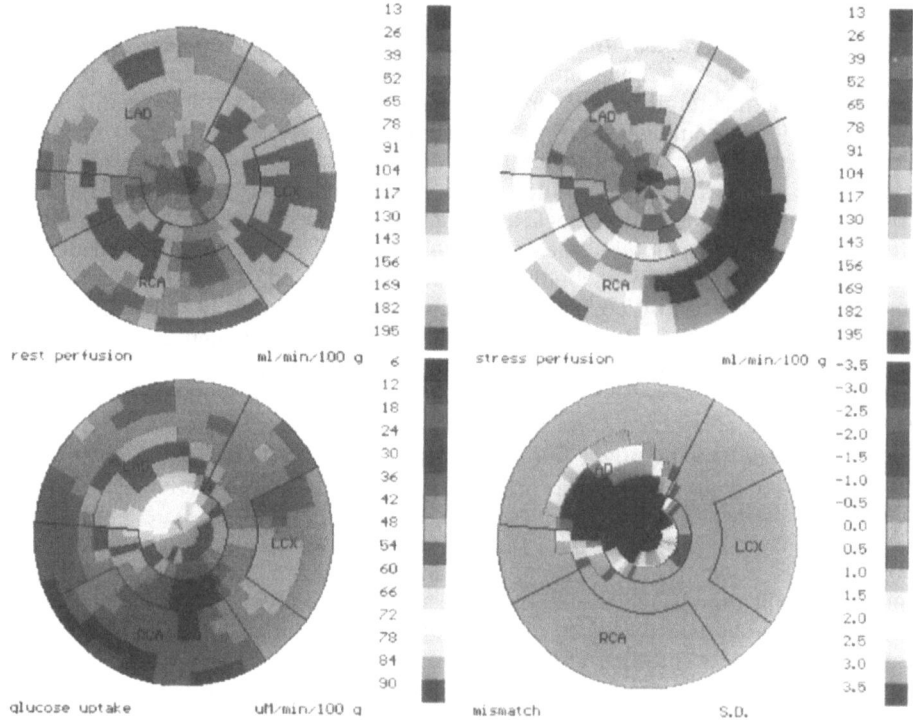

Figure 1. Paramap of glucose metabolism, perfusion, perfusion reserve and derived parameters. All polar maps are from a patient with reduced myocardial contractility in the mid and apical anterior region with uncertainty about myocardial viability in these regions. The left upper panel shows a polar map of the myocardial perfusion in rest. The right upper panel shows a polar map of the myocardial perfusion during vasodilation with dipyridamole iv. The left lower panel shows a polar map of the glucose uptake.

Note the almost evenly distributed perfusion during rest, not showing signs of chronic ischemia in rest. There is however an obvious reduction of perfusion in the left anterior descending coronary artery (LAD) mid and apical region under dipyridamole showing a reduced ability to raise the perfusion in these regions. The ¹⁸FDG extraction as a measure of glucose uptake, is enhanced in the same region. The right lower panel shows one of the derived parameters, ie. the mismatch pattern. The glucose uptake values exceeding the standard deviation of the average glucose uptake for the measured values of dipyridamole perfusion in that segment, is represented here. The colors represent the grade of deviation from the average with a range of 1 to 3.5 times the standard deviation.

In conclusion, the area of interest, mid and apical anterior, show normal perfusion in rest, reduced perfusion reserve and preserved viability. (see for colourplate of this figure page 241).

the uptake of glucose from blood across the cellular membrane into the myocardial Paramap of glucose metabolism, perfusion, perfusion reserve and derived parameterscell, where it is phosphorylated to ¹⁸FDG-6-phosphate with the help of hexokinase. This form cannot be metabolized further and therefore does not trace other steps in the glucose metabolism or glycogen synthesis and reflects only the rate of glucose uptake and subsequent hexokinase mediated phosphorylation. ¹⁸FDG-phosphate is trapped within the cell because it cannot pass the cell membrane. These qualities makes [18]FDG a suitable tracer to study glucose metabolism.[14] The studies in man are performed after glucose loading, for the glucose uptake under fasting condition is usually not enough to provide an image. Glucose is administered orally around one to one and a half hours before intravenous [18]FDG administration. In a dynamic study for quantification of glucose metabolism, several scans immediately hereafter would be made. The last scan is performed around 45 to 60 minutes after [18]FGD administration, when uptake of [18]FDG is sufficient to provide visualization of the myocardium.

Unfortunately, glucose uptake does not solely depend on preserved viability during substrate shift induced by ischemia. It also depends on flow, oxygenation, the arterial glucose concentration, and neurohumoral activity and may therefore show some variability. To reduce this variability, a euglycemic insulin clamp has been tried, whereby the patient is given insulin and glucose intravenously under rigorous control of arterial blood glucose levels, to ensure a constant blood glucose. Whether this will enhance a more accurate detection of viable myocardium remains unclear. A large cooperative European study group is currently testing this hypothesis. As insulin is necessary for the flux of glucose into the cell, shortage of insulin in diabetic patients will cause insufficient [18]FDG uptake. Therefore, a euglycemic insulin clamp is employed in diabetic patients. Encouraging results has recently been published, regarding to the use of a nicotinic acid derivative, acipimox, which rapidly reduces serum free fatty acids levels by inhibiting lipolysis in peripheral tissues and therefore promotes glucose metabolism.[15] Quantification of glucose uptake with mathematical modeling has already been tried to improve detection of viability. Probably due to the large endogenous regional variation in glucose uptake, this did not seem to contribute to a more accurate method in one published study.[16] The large regional variation in [18]FDG uptake is seen in healthy volunteers especially under fasting conditions. There are also some indications that under circumstances, such as early after an infarction and reperfusion, [18]FDG can be taken up by myocardial tissue without the ability to recover. An explanation may be that [18]FDG uptake in these circumstances reflects anaerobic metabolism and since anaerobic metabolism alone cannot sustain the myocardial cell long enough to remain viable, this signal of [18]FDG uptake will not predict viability. It is believed that this phenomenon does not appear in chronic dysfunction.

Because of the dependence of glucose uptake on perfusion, especially in areas of low perfusion, the uptake of glucose has been related to the perfusion in that segment. A pattern of enhanced glucose uptake more than a certain value relative to the perfusion in that segment may lift the sensitivity and specificity for detection of viability.[10]

Most studies reporting the use of [18]FDG for assessment of viability used qualitative [18]FDG uptake in relation with perfusion studies, performed with another tracer like ^{13}N-ammonia, ^{15}O-water or rubidium-82 ([82]Rb). In areas of contractile dysfunction three patterns of [18]FDG uptake relative to perfusion are described. Preserved glucose uptake combined with preserved perfusion or preserved glucose uptake combined with reduced perfusion, the "mismatch defect", both predicting viability, and reduced glucose uptake combined with reduced perfusion, the "match defect", predicting non-viability. These match and mismatch patterns were compared to improvement of contractility after revascularization. The caveats of a comparison with such a "gold standard" will be dealt with in the chapter concerning cost effectiveness of clinical viability assessment by Hunink. It suffices to mention here that the interposition of a treatment and time window between diagnostic method and verification and having a verification sometimes conditional on the diagnostic method, may give rise to some bias, making the reported predictive values somewhat unreliable.

Until now, glucose metabolism studies combined with perfusion measurements form the largest body of data concerning PET research for viability. Despite all the abovementioned limitations, all studies have shown excellent results. Mismatch defects predicted recovery of contractile function after revascularization in about 80% of segments and mismatch defects did not improve in contractile function in about 85% of segments.

However, a better measure of merit of detection of viability with a method, may be the effectiveness of the decision taken on the information provided through that method. At least, the outcome of interest to the patient will then be measured. For example, Eitzman et al.[17] have shown in a retrospective study, that the patients with preserved viability diagnosed with [18]FDG-PET but no revascularization, experienced 50% of events (death and reinfarction) in the first year. The patients with viability and subsequent revascularization experienced a low event rate of 12% comparable to the patients without viability as diagnosed with PET. It is conceivable therefore that, in a comparable group of patients, revascularization decisions taken with the information of PET viability studies will reduce the events in patients with preserved viability for about 38% in the first year. Of course, to measure such a difference reliably, a prospective, randomized, controlled trial with a follow up on events, comparing patients with a revascularization strategy based on one viability assessment method with a revascularization strategy based on another method, should be performed. The cost of the strategy should also be measured, as this would reflect the cost efficiency of the method. With such a study, methodological difficulties could be overcome and at the same time, an end point of interest to the patient and the public could be measured.

[11]C-acetate

In the light of the aforementioned obstacles of measuring myocardial viability using glucose metabolism, newer radiopharmaceuticals are being developed. ^{11}C-acetate as a tracer to measure the oxidative metabolism seems to be the most promising alternative.[18,19] Maintenance of oxidative metabolism seems to be essential for viability. It may therefore predict improvement of contractility after revascularization. Energy production in the mitochondrium starts with the citric acid cycle, where acetyl-CoA is metabolized, producing reducing equivalents. These are converted to high energy phosphate bonds through oxidative phosphorylation by the respiratory chain. Acetate, a direct precursor of acetyl-CoA, traces the citric acid flux the closest to the point of entry into the cycle. It therefore has the lowest chance to be metabolized through another pathway compared to other substrates. ^{11}C-acetate is oxidized to [11]CO_2 which then effluxes from the myocardium. The rate of decline of radioactivity in the heart correlates with oxidative metabolism and this in turn is proven to reflect the degree of oxygen consumption. It has been observed that, in dysfunctional but viable myocardium, the myocardial oxygen consumption calculated with ^{11}C-acetate is of a comparable level as in normal myocardium, but significantly higher than in non-viable myocardium. In one clinical study, directly comparing ^{11}C-acetate and [18]FDG in 34 patients, ^{11}C-acetate yielded significantly better results than [18]FDG for prediction of viability.[20] The initial results of ^{11}C-acetate based on the theoretical advantages look promising and certainly merits further confirmation. Another advantage of ^{11}C-acetate is the possibility to measure perfusion by the early washout time activity curves, obviating a perfusion measurement with another tracer. Table 1 shows the accuracies of [18]FDG-PET and ^{11}C-acetate for prediction of improvement of contractility after revascularization and after coronary occlusion.

Table 1. [18]FDG-PET and myocardial viability studies

Studies using [18]FDG-PET (in relation to perfusion) for prediction of improvement of contractility after revascularization	pts. n	pos pred value	neg pred value
Tillisch et al. Reversibility of cardiac wall-motion abnormalities predicted by PET. N Eng J Med 1986.[21]	17	85%	92%
Tamaki et al. PET using [18]FDG in evaluation of CABG. Am J Cardiol 1989.[22]	28	78%	87%
Marwick et al. Metabolic responses of hibernating and infarcted myocardium to revascularization. A follow up study of regional perfusion, function and metabolism. Circulation 1992.[23]	16	71%	76%
Lucignani et al. Presurgical identification of hibernating myocardium by combined use of ^{99m}Tc-MIBI SPECT and [18]FDG PET in patients with coronary artery disease. Eur J Nucl Med 1992.[24]	14	95%	80%
Gropler et al. Comparison of ^{11}C-acetate with [18]FDG for delineating viable myocardium by PET. J Am Coll Cardiol 1993.[20]	34	52%	81%

Studies using [18]FDG-PET (in relation to perfusion) for prediction of spontaneous recovery of contractility after acute coronary occlusion	pts. n	pos pred value	neg pred value
Piérard et al. Identification of viable myocardium by echocardiography during dobutamine infusion in patients with myocardial infarction after thrombolytic therapy: comparison with PET. J Am Coll Cardiol 1990;15:1021-31.[25]	17	55%	100%
Schwaiger et al. Regional myocardial metabolism in patients with acute myocardial infarction assessed by PET. J Am Coll Cardiol 1986;8:800-8.[26]	13	50%	100%

pts. n = number of patients; pos pred value = positive predictive value (true pos / true pos + false pos); neg pred value = negative predictive value (true neg / true neg + false neg)

Summary

PET research has already introduced the concept of viability to the daily clinical practice. Because of its ability to study metabolic processes in the intact human body, it will certainly deepen our understanding of (patho)physiological processes in the future, and therefore has become indispensable for the execution of state of the art research. Whether it can evolve from a sophisticated but expensive research tool to a useful clinical method in cardiology, still remains a question. It may very well be that only a well performed cost effectiveness study will be able to provide an answer to this question.

References

1. Rahimtoola SH. The hibernating myocardium. Am Heart J 1989;117:211-21.
2. Yusuf S, Zucker D, Peduzzi P et al. Effect of coronary artery bypass graft surgery on survival: overview of 10-years results from randomized trials by the Coronary Artery Bypass Graft Surgery Trialist Collaboration. Lancet 1994;344:563-70.
3. Unpublished experience of the Thoraxcenter of the University Hospital Groningen during 1993 and 1994. A centre with an estimated annual coronary angiogram review rate of 5000 resulting in a patient turnover of approximately 1200 CABG and 1200 PTCA per year.
4. Braunwald E, Kloner RA. The stunned myocardium: Prolonged, postischemic ventricular dysfunction. Circulation 1982;66:1146-9.
5. Zaret BL, Wackers FJ. Nuclear cardiology. Second of two parts. N Engl J Med 1993;329:855-63.
6. Matzusaki M, Gallagher KP, Kemper WS et al. Sustained regional dysfunction produced by prolonged coronary stenosis: Gradual recovery after reperfusion. Circulation 1987;68:170-82.
7. Fedele FA, Gerwitz H, Capone RJ et al. Metabolic response to prolonged reduction of myocardial blood flow distal to a severe coronary stenosis. Circulation 1988;78:729-35.
8. Opie LH. Effects of regional ischemia on metabolism of glucose and fatty acids. Circ Res 1976;38:152-74.
9. Vanoverschelde JL, Wijns W, Depre C et al. Mechanisms of chronic regional postischemic dysfunction in humans. New insights from the study of non infarcted collateral dependent myocardium. Circulation 1993;87:1513-23.
10. Borgers M, Ausma J, Wijffels M et al. Atrial fibrillation in the goat: a model for chronic hibernating myocardium. Circulation 1994;90:I-467 (Abstract).
11. Elsner D, Riegger GAJ. Animal models of heart failure. Curr Opin Cardiol 1991;6:334-40.
12. Blanksma PK, Willemsen ATM, Meeder JG et al. Quantitative myocardial mapping of perfusion and metabolism using parametric polar map display in cardiac PET. J Nucl Med 1995;36:153-58.
13. Yamamoto Y, De Silva R, Rhodes CG et al. A new strategy for the assessment of viable and regional myocardial blood flow using 15-O-water and dynamic positron emission tomography. Circulation 1992;86:167-78.
14. Phelps ME, Hoffman EJ, Selin CE et al. Investigation of ^{18}F-2-fluoro-2-deoxyglucose for the measure of myocardial glucose metabolism. J Nucl Med 1978;19:1311-9.
15. Knuuti MJ, Yki-Järvinen H, Voipio-Pulkki LM et al. Enhancement of myocardial (fluorine-18)fluorodeoxyglucose uptake by a nicotinic acid derivative. J Nucl Med 1994;35:989-98.
16. Knuuti MJ, Nuutila P, Ruotsalainen U et al. The value of quantitative analysis of glucose utilization in detection of myocardial viability by PET. J Nucl Med 1993;34:2068-75.
17. Eitzman D, Al-Aouar Z, Kanter HL et al. Clinical outcome of patients with advanced coronary artery disease after viability studies with positron emission tomography. J Am Coll Cardiol 1992;20:559-65.
18. Brown M, Marshall DR, Sobel BE et al. Delineation of myocardial oxygen utilization with carbon-11 labeled acetate. Circulation 1987;76:687-96.
19. Brown M, Myers DW, Bergmann SR et al. Noninvasive assessment of canine myocardial oxidative metabolism with carbon-11 acetate and positron emission

tomography. J Am Coll Cardiol 1988;12:1054-63.

20. Gropler RJ, Geltman EM, Sampathkumaran K et al. Comparison of carbon-11-acetate with fluorine-18-fluorodeoxyglucose for delineating viable myocardium by positron emission tomography. J Am Coll Cardiol 1993;22:1587-97.

21. Tillisch J, Brunken R, Marshall R et al. Reversibility of cardiac wall-motion abnormalities predicted by positron emission tomography. N Engl J Med 1986;314:884-8.

22. Tamaki N, Yonekura Y, Yamashita K et al. Positron emission tomography using fluorine-18-deoxyglucose in evaluation of coronary artery bypass grafting. Am J Cardiol 1989;64:860-5.

23. Marwick HT, MacIntyre WJ, Lafont A et al. Metabolic responses of hibernating and infarcted myocardium to revascularization. A follow up study of regional perfusion, function and metabolism. Circulation 1992;85:1347-53.

24. Lucignani G, Paolini G, Landoni C et al. Presurgical identification of hibernating myocardium by combined use of technetium-99m hexakis 2-methoxyisobutylisonitrile single photon emission tomography and fluorine-18 fluoro-2-deoxy-d-glucose positron emission tomography in patients with coronary artery disease. Eur J Nucl Med 1992;19:874-81.

25. Pierard LA, De Landsheere CM, Berthe C et al. Identification of viable myocardium by echocardiography during dobutamine infusion in patients with myocardial infarction after thrombolytic therapy: comparison with positron emission tomography. J Am Coll Cardiol 1990;15:1021-31.

26. Schwaiger M, Brunken R, Grover-McKay M et al. Regional myocardial metabolism in patients with acute myocardial infarction assessed by positron emission tomography. J Am Coll Cardiol 1986;8:800-8.

3   COMPARISON OF THALLIUM SCINTIGRAPHY AND POSITRON EMISSION TOMOGRAPHY

Menco G. Niemeyer, Joan G. Meeder, Aaf F.M. Kuijper,
Paul K. Blanksma, and Ernst E. van der Wall

Introduction

The conventional imaging techniques provide a clear means of evaluating the anatomy and function of the heart. However, these methods show limitations in answering questions regarding physiologic significance of given anatomy or of myocardial viability. Whereas planar imaging and single photon emission computed tomography (SPECT) have considerable practical advantages and can be applied in almost any hospital with current commercially available nuclear medicine equipment and radiopharmaceuticals, positron emission tomography (PET) theoretically offers major advantages in its potential to quantitatively study regional myocardial metabolism and blood flow because of its ability to correct for attenuation. PET measures local tissue concentrations of radioisotopes in the body which cannot be performed by other tomographic imaging techniques such as SPECT, computed tomography or magnetic resonance imaging.[1] In cardiac studies, PET can be used for the detection of myocardial ischemia, identification of tissue viability, and pathophysiologic assessment of various myocardial diseases, such as hypertrophic cardiomyopathy.[2-4] With diffusible tracers such as nitrogen-13 (^{13}N) and rubidium-82 (^{82}Rb) it is possible to measure myocardial blood flow with PET. In addition to its ability to measure myocardial perfusion, PET is currently the only available technique that can assess cardiac metabolism in humans quantitatively. To study metabolism of myocardial tissue with PET, several different types of metabolic compounds are available: fluorine-18 (^{18}F)-labeled fluorodeoxyglucose (^{18}FDG), and carbon-11 (^{11}C) labeled palmitic acid, and recently ^{11}C acetate.[6,7] The combined evaluation of cardiac metabolism and perfusion enables detection of viable myocardium, which is crucial for determination of appropriate therapy. In this respect ^{13}N ammonia and ^{18}FDG were preferred imaging agents in the majority of studies addressing myocardial viability. Additionally, modifications of the standard exercise- redistribution thallium protocol may also produce accurate results. These modifications include late thallium-201 (^{201}Tl) redistribution imaging, performed 8-72 hours following initial ^{201}Tl injection, and ^{201}Tl

37

E. E. van der Wall et al. (eds.), Cardiac Positron Emission Tomography, 37–50.
© 1995 Kluwer Academic Publishers.

reinjection at rest after (3-4 hours) or late (8-72 hours) redistribution imaging. These methods can identify viable myocardium in many ^{201}Tl defects that appear to be irreversible on standard 3-4 hour redistribution imaging.[7]

Assessment of perfusion and viability by [201]Tl

In single photon imaging two main groups of tracers are used: the potassium analogues, of which ^{201}Tl has gained the most extensive use in the last two decades, and the technetium (^{99m}Tc) labeled compounds.

The uptake of ^{201}Tl in the myocardial cell is mainly controlled by passive transport over the intact cell membrane and is proportional to myocardial blood flow under physiologic conditions.[8,9] The efficacy of the radiopharmaceutical to detect coronary artery disease is hampered by relatively low emitted energy of 80 KeV and the three-day half-life which limits the administration of a sufficiently high dose to improve imaging quality.

The overall sensitivity and specificity of exercise ^{201}Tl scintigraphy using qualitative techniques range from 68-83% and 75-90%, respectively.[10,11] By using quantitative computer-assisted techniques, both the sensitivity and specificity of ^{201}Tl scintigraphy increased to the 90% or greater range.[12]

For the sole detection of myocardial ischemia the administration of ^{201}Tl at maximal stress with subsequent recording of one single imaging sequence is sufficient: a hemodynamically significant stenosis in one of the epicardial coronary arteries causes a perfusion defect. A good correlation between measured transstenotic pressure drop, calculated coronary flow reserve derived from quantitatively assessed angiographic anatomic variables and scintigraphic results has been reported.[13]

However, the single stress images cannot distinguish ischemia from myocardial infarction and therefore Pohost et al.[14] introduced a second imaging sequence after redistribution of ^{201}Tl from normal to hypoperfused myocardium. Normal ^{201}Tl uptake with exercise and ^{201}Tl defects that redistribute on 3-4 hour delayed images are accurate indicators of viable myocardium. However, reduced or absent ^{201}Tl uptake during stress and lack of redistribution on delayed images does not necessarily indicate myocardial scar, because severely ischemic but viable myocardium as well as a mixture of scar and viable myocardium may also produce an irreversible defect.[15]

Additional filling-in of defects with incomplete resolution after 4 hour redistribution was observed after 8-24 hour delayed imaging.[16,17] Dilsizian et al.[18] were the first to underscore the value of optimizing the ^{201}Tl stress testing protocol by means of a second injection (reinjection) of ^{201}Tl after redistribution imaging. It is assumed that as many as 50% of myocardial regions with apparently irreversible perfusion defects after stress-redistribution ^{201}Tl scintigraphy show improved ^{201}Tl uptake after reinjection and subsequent improvement in wall motion after revascularization.[19,20] Thus, since the introduction of the reinjection technique, the interest in ^{201}Tl imaging is shifting from the ability to detect myocardial ischemia towards the ability to detect myocardial viability.

In summary, different study protocols may have advantages and disadvantages depending on the specific situation in different imaging laboratories. However, it has to be emphasized that there are two rational and proven protocols: 1) exercise/3-hour redistribution/reinjection imaging,[18] and 2) rest-3 hour redistribution imaging[21]. A third recently proposed time-saving patient convenient protocol is the exercise/immediate reinjection procedure[22] (Figure 1).

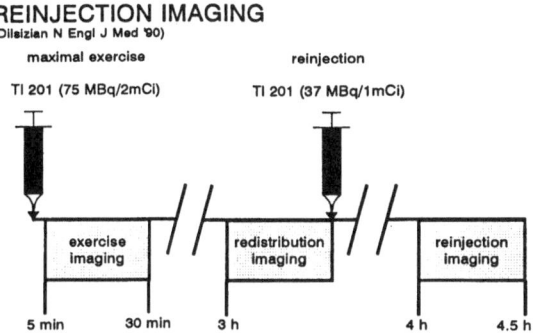

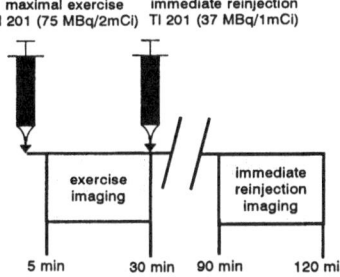

Figure 1. Currently established protocols (1A, 1B) and proposed (1C) protocol for detection of myocardial viability by [201]Tl.

Positron-emitting agents

Radioactive isotopes of oxygen, nitrogen, and carbon can be made and substituted for the same stable elements in the molecules to be studied. The use of these 'natural' radioactive constituents avoids alterations of the normal metabolic pattern that may result from the use of 'foreign' isotopes such as ^{201}Tl or [99m]Tc. The activity passing through a volume of scanned tissue can then be measured. Although some radiopharmaceuticals can almost be used as they are produced by the cyclotron such as oxygen-15 (^{15}O), or generator-produced compounds such as [82]Rb, they still require some form of radiosynthesis. For [15]O the actual product of the cyclotron is [15]O carbon dioxide, and synthesis is needed to measure perfusion with ^{15}O-labeled water. For ^{13}N, ^{13}N ammonia must be synthesized. The variety of functions that can be assessed and imaged is limited by the availability of tracers that can be rapidly labeled chemically with the isotopes, which have extremely short half-lives. For example, the half-life of [15]O is 2.07 minutes and that of [13]N 9.96 minutes. Measuring the amount of labeled molecule in the tissues depends on several chemical, physical, and biological factors, any of which may be the focus of primary, clinical, or biological interest. Because of the short half-lives of the positron-emitting radionuclides, the synthesis must be performed expeditiously. Work is progressing to automate and make routine the synthesis of PET radiopharmaceuticals. The short half-lives permit serial studies at short time intervals. Three positron-emitting tracers have been shown to have clinical value as markers of myocardial perfusion: [82]Rb, [15]O labeled water, and most frequently ^{13}N ammonia.

Measurement of regional myocardial blood flow by ^{13}N ammonia

Tracers of blood flow may be classified as extractable particles and extractable diffusion indicators. Labeled albumin microspheres are the most widely used agents in the first group. Inasmuch as they are extracted almost 100% during a single capillary transit, the local deposited activity reflects local capillary blood flow. [13]N ammonia as an indicator of myocardial blood flow appears to diffuse across capillary and cellular membranes and becomes metabolically trapped in the myocardium. Excellent correlation between the ^{13}N ammonia method and the microsphere technique has been demonstrated in animal models, although at high rates flow will be underestimated by ^{13}N ammonia.[23] This requires the inclusion of multicompartment analysis to model high levels of flow. The ^{13}N ammonia method has been studied in humans by investigators from the UCLA group.[24,25] By use of a multicompartment model they found in human volunteers that the average blood flow reserve of 2.2 with exercise correlated well with invasively established values.[24] These investigators concluded that ^{13}N ammonia may be used to determine absolute flow in patients with coronary artery disease.

The advantages of ^{13}N ammonia include rapid clearance from blood and high myocardial extraction (80-90%) and retention (82%), which results in high contrast myocardial images.[26] A linear relationship was observed between microspheres and ^{13}N ammonia for myocardial blood flow at low to moderately high flow rates. A potential disadvantage of ^{13}N ammonia is its retention in the myocardium by metabolic trapping mainly by the glutamic acid-glutamine pathway.[27] Therefore ^{13}N ammonia may not accurately reflect blood flow during conditions such as extremely low pH or reduced intracellular adenosine triphosphate. In addition, after intravenous injection ^{13}N ammonia is rapidly converted to metabolic intermediates making quantitation problematic.

Assessment of perfusion and function by PET imaging

Coronary artery disease

PET imaging of the heart with cyclotron-produced ^{13}N ammonia, preferably in conjunction with [18]FDG when information on viability is needed may be desirable for 1) accurate noninvasive diagnosis of coronary artery disease in symptomatic or asymptomatic patients,[28-32] 2) assessing physiologic stenosis severity,[33] 3) imaging myocardial infarction and determining myocardial viability,[34-38] 4) assessing effects of interventions such as thrombolysis on metabolism,[39] percutaneous transluminal coronary angioplasty (PTCA) on coronary flow reserve,[40] and bypass surgery on function and metabolism,[41] 5) following the progression or regression of coronary artery disease during risk factor modification, and 6) evaluating collateral function noninvasively.[42]

Accurate detection of coronary artery disease by means of PET is possible by evaluation of blood flow at rest compared with images after either intravenous dipyridamole or exercise. The assessment of extent of myocardial infarction, ischemia, and/or viability by PET seems promising in clinical cardiology. In patients with sustained myocardial infarction two patterns can be observed when comparing cardiac PET by use of ^{13}N ammonia and [18]FDG: 1) a concordant decrease in ^{13}N ammonia and [18]FDG uptake, and 2) a relative increase in [18]FDG uptake compared with blood flow. This latter pattern is observed predominantly with patients with persistent symptoms and signs of ischemia and is thought to represent viable myocardial tissue that is still able to metabolize glucose anaerobically.[43] In the presence of injured or ischemic but viable myocardial cells, myocardial metabolism is shifted towards anaerobic glycolysis. [18]FDG uptake then increases relative to the rest of the myocardium, thereby identifying ischemic viable tissue since necrotic myocardium does not extract FDG. In patients with chronic coronary artery disease and acute myocardial infarction, myocardial areas with a ^{13}N ammonia resting perfusion defect and normal [18]FDG uptake after oral glucose loading (flow-metabolism mismatch) are considered to be viable and may demonstrate improved left ventricular function after revascularization.[41] Studies have suggested further that the blood flow-metabolism mismatch may reflect different states of ischemia such as 'stunned myocardium' (i.e. complete restoration of blood flow after a transient ischemic event but delayed metabolic and functional recovery) and, 'hibernating myocardium' (i.e., persistently reduced flow).[44]

Dilated cardiomyopathy

This condition is unrelated to coronary artery disease and may also be diagnosed by positron imaging as an enlarged, poorly functioning heart with no resting or stress perfusion defects typical of ischemic cardiomyopathy due to coronary artery disease.[5] In cases of dilated congestive cardiomyopathy, PET has been found to accurately distinguish between idiopathic and ischemic types of cardiomyopathy.[45,46] Idiopathic dilated cardiomyopathy characteristically exhibits homogeneous blood flow, homogeneous glucose utilization, and diffusely heterogenous fatty acid uptake and metabolism. In contrast, ischemic types of dilated cardiomyopathy characteristically exhibit large discrete reductions in regional myocardial blood flow, corresponding to well-defined vascular territories. Relative increases in glucose utilization in such segments identify myocardium as viable and predict a potential functional improvement after interventional revascularization. Loss of metabolic activity, on the other hand, defines such hypoperfused regions as irreversibly injured without the potential for functional recovery.[44]

Duchennes's muscular dystrophy has been shown to selectively involve the posterolateral wall of the left ventricle as the initial and primary site of myocardial dystrophy.[47] Electrocardiography changes in this patient population suggest myocardial damage in corresponding ventricular segments. Perloff et al.[48] investigated 15 patients with Duchenne's muscular dystrophy and reported decreased ^{13}N ammonia uptake but maintained or increased [18]FDG uptake in the posterolateral wall.

Hypertrophic cardiomyopathy

Patients with classic hypertrophic cardiomyopathy have been studied with ^{13}N ammonia PET.[49-51] By gating the positron-emission tomograms with the electrocardiography, left ventricular function and wall thickening may be assessed regionally in three dimensions.[52] Grover-McKay et al.[3] found a homogeneous tissue distribution of ^{13}N ammonia. In contrast, reduced [18]FDG concentration in the septum was observed as compared with that in the free wall of the left ventricle. Camici et al.[51] showed in patients with hypertrophic cardiomyopathy using ^{13}N ammonia PET that coronary vasodilator reserve is abnormal not only in the hypertrophied interventricular septum, but also in the free wall of the left ventricle. This finding suggests that the reduction in coronary flow reserve is not necessarily the result of myocardial hypertrophy, but may be a primary defect.

Comparison of ^{201}Tl scintigraphy with perfusion and/or metabolic PET imaging

Bonow et al.[38] and Tamaki et al.[53] were able to show that the ^{201}Tl reinjection method yields nearly the same results as [18]FDG PET. Bonow et al.[38] performed a comparison of ^{201}Tl reinjection SPECT imaging and [18]FDG PET imaging in 16 patients (432 segments) with chronic ischemic heart disease and left ventricular dysfunction. Of the 432 segments, 166 (38%) had an irreversible ^{201}Tl defect on standard redistribution images. [18]FDG uptake could be demonstrated in 73% of these 166 segments. When irreversible ^{201}Tl defects were subgrouped into segments with mild (60-85% of peak activity) moderate (50-59%) or severe (<50%) defects, [18]FDG uptake was present in 91%, 88% and 51% of the segments. [201]Tl reinjection was routinely performed. The authors reported a 88% concordance between ^{201}Tl reinjection and [18]FDG imaging regarding myocardial viability: 45% of segments were identified as viable and 43% as scar in both studies. The following conclusions could be made:
1) Irreversible ^{201}Tl defects with >50% of peak activity contain a significant amount of viable myocardium (84%-91% of segments viable as assessed by [18]FDG PET):

therefore ^{201}Tl reinjection is not necessary.
2) In case of irreversible ^{201}Tl defects with <50% of peak activity, ^{201}Tl reinjection shows excellent concordance with [18]FDG PET with regard to myocardial viability (Figure 2). Therefore in cases of doubt (e.g. whether to revascularize or not), reinjection should be performed routinely.

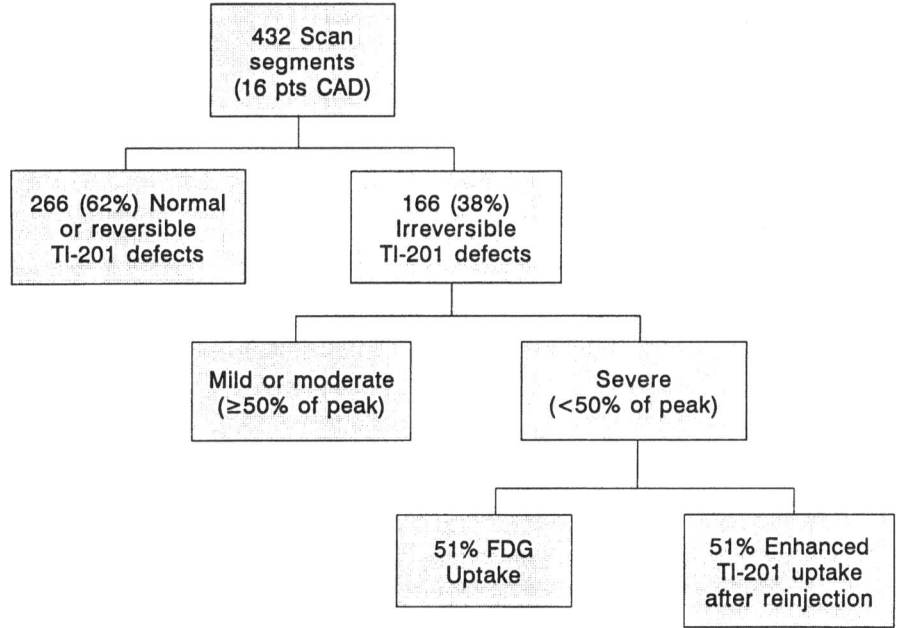

Figure 2. Comparison of [18]FDG-PET with ^{201}Tl reinjection in severe irreversible perfusion defects. CAD = coronary artery disease. Adapted from Bonow RO et al., Circulation 1991;83:26-37.

Tamaki et al.[53] confirmed these findings in a study of 18 patients with chronic congestive heart failure or recent myocardial infarction, 11 of whom underwent bypass surgery. Most segments assessed as viable by ^{201}Tl redistribution and reinjection showed an improvement in regional wall motion. In summary these authors reported 85% concordance between ^{201}Tl reinjection and [18]FDG PET imaging with respect to viable myocardial segments. [18]FDG uptake in the PET study had a slightly higher predictive value regarding viable tissue. In a later study, that was undertaken to evaluate the prognostic value, Tamaki et al.[54] showed that [18]FDG PET was the best predictor of a future event among all clinical, angiographic and radionuclide variables in stable patients with previous myocardial infarction. More important, even when stress ^{201}Tl scintigraphy did not show any redistribution, those patients who had an increase in [18]FDG uptake appeared to be likely to have a future cardiac event. Their conclusion was, that [18]FDG PET is capable of playing an important prognostic role in the study of patients with myocardial infarction. When an increase in [18]FDG uptake is observed, such patients may need aggressive treatment to prevent cardiac events (see also chapter by van der Wall).

There is evidence that concordance between ^{201}Tl reinjection and [18]FDG PET depends on the myocardial region studied. Altehoefer et al.[55] showed a close correlation in the anterior wall (r = 0.79) and in the lateral wall (r = 0.77), while the correlation in the posterior region was considerably lower (r = 0.52).

Dreyfus et al.[56] studied 50 patients with ischemic heart disease, congestive heart failure, and low ejection fraction who were initially referred for heart transplantation. Whenever myocardial viability was detected by ^{201}Tl scintigraphy or PET imaging coronary artery bypass grafting (CABG) as an alternative to orthotopic heart transplantation was performed. Myocardium was considered viable by ^{201}Tl scintigraphy when uptake improved in at least two different areas. When ^{201}Tl scintigraphy was noncontributory, patients underwent [15]O labeled water/ [18]FDG PET imaging (flow-metabolism mismatch was represented by the absence of flow in contrast to active metabolism and uptake of FDG). Myocardial viability assessment was carried out in 48 patients. Based on their criteria, 28 (58.3%) were positive at ^{201}Tl scintigraphy. The 20 considered negative at ^{201}Tl scintigraphy underwent PET. Eighteen of them were graded positive at PET imaging, and only 2 (10%) had a negative grade for [18]FDG uptake and therefore were treated by orthotopic heart transplantation. Perioperative mortality was 2.17% (1/46) in the patients undergoing CABG. They recommended CABG as an alternative to orthotopic heart transplantation whenever myocardial viability was detected by ^{201}Tl scintigraphy or PET scintigraphy. Figure 3 shows the proposed algorithm for detection of myocardial viability as performed by the authors.[56]

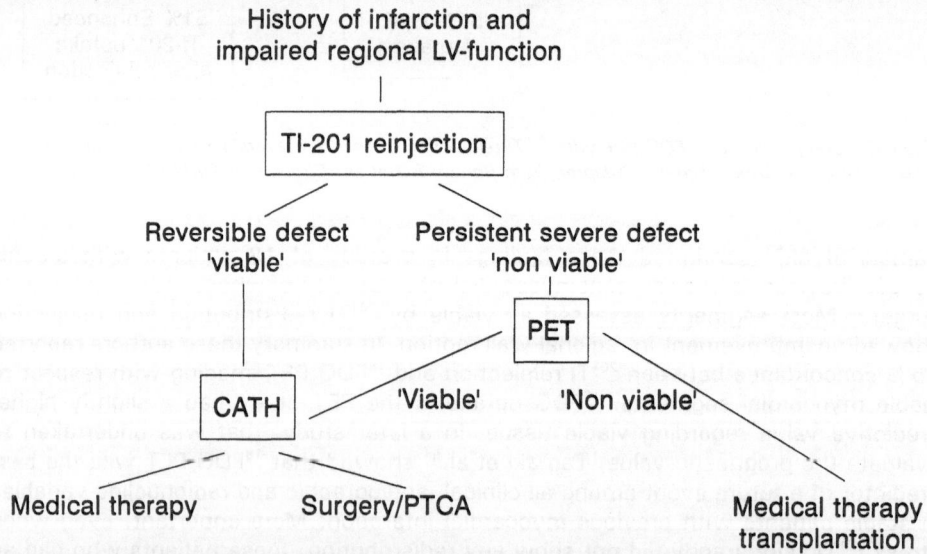

Figure 3. Diagnostic approach in patients with the clinical question of tissue viability. LV = left ventricle; TI-201 = thallium-201; PET = positron emission tomography; CATH = catheterization; PTCA = coronary angioplasty. Adapted from Dreyfus GD et al., Ann Thorac Surg 1994;57:1402-8, and Schwaiger M et al., Eur Heart J 1994;15(Suppl D):14-9.

In a study by Go et al.,[57] for a population of 202 patients studied, the sensitivity of [82]Rb PET imaging for the diagnosis of coronary artery disease was demonstrated to be significantly higher than the sensitivity of ^{201}Tl SPECT imaging in patients with and without previous bypass surgery or PTCA (93% vs 76%), whereas the difference in specificity was slight (78% vs 80%). In a study of 81 patients Stewart et al.[58] the overall sensitivity, specificity and accuracy of [82]Rb PET were 84%, 88% and 85%, respectively, whereas, SPECT imaging revealed a sensitivity of 84%, specificity of 53% ($p < 0.05$ vs PET) and accuracy of 79%.

Wackers[59] stated in his editorial that the comparative studies such as described by Go et al.[57] and Stewart et al.[58] demonstrate that with optimal imaging techniques it is possible to avoid artifacts that haunt ^{201}Tl SPECT imaging. PET has an important role in showing the way and direction for conventional imaging techniques. The recent modification of ^{201}Tl imaging protocols is an example of crossfertilization by PET.[18] When the limitations of conventional exercise/3-4 hour delayed ^{201}Tl imaging for complete visualization of viable myocardium were recognized,[16,17] PET provided a benchmark for differentiation between viable and infarcted tissue.[41]

Perrone-Filardi et al.[60] compared ^{201}Tl scintigraphy with PET and magnetic resonance (MR) imaging. Comparison of regional ^{201}Tl activity, before and after ^{201}Tl reinjection, with indices of regional systolic wall thickening by MR imaging, indicated that the majority of regions identified as viable by ^{201}Tl scintigraphy have preserved wall thickening, which is an accepted standard for viability. Importantly, in regions with absent wall thickening, in which the myocardium was either fibrotic or hibernating, there was an excellent concordance regarding the presence or absence of tissue viability between the results of ^{201}Tl reinjection and assessment of metabolic activity by PET. These data indicate that ^{201}Tl reinjection is a convenient, clinically accurate, and relatively inexpensive method with which to identify viable myocardium in patients with chronic coronary artery disease and left ventricular dysfunction.

Conclusion

PET provides an advanced imaging technology that permits the accurate definition of regional tracer distribution. Results of several studies indicate the superiority of PET compared with standard ^{201}Tl tomographic imaging. In addition, regional blood flow can be accurately measured with ^{13}N ammonia PET, and this approach can be used in conjunction with pharmacologic stress imaging to quantify regional flow reserve. In combination with metabolic markers, ^{13}N ammonia is capable of assessing myocardial viability. Furthermore, the ^{13}N ammonia PET approach may differentiate among various forms of cardiomyopathy. PET viability studies with perfusion agents as ^{13}N ammonia in conjunction with [18]FDG are valuable in patients with severely impaired regional or global function, with coronary anatomy suitable for revascularization regions of wall motion abnormality, and in the absence of reversible perfusion abnormalities on ^{201}Tl imaging after reinjection. The advantages of advanced PET technology are best observed for intermediate disease prevalence (<60% of the study population), moderate to less severe coronary artery disease, or both, in which the question of medical or mechanical intervention is unclear and ^{201}Tl stress testing is least accurate. The cost of providing PET imaging in a medical center is, however, high. Such facilities require an investment for a cyclotron and a PET imaging device and also the services of both well-trained radiochemists and physicists for maintenance and operation. More studies are needed to define the cost-benefit ratio of PET techniques for the management of patients with coronary artery disease or cardiomyopathy.

References

1. Phelps ME, Mazziotta JC, Schelbert HR. Positron emission tomography and autoradiography: principles and applications for the brain and heart. New York: Raven Press, 1986.
2. Yamashita K, Tamaki N, Yonekura Y et al. Regional wall thickening of left ventricle evaluated by gated positron emission tomography in relation to myocardial perfusion and glucose metabolism. J Nucl Med 1991;32:679-85.
3. Grover-McKay M, Schwaiger M, Krivokapich J, Perloff JK, Phelps ME, Schelbert HR. Regional myocardial blood flow and metabolism at rest in mildly symptomatic patients with hypertrophic cardiomyopathy. J Am Coll Cardiol 1989;13:317-24.
4. Niemeyer MG, Kuijper AFM, Gerhards LJ, D'haene EG, van der Wall EE. Nitrogen-13 ammonia perfusion imaging: relation to metabolic imaging. Am Heart J 1993;125:848-54.
5. Walsh MN, Geltman EM, Brown MA et al. Noninvasive estimation of regional myocardial oxygen consumption by positron emission tomography with carbon-11 acetate in patients with myocardial infarction. J Nucl Med 1989;30:1798-808.
6. Armbrecht JJ, Buxton DB, Schelbert HR. Validation of carbon-11 acetate as a tracer for noninvasive assessment of oxidative metabolism with positron emission tomography in normal, ischemic, postischemic, and hyperemic canine myocardium. Circulation 1990;81:1594-605.
7. Bonow RO, Dilsizian V. Assessing viable myocardium with thallium-201. Am J Cardiol 1992;70:10E-7E.
8. Nielsen AP, Morris KG, Murdock R, Bruno FP, Cobb FR. Linear relationship between the distribution of thallium-201 and blood flow in ischemic and nonischemic myocardium during exercise, Circulation 1980;61:797-801.
9. Melin JA, Becker LC. Quantitative relationship between global left ventricular thallium uptake and blood flow: effects of propranolol, ouabain, dipyridamole, and coronary occlusion. J Nucl Med 1986;27:641-52.
10. Kuijper AFM, van Eck-Smit BLF, Niemeyer MG, Bruschke AVG, Pauwels EKJ, van der Wall EE. The role of scintigraphic techniques in the evaluation of functional results of coronary bypass grafting and percutaneous transluminal coronary angioplasty. Int J Card Imaging 1993;9:49-58.
11. Beller GA, Gibson RS. Sensitivity, specificity and prognostic significance of noninvasive testing for occult or known coronary disease. Prog Cardiovasc Dis 1987;29:241-70.
12. Wackers FJ, Fetterman R, Mattera JA, Clements JP. Quantitative planar thallium-201 stress scintigraphy: a critical evaluation of the method. Semin Nucl Med 1985;1546-66.
13. Zijlstra F, Fioretti P, Reiber JH, Serruys PW. Which cineangiographically assessed anatomic variable correlates best with functional measurements of stenosis severity? A comparison of quantitative analysis of the coronary cineangiogram with measured coronary flow reserve and exercise/redistribution thallium-201 scintigraphy. J Am Coll Cardiol 1988;12:686-91.
14. Pohost GM, Zir LM, Moore RH, McKusick KA, Guiney TE, Beller GA. Differentiation of transiently ischemic from infarcted myocardium by serial imaging after a single dose of thallium-201. Circulation 1977;55:294-302.
15. Dilsizian V, Bonow RO. Current diagnostic techniques of assessing myocardial viability in patients with hibernating and stunned myocardium. Circulation 1993;87:1-20.
16. Cloninger KG, DePuey EG, Garcia EV, Roubin GS, Robbins WL, Nody A. Incomplete redistribution in delayed thallium-201 single photon emission computed tomographic (SPECT) images: an overestimation of myocardial scarring. J Am Coll Cardiol 1988;12:955-63.

17. Kiat H, Berman DS, Maddahi J, de Yang L, van Train K, Rozanski A. Late reversibility of tomographic myocardial thallium-201 defects: an accurate marker of myocardial viability. J Am Coll Cardiol 1988;12:1456-63.
18. Dilsizian V, Rocco TP, Freedman NMT, Leon MB, Bonow RO. Enhanced detection of ischemic but viable myocardium by reinjection of thallium after stress-redistribution imaging. N Engl J Med 1990;323:141-6.
19. Dilsizian V, Bonow RO. Differential uptake and apparent thallium-201 "washout" after thallium reinjection options regarding early redistribution imaging or late redistribution imaging after reinjection. Circulation 1992;85:1032-8.
20. Schoeder H, Friedrich M, Topp H. Myocardial viability; what do we need? Eur J Nucl Med 1993;20:792-803.
21. Ragosta M, Beller GA, Watson DD, Kaul S, Gimple LW. Quantitative planar rest-redistribution ^{201}Tl imaging in detection of myocardial viability and prediction of improvement in left ventricular function after coronary bypass surgery in patients with severely depressed left ventricular function. Circulation 1993;88:941-52
22. van Eck-Smit BLF, van der Wall EE, Kuijper AFM, Zwinderman AH, Pauwels EKJ. Immediate thallium-201 reinjection following stress imaging: a time saving approach for detection of myocardial viability. J Nucl Med 1993;34:737-43.
23. Shah A, Shelbert HR, Schwaiger M et al. Measurement of regional myocardial blood flow with ^{13}N ammonia and positron emission tomography in intact dogs. J Am Coll Cardiol 1985;5:92-100.
24. Krivokapich J, Smith GT, Huang S-C et al. 13-N ammonia myocardial imaging at rest and exercise in normal volunteers. Quantification of absolute myocardial perfusion with dynamic positron emission tomography. Circulation 1989;80:1328-37.
25. Hutchins GD, Schwaiger M, Rosenspire KC, Krivokapich J, Schelbert HR, Kuhl DE. Noninvasive quantification of regional blood flow in the human heart using ^{13}N ammonia and dynamic positron emission tomographic imaging. J Am Coll Cardiol 1990;15:1032-42.
26. Schelbert HR, Phelps ME, Huang SC et al. ^{13}N ammonia as an indicator of myocardial blood flow. Circulation 1981;63:1259-72.
27. Rauch B, Helus F, Grunze M et al. Kinetics of 13-N ammonia uptake in myocardial single cells indicating potential limitations in its applicability as a marker of myocardial blood flow. Circulation 1985;71:387-93.
28. Kambara H, Fudo T, Hashimoto T et al. Silent myocardial ischemia in patients with myocardial infarction: evaluation with positron emission computed tomography. Jpn Circ J 1989;53:1437-43.
29. Gould KL. Clinical cardiac positron emission tomography: state of the art. Circulation 1991;84(Suppl I):I-22-I-36.
30. Schelbert HR, Wisenberg G, Phelps ME et al. Non-invasive assessment of coronary stenosis by myocardial imaging during pharmacologic coronary vasodilation. VI. Detection of coronary artery disease in man with intravenous ^{13}N ammonia and positron computed tomography. Am J Cardiol 1982;49:1197-207.
31. Yonekura Y, Tamaki N, Senda M et al. Detection of coronary artery disease with 13-N-ammonia and high resolution positron emission computed tomography. Am Heart J 1987;113:645-54.
32. Zimmermann R, Tillmans H, Knapp WH et al. Regional myocardial nitrogen-13 glutamate uptake in patients with coronary artery disease: inverse post-stress relation to thallium-201 uptake in ischemia. J Am Coll Cardiol 1988;11:549-56.
33. Gould KL. Percent coronary stenosis: Battered gold standard pernicious relic, or clinical practicality? J Am Coll Cardiol 1988;11:886-8.

34. Schwaiger M, Brunken RC, Krivokapich J et al. Beneficial effect of residual anterograde flow on tissue viability as assessed by positron emission tomography in patients with myocardial infarction. Eur Heart J 1987;8:981-8.
35. Brunken K, Schwaiger M, Grover-McKay M, Phelps M, Tillisch J, Schelbert HR. Positron emission tomography detects tissue metabolic activity in myocardial segments with persistent thallium perfusion defects. J Am Coll Cardiol 1987;10:557-67.
36. Marshall RC, Tillisch JH, Phelps ME et al. Identification and differentiation of resting myocardial ischemia and infarction in man with positron computed tomography. ^{18}F-labeled fluorodeoxyglucose and ^{13}N ammonia. Circulation 1983;67:766-78.
37. Williams BR. Positron emission tomography for the assessment of ischemia and myocardial viability. J Myocardial Ischemia 1990;2:33-64.
38. Bonow RO, Dilsizian V, Cuocolo A, Bacharach SL. Identification of viable myocardium in patients with chronic coronary artery disease and left ventricular dysfunction. Comparison of thallium scintigraphy with reinjection and PET imaging with ^{18}F-Fluorodeoxyglucose. Circulation 1991;83:26-37.
39. Sobel BE, Geltman EM, Tiefenbrunn AJ et al. Improvement of regional myocardial metabolism after coronary thrombolysis induced with tissue-type plasminogen activator or streptokinase. Circulation 1984;69:983-90.
40. Goldstein RA, Kirkeeide R, Smalling RW et al. Changes in myocardial perfusion reserve after PTCA: Non-invasive assessment with positron tomography. J Nucl Med 1987;28:1262-7.
41. Tillisch J, Brunken R, Marschall R et al. Reversibility of cardial wall-motion abnormalities predicted by positron tomography. N Engl J Med 1986;314:884-8.
42. Demer LL, Gould KL, Goldstein R, Kirkeeide L. Non-invasive assessment of coronary collaterals in man by PET perfusion imaging. J Nucl Med 1990:31:259-70.
43. Brunken K, Kottou S, Nienaber CA et al. PET detection of viable tissue in myocardial segments with persistent defects at TI-201 SPECT. Radiology 1989;172:65-73.
44. Schelbert HR. Positron emission tomography for the assessment of myocardial viability. Circulation 1991;84(Suppl I):I-122-I-131.
45. Vaghaiwalla-Mody FV, Brunken RC, Warner Stevenson L, Nienaber CA, Phelps ME, Schelbert HR. Differentiating cardiomyopathy of coronary artery disease from nonischemic dilated cardiomyopathy utilizing positron tomography. J Am Coll Cardiol 1991;17:373-83.
46. Geltman EM, Smith JL, Beecher D, Ludbrook PA, Ter-Pogossian MM, Sobel BE. Altered regional myocardial metabolism in congestive cardiomyopathy detected by positron tomography. Am J Med 1983;74:773-85.
47. Perloff JK, Roberts WC, Deleon ACJ, O'Doherty D. The distinctive electrocardiogram of Duchenne's progressive muscular dystrophy. An electrocardiographic pathologic correlative study. Am J Med 1967;42:179-88.
48. Perloff JK, Henze E, Schelbert HR. Alterations in regional myocardial metabolism perfusion, and wall motion in Duchenne's muscular dystrophy studied by radionuclide imaging. Circulation 1984;69:33-42.
49. Endo M, Yoshida K, Iinuma TA et al. Noninvasive quantification of regional myocardial blood flow and ammonia extraction fraction using nitrogen-13 ammonia and positron emission tomography. Ann Nucl Med;1987:1:1-6.
50. Yoshida K, Endo M, Himi T et al. Measurement of regional myocardial blood flow in hypertrophic cardiomyopathy: application of the first-pass flow model using ^{13}N-ammonia and PET. Am J Physiol Imaging 1989;4:97-104.
51. Camici P, Chiriatti G, Lorenzoni R et al. Coronary vasodilatation is impaired in both hypertrophied and nonhypertrophied myocardium of patients with hypertrophic cardiomyopathy: a study with nitrogen-13 ammonia and positron emission tomography.

J Am Coll Cardiol 1991;17:879-86.
52. Kehtarnavaz N, Defigueiredo RJP. A novel surface reconstruction and display method for cardiac PET imaging. IEEE Trans Med Imaging 1984;MI-3:108-15.
53. Tamaki N, Ohtani H, Yamashita K et al. Metabolic activity in the areas of new fill-in after thallium-201 reinjection: comparison with positron emission tomography using fluorine-18-deoxyglucose. J Nucl Med 1991;32:673-8.
54. Tamaki N, Kawamoto M, Takahashi N et al. Prognostic value of an increase in fluorine-18 deoxyglucose uptake in patients with myocardial infarction: comparison with stress thallium imaging. J Am Coll Cardiol 1993;22:1621-7.
55. Altehoefer C, Dahl J vom, Buell U, Uebis R, Kleinhans E, Hanrath P. Comparison of thallium-201 single-photon emission tomography after rest injection and fluorodeoxyglucose positron emission tomography for assessment of myocardial viability in patients with chronic coronary artery disease. Eur J Nucl Med 1994;21:37-45.
56. Dreyfus GD, Duboc D, Blasco A et al. Myocardial viability assessment in ischemic cardiomyopathy: benefits of coronary revascularization. Ann Thorac Surg 1994;57:1402-8.
57. Go RT, Marwick TH, MacIntyre WJ et al. A prospective comparison of rubidium-82 PET and thallium-201 SPECT myocardial perfusion imaging utilizing a single dipyridamole stress in the diagnosis of coronary artery disease. J Nucl Med 1990;31:1899-905.
58. Stewart RE, Schwaiger M, Molina E et al. Comparison of rubidium-82 positron emission tomography and thallium-201 spect imaging for detection of coronary artery disease. Am J Cardiol 1991;67:1303-10.
59. Wackers FJTh. Planar, SPECT, PET: the quest to predict the unpredictable? J Nucl Med 1990;31:1906-9.
60. Perrone-Filardi P, Bacharach SL, Dilsizian V, Maurea S, Frank JA, Bonow RO. Regional left ventricular wall thickening: relation to regional uptake of ^{18}F-fluorodeoxyglucose and ^{201}Tl in patients with chronic coronary artery disease and left ventricular dysfunction. Circulation 1992;86:1125-37.

4   CARDIAC METABOLISM: POSITRON EMISSION TOMOGRAPHY VERSUS SINGLE PHOTON EMISSION COMPUTED TOMOGRAPHY

Ernst E. van der Wall

Introduction

Many noninvasive methods for imaging cardiac metabolism have been developed in the past decades. Initially, these methods were mainly used for research purposes, but they are now increasingly used in clinical practice for assessment of viable cardiac tissue. The key issue is to detect potentially salvageable tissue in jeopardized areas, predominantly pertaining to infarct zones and areas supplied by critically stenosed arteries.[1] The correct identification of hibernating and stunned myocardium in patients with severely depressed cardiac function can have vital therapeutic consequences for the patient. Changes in myocardial fatty acid and glucose metabolism during acute and prolonged ischemia can be traced by positron emitting or gamma emitting radiopharmaceuticals. Positron emission tomography (PET) that uses combinations of flow tracers and metabolic tracers offers unique opportunities for quantification and high-resolution static and rapid dynamic studies. Currently, assessment of glucose metabolism with fluorine-18-fluorodeoxyglucose ([18]FDG) is regarded as the gold standard for myocardial viability and for prediction of improvement of impaired contractile function after revascularization. However, preserved oxidative metabolism may be required for potential functional improvement and therefore, assessment of residual oxidative metabolism by carbon-11(^{11}C)-acetate PET may prove to be more accurate than [18]FDG PET which reflects both anaerobic and oxidative metabolism. Moreover, because fatty acids are metabolized only aerobically, they are excellent candidates for clinical assessment of myocardial viability and prediction of functional improvement after revascularization. Apart from positron emission agents for studying cardiac metabolism, single photon agents have gained renewed interest. In this regard, radioiodinated free fatty acids have been shown to be valuable alternative tracers for studying cardiac metabolism and viability. Especially derivatives of radioiodinated free fatty acids which are not metabolized but accumulate in the myocyte are attractive for myocardial imaging. Examples are [123]I-ß-methyl-p-iodophenyl pentadecanoic acid (^{123}I-BMIPPA) and 15-(o-^{123}I-phenyl)-pentadecanoic acid (^{123}I-oIPPA). These tracers can be

E. E. van der Wall et al. (eds.), Cardiac Positron Emission Tomography, 51–73.
© 1995 *Kluwer Academic Publishers.*

detected by planar scintigraphy and single photon emission computed tomography (SPECT), which are more economical and more widely available techniques than PET. In addition, 511 keV collimators have been developed recently, making the detection of positron emitters by planar scintigraphy and SPECT feasible. The purpose of this chapter is to explore the properties of myocardial metabolism that offer opportunities for imaging and to discuss how different imaging modalities are capable to translate changes in metabolism into clinically useful information.

Modalities for imaging of cardiac metabolism

Generally, several different approaches are available for noninvasive direct assessment of metabolism (Figure 1). The first option is to use radioactive tracer molecules that are chemically indistinguishable from their native counterparts. Since most of life's molecules contain predominantly carbon, hydrogen and oxygen, and radioactive isotopes of these elements ^{11}C and oxygen-15(^{15}O) are positron-emitters, they can be used in tracer molecules for diagnostic imaging by PET. The second option is to use chemically modified molecules labeled with either gamma- or positron-emitting radionuclides, which can be detected by planar scintigraphy, SPECT or PET imaging. The metabolism of such molecules can be different from their native counterparts,

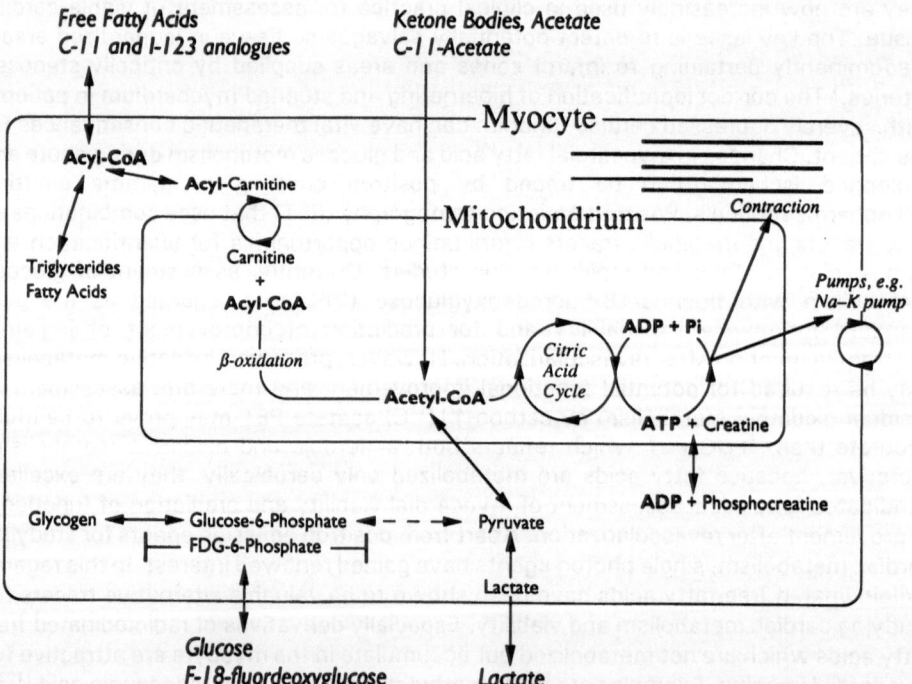

Figure 1. Schematic outline of cardiac metabolic pathways and entry points for various noninvasive diagnostic methods (From Valkema R et al, J Nucl Cardiol 1994;1:546-60. Reproduced with permission).

offering opportunities for "tailor-made" molecules for assessment of specific aspects of myocardial metabolism. Examples are the glucose analogue [18]FDG and the various radioiodinated fatty acid analogues. The third option is to use the molecules that are already present in the cells. The only technique to exploit this option is magnetic resonance spectroscopy. However, magnetic resonance spectroscopy falls beyond the scope of this chapter and we will only address the appropriate scintigraphic techniques for detection of cardiac metabolism. The most important approaches for noninvasive assessment of cardiac metabolism are listed in Table 1.

Table 1. Major current and potential noninvasive modalities for clinical evaluation of cardiac metabolism

Applications	Modality	Substance used for evaluation
Glucose utilization	PET, SPECT, planar scintigraphy	[18]FDG
Free fatty acid metabolism	PET	^{11}C-palmitate
	SPECT, planar scintigraphy	^{123}I-labeled fatty acid analogs
Oxidative metabolism	PET	^{11}C-acetate
Phosphate metabolism	Magnetic resonance spectroscopy	Intracellular ^{31}P-containing molecules
Perfusion	PET, with metabolic tracer	^{15}O-labeled water
	PET, with metabolic tracer	^{13}N-labeled ammonia
Ischemia	PET	^{18}F-fluoromisonidazole
	SPECT, planar scintigraphy	[123]I- and [99m]-Tc-labeled misonidazole
Na/K-ATP-ase pump	SPECT, planar scintigraphy	[201]Tl

Metabolism of glucose: [18]FDG

The most widely used metabolic tracer for PET studies of the heart is [18]FDG. The cardiac metabolism of glucose has already been extensively described in the chapters by Camici and Tan. Briefly, [18]FDG is taken up by the myocyte and phosphorylated to [18]FDG-6-phosphate analogous to glucose. After this process it accumulates in the myocytes, since it cannot enter glycolysis or glycogen synthesis reactions. This allows static imaging for qualitative and quantitative assessment of exogenous glucose utilization.[2-6]

The uptake of glucose (and [18]FDG) increases with ischemia, when oxidation of fatty acid is impaired, parallel with increased aerobic and anaerobic glycolysis. It was demonstrated in dogs that specific identification of ischemically injured myocardium was possible by [18]FDG PET.[7] Methods for quantification of myocardial glucose metabolism with PET use multi-compartmental modeling or Patlak graphic analysis.[8] For a long time it has remained controversial whether [18]FDG should be injected in the fasting state or glucose loading state for PET imaging. Under fasting conditions, the contribution of glucose to total energy production in the myocardium is decreased.[9] Gropler et al.[10] and Choi et al.[11] demonstrated that glucose metabolism is depressed in the fasting state which can lead to inhomogeneous distribution of [18]FDG, whereas oxidative metabolism, assessed by ^{11}C-acetate, is not impaired. The fasting technique may be useful for detecting ischemic and perhaps jeopardized myocardium as areas of increased accumulation of [18]FDG. In contrast, after glucose loading the regional distribution of myocardial [18]FDG became more homogeneous, resulting in a better [18]FDG image quality.[12] For absolute quantitations of glucose uptake as an accurate measure of myocardial viability, the use of a hyperinsulinemic euglycemic clamp appears appropriate.[13] In most institutions, the latter technique is now routinely being used for identifying viable myocardium.

[18]FDG-PET:assessment of viability
The combined evaluation of cardiac metabolism and perfusion enables detection of residual viability in myocardial segments with decreased perfusion.[14,15] Marshall et al.[16] showed that a mismatch pattern of regional concentrations of [18]FDG and ^{13}N-ammonia - i.e. reduced coronary perfusion with preserved metabolic activity - in patients with a recent myocardial infarction, was consistent with increased glucose consumption and hence indicative of jeopardized but viable tissue. Necrosis was compatible with a concordant decreased glucose utilization and flow (match pattern). Tillisch et al.[17] assessed myocardial viability with [18]FDG in 17 patients to predict recovery of regional wall motion after revascularization. Of 41 viable segments according to [18]FDG PET criteria, 35 (85%) showed improvement of regional wall motion after coronary artery bypass surgery. Persistent abnormal contraction was correctly predicted in 24 (92%) of 26 nonviable regions. These initial findings have been corroborated by a vast amount of subsequently performed studies,[18-25] which showed positive predictive values from 78% to 85% (average 82%) and negative predictive values from 78% to 92% (average 83%). A recent study by vom Dahl et al.[26] who studied 37 patients with impaired left ventricular function, showed a negative predictive value for functional recovery of 86%, but a positive predictive value of only 53%; if only regions with marked left ventricular dysfunction were taken into consideration, the positive predictive value increased to 75%.

[18]FDG-uptake:prognostic significance
Apart from the capability of [18]FDG-PET to demonstrate myocardial viability and to predict functional recovery following revascularization, there are now concordant data from several institutions regarding the long-term prognostic significance of demonstrating viable myocardium using [18]FDG-PET in patients with left ventricular dysfunction.[27-31] Eitzman et al.[27] reported a retrospective 12-month follow-up study with [18]FDG PET in 82 patients with myocardial infarction who underwent coronary bypass surgery. They were the first to point out that augmented [18]FDG uptake in hypoperfused areas (mismatch) was a potential prognostic indicator; patients with an increase in 18FDG-uptake in the infarcted region were more likely to have future cardiac events than patients without any [18]FDG uptake (match). In addition they found that patients with a mismatch had a significantly lower event rate if they were revascularized (13%) compared to patients with a mismatch who were not revascularized (50%) or patients with a match. The authors concluded that [18]FDG uptake in the infarcted area was the best predictor of future cardiac events. Similarly, Tamaki et al.,[28] in 84 patients with myocardial infarction (> 1 month old), showed that

a regional increase in [18]FDG-PET uptake was the best predictor of a future cardiac events over a 2-year follow-up. Yoshida and Gould[29] showed that myocardial viability by [18]FDG-PET and infarct size (> 23% of the left ventricle) are better prognostic indicators than left ventricular ejection fraction in a 3-year follow-up study in 35 patients following myocardial infarction. They concluded that PET imaging using [18]FDG may be useful in selecting patients for revascularization, especially in those patients with impaired left ventricular function. A 1-year follow-up of 79 patients with severe left ventricular dysfunction presented by DiCarli et al.,[30] suggested that unrevascularized patients with hibernating myocardium ([18]FDG mismatch) showed an excessive prevalence of cardiac death; the survival rate of the revascularized patients was higher than those treated medically (88% versus 59%). Finally, Lee et al.,[31] who studied 129 patients with myocardial infarction over a 2-year follow-up, reported an occurrence rate of nonfatal ischemic events of 48% in medically treated patients showing a mismatch compared with 8% of revascularized patients showing a mismatch. To conclude, these prognostic studies suggested that metabolically active, dysfunctional myocardium is an unstable substrate after myocardium which is likely to lead to ischemic events if left unrevascularized. However, one should bear in mind that these studies were retrospective and larger prospective studies are therefore warranted to provide the final answer.

[18]FDG-PET:gold standard of viability?
The relation between preserved glucose metabolism and functional recovery after revascularization of akinetic myocardial segments has now been clearly established and [18]FDG PET is considered to be the gold standard of assessment of viability.[32] However, [18]FDG PET may overestimate the extent of tissue viability in as many as 32% of myocardial segments and underestimates tissue viability in up to 22% of segments.[17-26] This suggests that not only glucose utilization but also other factors such as the level of perfusion may be an important prognostic factor. Takahashi et al.[33] showed that a miminum threshold of perfusion (45% of normal) for the maintenance of glucose metabolism must exist under both fasting and glucose loading conditions. Below this threshold, irreversible damage may occur in the myocardium. Above the threshold, calculation of the regional metabolic rate of glucose may allow differentiation of reversibly ischemic from necrotic myocardium. As the authors[33] showed a very wide scatter even under the glucose loading condition, quantitative analysis of glucose metabolism rather than relative [18]FDG display is required. Alternative explanations for the less than optimal correlation between the uptake of [18]FDG and functional recovery after revascularization include the inability of the technique to distinguish between anaerobic and aerobic glucose utilization, the changing pattern in time of glucose utilization in reperfused myocardium, or some degree of [18]FDG accumulation in necrotic myocardium.[34] Alternatively, the use of ^{11}C-acetate may provide more accurate information on cardiac metabolism and viability[35] (See section on ^{11}C-acetate).

[18]FDG-SPECT: alternative to [18]FDG-PET?
Although PET has many technical features to make it the technique of choice,[36] it is relatively expensive and not widely available in clinical practice. On the other hand, standard planar and SPECT gamma cameras are widely available but less suitable for

imaging gamma energies of 511 keV. Recently, a special collimator was developed and tested for the imaging of positron emitters with a planar gamma camera by researchers from the Free University Hospital, Amsterdam, The Netherlands, and they evaluated this system for SPECT acquisition of 511 keV photons.[37] This study showed, that positron emitters can be effectively imaged with the generally available planar and SPECT gamma cameras if absolute quantification is not necessary. Of the clinically useful positron emitters only ^{18}F lends itself for planar imaging because of its half life of 110 minutes, whereas the half-life of ^{11}C and other positron emitters is too short. Clinical studies using [18]FDG with planar scintigraphy are now appearing.[38-41] Williams et al.[38] studied 32 patients with previous myocardial infarction and compared [18]FDG with ^{201}Tl exercise/24 hour redistribution scintigraphy. A subset of 14 patients underwent serial exercise ^{201}Tl scintigraphy or gated equilibrium radionuclide angiography after revascularization or medical therapy. Thirty of the 46 fixed ^{201}Tl defects demonstrated serial scintigraphic improvement. [18]FDG-^{201}Tl mismatch was present in 81% of these segments, but was absent in the majority of the unimproved segments, suggesting that planar scintigraphy with [18]FDG can detect clinically important residual viability. Preliminary results with [18]FDG SPECT and ^{201}Tl in patients with ischemic heart disease studied by Bax et al.[39-41] have confirmed the practical applicability of this technique. The current developments with the newly developed collimators for planar and SPECT scintigraphy have demonstrated that imaging of positron emitters is an attractive option, but widespread use of these techniques may still be hampered because of the requirement of a nearby cyclotron for the production of [18]F. The issue of [18]FDG-PET versus [18]FDG-SPECT will be discussed in more detail in the chapter written by Bax et al.

Oxidative metabolism: ^{11}C-Acetate

PET scintigraphy using ^{11}C-acetate provides a noninvasive method of measuring overall myocardial oxygen consumption. Because of the short half-life of [11]C (20.3 minutes) and the rapid metabolism of ^{11}C-acetate, dynamic PET imaging is required. ^{11}C-acetate readily enters the mitochondria of the myocyte, is quickly converted to acetyl coenzyme A, and is oxidized further in the citric acid cycle with clearance in the form of [11]CO$_2$. All substrates that are metabolized aerobically, including fatty acids, glucose, lactate, pyruvate and ketone bodies, are eventually converted to acetyl coenzyme A before entering the citric acid cycle.[42] There is a close correlation between the turnover rate constant (k1) which describes the rapid phase of myocardial clearance of ^{11}C-acetate after administration, and myocardial oxygen consumption.[43,44] This relationship of ^{11}C-acetate turnover to overall oxidative metabolism is relatively insensitive to variations in the kinds of substrate available for oxidation, so standardization in this respect is not necessary.[45,46]

In recent experimental studies in dogs it has been demonstrated that recovery of myocardial oxidative metabolism, assessed by sequential PET with ^{11}C-acetate, is a prerequisite for recovery of contractile function following reperfusion;the time course for recovery of oxidative metabolism and function is similar.[47,48] In 16 patients with chronic coronary artery disease, studied with PET using labeled water (H$_2$[15]O), [18]FDG and ^{11}C-acetate before revascularization, Gropler et al.[49] found that preservation of

Alkyl fatty acids

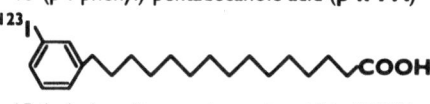

I-^{11}C-palmitate

Iodo-alkyl fatty acids

^{123}I∿∿∿∿∿COOH

17-I-heptadecanoic acid (**IHDA**)

Terminal iodo-phenyl fatty acids

^{123}I—⟨benzene⟩∿∿∿∿∿COOH

15-(p-I-phenyl)-pentadecanoic acid (**p-IPPA**)

^{123}I⟨benzene⟩∿∿∿∿∿COOH

15-(o-I-phenyl)-pentadecanoic acid (**o-IPPA**)

Methyl branched iodo-phenyl fatty acids

^{123}I—⟨benzene⟩∿∿∿∿ᴄʜ₃COOH
CH₃

15-(p-I-phenyl)-3-R,S-methyl pentadecanoic acid (**3-BMIPPA**)

^{123}I—⟨benzene⟩∿∿∿ CH₃ COOH CH₃

15-(p-I-phenyl)-3,3-dimethyl pentadecanoic acid (**DMIPPA**)

Figure 2. Chemical structures of various labeled fatty acids and fatty acid analogues (From Valkema R et al, J Nucl Cardiol 1994;1:546-60. Reproduced with permission).

oxidative metabolism in dysfunctional myocardial segments was a necessary condition for recovery of function after revascularization. Recently, the same group of investigators concluded from comparative PET studies with ^{18}FDG and ^{11}C-acetate before revascularization in 34 patients that the extent of functional recovery can be anticipated more accurately by quantification of regional oxidative metabolism using ^{11}C-acetate than by assessment of glucose utilization using ^{18}FDG.[25] Because glucose is metabolized both aerobically and anaerobically, ^{18}FDG studies yield different information than do studies with ^{11}C-acetate, which may explain the lower accuracy of ^{18}FDG compared with ^{11}C-acetate. Walsh et al.[50] showed in patients with recent myocardial infarction, who were not treated with thrombolytic agents, that myocardial oxidative metabolism measured with ^{11}C-acetate was clearly reduced in the center of the infarct zone 48 hours after the acute event, and that it had not changed at more than 7 days after the event. In contrast, in patients with evolving myocardial infarction who were treated with thrombolytic agents, successful restoration of perfusion within 24 hours was associated with improvement of regional oxidative metabolism and contractile function by 1 week after the acute event.[51] Based on these studies it seems that preserved oxidative metabolism, as assessed by ^{11}C-acetate, and not glucose utilization is the key factor that determines whether a particular myocardial area can benefit from revascularization.

Metabolism of fatty acids: ^{11}C-palmitate and ^{123}I-labeled analogues

Free fatty acids are the preferred substrates for cardiac metabolism when no or mild ischemia is present. In severe ischemia the level of fatty acid metabolism is greatly reduced. Therefore, radioactive fatty acid analogues can be used for noninvasive assessment of ischemia and viability (Figure 2). The first efforts with radiolabeled free fatty acids were aimed at the search for myocardial imaging agents. Only recently, the noninvasive evaluation of regional metabolic turnover rates in the myocardium has become an issue. For quantification of metabolic turnover rates the myocardial uptake and clearance of these tracers in relation to the local biochemical processes must be known. Previous experimental studies[52,53] have demonstrated a similar type of myocardial pharmacokinetics for ^{11}C-palmitate and various radioiodinated fatty acid analogs (Figure 3). The radioiodinated fatty acids were mainly studied by European and Japanese researchers, in contrast to ^{11}C-palmitate, that was predominantly studied in the United States.

[11]C-palmitate

Carbon-11-palmitate was one of the initial tracers of cardiac metabolism.[54-56] This radiopharmaceutical has complex kinetics and intracellular metabolism.[57-59] ^{11}C-palmitate is avidly taken up by the myocardium after intravenous administration with rapid blood clearance, permitting clear delineation of the myocardium on PET images after 5 minutes.[60] Initial myocardial distribution roughly correlates with myocardial perfusion. Clearance from the myocardium follows then a biexponential pattern. The first rapid phase corresponds with ß-oxidation of ^{11}C-palmitate with release of [11]CO_2, while the second, slower phase corresponds with incorporation of ^{11}C-palmitate in the intracellular lipid pool.[61] These observations in animal studies have been confirmed in human studies.[62,63] In these studies, clearance half-time of ^{11}C-palmitate was increased after ingestion of glucose and decreased during atrial pacing. Circulating substrate levels and other conditions as well have effects on the kinetics and metabolic fate of ^{11}C-palmitate. Experimental studies showed that back-diffusion of the unaltered tracer increases during myocardial ischemia and would be falsely reflected as enhanced oxidative metabolism.[64] Therefore, the diagnostic application of this agent has remained limited in the clinical setting.

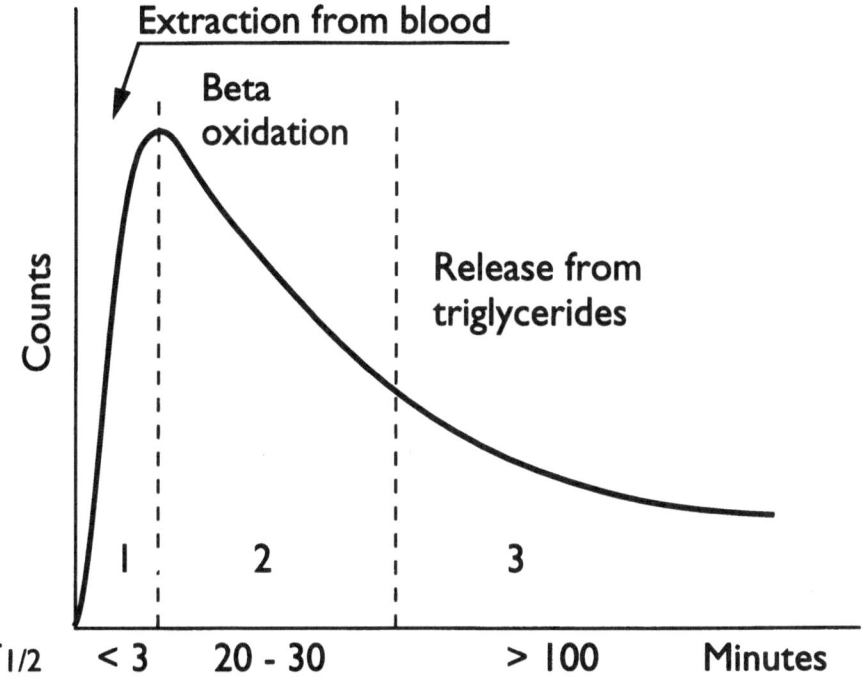

Figure 3. Schematic illustration of the characteristic time-activity curve of clinically used radiolabeled free fatty acids in the myocardium. Three different phases are recognized. (From van der Wall, EE. in: van der Wall EE., ed. Noninvasive imaging of cardiac metabolism. Dordrecht: Martinus Nijhoff, 1987:39-59. Reproduced with permission).

Radioiodinated fatty acid analogues

Free fatty acids can be labeled with gamma emitting isotopes of iodine (^{123}I or ^{131}I), so their metabolism can be studied both with planar and SPECT imaging which are less expensive and more widely available than PET. To be useful in a clinical setting these compounds have to be taken up by the myocardium and metabolized in essentially the same way as their native counterparts. While ^{11}C-palmitate is chemically indistinguishable from normal palmitate, the radioiodinated fatty acids are all more or less different from the native compound (Figure 2).

Iodoalkyl fatty acids
Evans et al.[65] were the first to use radioiodinated fatty acids, ^{131}I labeled oleic acid, in dogs. This substance had a low specific activity, poor imaging quality, and unfavorable radiation dosimetry (half-life of [131]I 8.06 days), which never became clinically useful. The first useful substrate was 16-iodo-hexadecanoic acid (^{123}I-HA), which behaves like heptadecanoic acid. Poe et al.[66] postulated that the terminal iodine maintains a configuration similar to a methyl group and the compound is therefore is metabolized

as though it had an extra carbon atom. Terminally radioiodinated hexadecanoic acid has an initial myocardial distribution proportional to blood flow, similar to potassium-43 (^{43}K) and ^{201}Tl.[67] From these results it was concluded that ^{123}I-labeled free fatty acids are distributed according to myocardial blood flow and metabolized by known metabolic pathways. The clearance rates of the iodoalkyl fatty acids ^{123}I-HA and ^{123}I-17-heptadecanoic acid (^{123}I-HDA) are slower in ischemic regions than in normal regions, but consistently faster in infarcted regions compared to normal.[68-70]

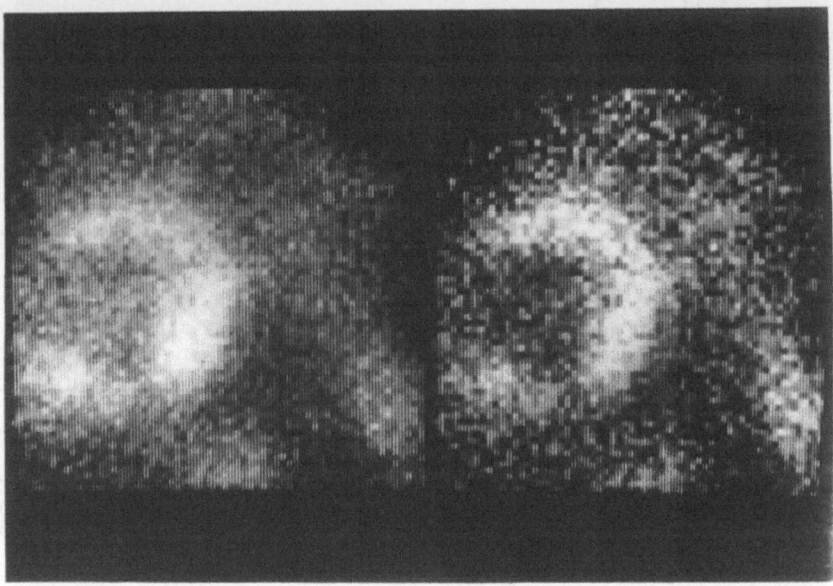

Figure 4.   Myocardial ^{123}I-heptadecanoic acid scintigram before (left) and after (right) background correction in a patient with anteroseptal infarction. (From van der Wall, EE. in: van der Wall EE., ed. Noninvasive imaging of cardiac metabolism. Dordrecht: Martinus Nijhoff, 1987:39-59. Reproduced with permission).

Comparison of radioiodinated I-HA and I-HDA in dogs showed that I-HDA is a better indicator of myocardial metabolism, because of higher uptake in normal myocardium and lower uptake in ischemic areas.[71] After uptake, a major part of the fatty acids is immediately oxidized via ß-oxidation. A small amount is stored into lipids, mainly phospholipids. The iodide ion is split off and probably diffuses out of the cell, contributing to the background activity. The problem of high background activity can be alleviated by special background subtraction algorithms[69] (Figure 4). For kinetic study of free fatty acid metabolism using iodoalkyl fatty acids, serial planar imaging is required. Time-activity curves over defined regions of interest are generated from the serial images. Due to the rapid clearance of the tracer from normal myocardium, SPECT is not feasible with these tracers. Additionally, carefully conducted studies in dogs by Visser et al.[72] using ^{123}I-HDA have shown that washout of free radioiodide and not ß-oxidation determines the myocardial elimination rate of ^{123}I-HDA. In a subsequent study, van Eenige et al.[73] demonstrated that myocardial time-activity curves obtained from ^{123}I-HDA studies, using monoexponential curve fitting (plus a constant), allowed the appreciation of fatty acid oxidation and storage. In occlusion/reperfusion experiments in dogs, Chappuis et al.[74] found that the regional concentration of ^{123}I-HDA reflects viability as assessed by TTC staining and its clearance is prolonged in viable myocardium compared to infarcted myocardium. In their experiment, ^{201}Tl acted as a flow tracer while ^{123}I-HDA acted as a viability tracer.

Iodophenyl fatty acids
Several modified fatty acid analogues labeled with ^{123}I have been studied in animals and humans. Terminal iodophenyl fatty acids and methyl branched fatty acids have different kinetics and metabolism compared to the iodoalkyl fatty acids. Machulla et al.[75] introduced 15-(para-^{123}I-phenyl)-pentadecanoic acid (^{123}I-pIPPA). ^{123}I-pIPPA is catabolized to para-iodobenzoic acid rather than free iodide. Its metabolites are excreted via the liver and kidneys, leading to lower blood levels than with iodoalkyl fatty acids, with more favorable heart to background levels.[76,77] Reske et al.[78] showed in an experimental study in mice that ^{123}I-pIPPA was metabolized very similarly to ^{14}C-palmitic acid. While in the human myocardium the metabolism of ^{123}I-pIPPA is comparable with that of iodoalkyl fatty acids, the metabolism of 15-(ortho-^{123}I-phenyl)-pentadecanoic acid (^{123}I-oIPPA) is quite different.[79-82] Kaiser et al.[81] found that ^{123}I-oIPPA is bound to coenzyme A and is retained in the cytosolic lipid pool, while ^{123}I-pIPPA is metabolized by mitchondrial ß-oxidation. This results in nearly irreversible retention of ^{123}I-oIPPA in human myocardium, making this tracer suitable for measurement of uptake differences between normal and diseased myocardium.

Methyl-branched fatty acids
The methyl-branched fatty acids have been specifically developed to overcome the problem of rapid clearance of radioactivity of the iodoalkyl fatty acids through oxidation (Figure 5). The methyl-branched analogues which have been used in clinical

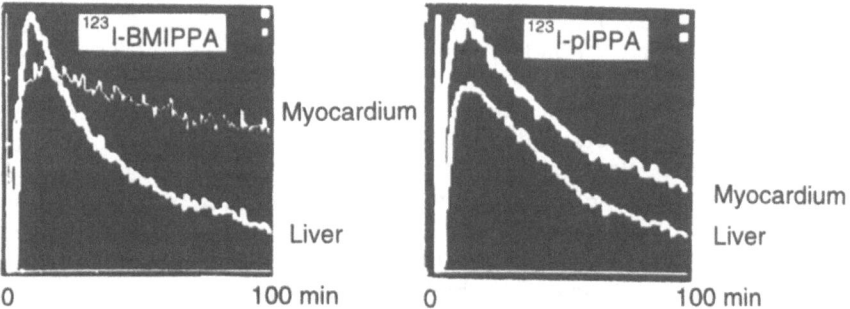

Figure 5. Time-activity curves of ^{123}I-BMIPPA uptake (left) and of ^{123}I-pIPPA uptake (right) in the myocardium and liver in a patient with normal coronary arteries. Note relatively long myocardial retention of ^{123}I-BMIPPA compared with ^{123}I-pIPPA. (From Knapp FF, et al. In: Van der Wall EE, ed. Noninvasive imaging of cardiac metabolism. Dordrecht: Martinus Nijhoff, 1987:159-201. Reproduced with permission).

studies are comparably metabolized in the myocardium.[83,84] Recent studies have shown that [123]I-ß-methyl-p-iodophenyl pentadecanoic acid (^{123}I-BMIPPA) undergoes initial α-oxidation and subsequent ß-oxidation to p-iodophenylacetic acid, which remains in the cytosol.[85,86] Knapp et al.[87] have designed 15-(p-iodophenyl)-3,3-dimethylpentadecanoic acid (^{123}I-DMIPPA) to block catabolism. In a recent study by Sloof et al.,[88], the kinetics and myocardial metabolism of ^{123}I-HDA, ^{123}I-pIPPA and ^{123}I-DMIPPA were compared. The authors found significant differences in the myocardial uptake, oxidation and lipid distribution of ^{123}I-HDA, ^{123}I-pIPPA and ^{123}I-DMIPPA. They concluded that ^{123}I-DMIPPA is a promising tracer for fatty acid uptake studies with SPECT because of its prolonged retention and high myocardium-to-blood ratios. Several authors[98,90] observed increased uptake of ^{123}I-BMIPPA in excess of flow measured with microspheres or ^{201}Tl in reperfused viable myocardium. Due to the prolonged myocardial retention of ^{123}I-BMIPPA, this type of modified free fatty acid is more suited for cardiac SPECT than a straight-chain fatty acid such as ^{123}I-HDA or ^{123}I-IPPA.

Radioiodinated fatty acids: clinical findings in ischemic heart disease
Clinical studies with various radioiodinated fatty acids demonstrated that the normal pattern of uptake, distribution and turnover was disturbed in patients with coronary artery disease.[91-100] Van der Wall et al.[68-70,94] were the first to apply these compounds (^{123}I-HA, ^{123}I-HDA) in patients with angiographically documented coronary artery disease. They reported that increased elimination of the tracer, as compared to normal myocardium, was associated with scar tissue and that decreased elimination was associated with reversible ischemia. The authors also showed a good comparison between the fatty acid images and the ^{201}Tl images in a similar group of patients. These findings are in line with the data of Hansen et al.,[99] who reported that ^{123}I-IPPA provided similar information as ^{201}Tl in 33 patients with stable coronary artery disease indicating that ^{123}I-IPPA can be used to identify patients with ischemic heart disease. Chouraqui et al.[100] compared ^{123}I-iodophenyl-methyl-pentadecanoic acid (DMIPPA) with ^{201}Tl in patients during stress-induced ischemia and they observed a good agreement with both tracers in terms of initial poststress myocardial uptake and defect reversibility. Conversely, recent studies using ^{123}I-IPPA and ^{123}I-BMIPPA have shown a dissociation between ^{123}I-BMIPPA uptake and ^{201}Tl uptake.[101-103] Pippin et al.[101] studied prospectively 55 patients with both ^{201}Tl and ^{123}I-IPPA and showed, despite a similar detection rate for initial stress-induced defects, an increased sensitivity for reversible ischemic defects with ^{123}I-IPPA. Tamaki et al.,[102] in 28 patients with myocardial infarction, clearly showed that uptake of ^{123}I-BMIPPA was independent of myocardial perfusion; BMIPP uptake was decreased compared to ^{201}Tl uptake in 61% of patients and in 25% of segments. Matsunari et al.,[103] who compared the myocardial kinetics of ^{123}I-BMIPPA with ^{201}Tl in 26 patients with prior myocardial infarction, observed significant clearance of ^{123}I-BMIPPA from myocardium with reversible ^{201}Tl defects suggesting enhanced contribution of back diffusion from ^{123}I-BMIPPA in ischemic myocardium. They also showed that the stress ^{123}I-BMIPPA images showed more severe defects than the stress ^{201}Tl images, which may be due to both decreased coronary blood flow and impaired fatty acid uptake by exercise-induced ischemia.

Radioiodinated fatty acids: assessment of myocardial viability

Myocardial tissue viability has also been investigated using radioiodinated fatty acids.[104] Murray et al.[105] studied 15 patients with coronary disease and depressed left ventricular function with ^{123}I-pIPPA. Despite resting akinesis or dyskinesis in 20/22 (91%) infarcted territories, 16/22 (73%) of these territories were metabolically viable. Transmural myocardial biopsies in all patients (43 sites, 42 vascular territories) during coronary bypass surgery confirmed ^{123}I-pIPPA results in 39/43 territories (91%). When compared to biopsy, ^{123}I-pIPPA scan sensitivity for viability was 33/36 (92%) with a specificity of 6/7 (86%). Furthermore, 80% of infarcted but ^{123}I-pIPPA viable segments which were revascularized demonstrated improved regional systolic wall motion postoperatively. Additional comparative studies by Murray et al.[106] in 30 patients with myocardial infarction showed viability in 18 of 35 (51%) segments with ^{201}Tl stress-reinjection SPECT, while ^{123}I-pIPPA showed viability in 26 of 35 (74%) of segments. From their studies, they concluded that ^{123}I-pIPPA cardiac viability imaging is a safe, inexpensive technique that may be a useful alternative to PET. Kuikka et al.[107] compared ^{123}I-pIPPA SPECT and ^{99m}Tc-sestamibi SPECT in 31 patients with coronary artery disease. With ^{99m}Tc-sestamibi they found 57 persistent defects in a total of 124 segments. All patients had at least 1 persistent defect. In 14 (25%) of these segments ^{123}I-pIPPA activity was normal and in 22 (39%) segments ^{123}I-pIPPA activity was "partially" preserved, suggesting residual viability. However, no confirmation of viability after revascularization was available. Henrich et al.[108] compared SPECT with ^{123}I-oIPPA and [18]FDG PET in 32 patients with chronic myocardial infarction who showed persistent ^{201}Tl defects at redistribution. Of the 408 segments with a persistent ^{201}Tl defects, 51% had a decreased uptake of both [18]FDG and ^{123}I-oIPPA; in 22% of the segments [18]FDG and ^{123}I-oIPPA uptake was normal. Thus, a substantial fraction of persistent thallium-defects after healed myocardial infarction exhibited [18]FDG as well as ^{123}I-oIPPA uptake, suggesting that viability can be demonstrated with radioiodinated fatty acids. The potential role of ^{123}I-HDA, ^{123}I-oIPPA and ^{123}I-BMIPPA for the assessment of viability in reperfused myocardium has been investigated by Visser et al.,[109] Franken et al.,[110] and De Geeter et al.[111] Visser et al.,[109] in acute infarct patients, showed restored fatty acid metabolism in myocardial areas that were successfully reperfused. Franken et al.[110] studied 9 patients with ^{123}I-oIPPA and ^{99m}Tc-sestamibi SPECT within 2 weeks after acute myocardial infarction and thrombolysis; in 15 myocardial segments metabolic defects were more severe than perfusion defects while wall motion was improved or normal in 12 segments. The authors concluded that metabolic abnormalities often persist longer than perfusion disturbances after reperfusion, and that such ^{123}I-oIPPA abnormalities reflect the salvaged areas. The same group[111] studied 26 patients with subacute myocardial infarction, 14 of whom were treated with streptokinase within 6 hours after the onset of chest pain. All patients underwent ^{99m}Tc-sestamibi and ^{123}I-BMIPPA SPECT. Results obtained were similar to those in their study with ^{123}I-oIPPA,[110] illustrating the similar characteristics of ^{123}I-OIPPA and ^{123}I-BMIPPA in clinical practice, as could be expected from experimental metabolic studies. Although patient numbers in the above-mentioned studies are relatively small, the data clearly indicate that radioiodinated fatty acid scintigraphy holds significant potential for the assessment of myocardial viability.

Metabolism versus flow

When considering tracer techniques to investigate myocardial metabolism in ischemic areas, one must bear in mind that blood flow influences myocardial tracer distribution independent of metabolism. To assess changes in metabolism the tracers must arrive in the ischemic area. The tracer distribution is dependent on blood flow, especially in case of a high first-pass extraction. Theoretically, diminished uptake of a metabolic tracer in an area with impaired blood flow can at least in part be caused by insufficient amounts of tracer arriving in myocytes and does not necessarily reflect a pure change in metabolism. Conversely, imaging with many so-called "perfusion" tracers relies on active extraction by the myocardium, which is only possible in the presence of an intact cellular membrane and some degree of metabolism. In cases of well perfused, but necrotic myocardium after reperfusion no uptake will occur and perfusion will be underestimated with these actively extracted tracers. Well known examples of this class of tracers are ^{201}Tl and ^{99m}Tc-sestamibi.

The myocyte extracts the potassium analogue ^{201}Tl from the extracellular fluid via the sodium-potassium pump which is constantly active to maintain the difference in intracellular and extracellular concentrations of sodium and potassium, essential for survival of the cell. Energy in the form of ATP is required for this process. Therefore, uptake of ^{201}Tl via the sodium-potassium pump is tightly coupled to myocardial metabolism and may be considered as an indirect marker of it. With the advent of new imaging protocols with ^{201}Tl, such as the so-called "reinjection" of a second smaller dose of ^{201}Tl at rest after the stress study, myocardial viability may be assessed reliably, and functional improvement after revascularization may be predicted by ^{201}Tl SPECT and planar scintigraphy with comparable sensitivity and specificity as provided by [18]FDG PET.[112-119]

Myocardial cell viability is essential for ^{99m}Tc-sestamibi uptake and retention.[120] After passive diffusion into the myocardial cell, ^{99m}Tc-sestamibi binds to mitochondrial membranes.[121,122] Therefore, ^{99m}Tc-sestamibi can certainly also be considered as a marker of metabolism as well as a marker of flow. However, ^{99m}Tc-sestamibi substantially underestimates the amount of viable myocardium in comparison with [18]FDG PET[123,124] and ^{201}Tl scintigraphy,[125,126] because mitochondrial binding can be impaired in ischemic but still viable cells.[127] Consequently, ^{201}Tl is currently regarded as a better marker of myocardial viability than ^{99m}Tc-sestamibi (See also chapter by Niemeyer et al).

Conclusions

In acute and prolonged ischemia the metabolism changes profoundly and these changes can be detected noninvasively to give important diagnostic information which is needed to select the most appropriate therapy. As indicated in this chapter, several techniques are available in the clinical setting now or they will be in the near future.[127,128]

PET scintigraphy using [18]FDG is nowadays considered to be the gold standard for the detection of ischemic but viable myocardium. This status has been challenged by Gropler et al.[25] who used ^{11}C-acetate for the assessment of oxidative myocardial metabolism, independent of the substrates available to the myocyte. From their studies it seems that preserved oxidative metabolism and not glucose utilization, which reflects a mixture of anaerobic and aerobic metabolism, is the key factor that determines whether a particular area of myocardium can benefit from revascularization. Whether this is true remains to be confirmed. If preserved oxidative metabolism is indeed the main determinant for functional improvement after successful revascularization, then it should be detectable with carefully chosen labeled fatty acid analogues using SPECT. In this regard, especially ^{123}I-olPPA and the methyl-branched fatty acid analogues may emerge as the optimal noninvasive markers of myocardial metabolism and viability for use in clinical practice. At present, PET imaging remains the mainstay in the evaluation of cardiac metabolism.

Acknowledgements
Dr. R. Valkema is gratefully acknowledged for his valuable contribution to this chapter

References

1.   Gropler RJ, Bergmann SR. Myocardial viability—what is the definition? J Nucl Med 1991;32:10-2.
2.   Gallagher BM, Fowler JS, Gutterson NI, MacGregor RR, Wan CN, Wolf AP. Metabolic trapping as a principle of radiopharmaceutical design: some factors responsible for the biodistribution of [18F]2-fluoro-2-deoxy-D-glucose. J Nucl Med 1978;19:1154-61.
3.   Ratib O, Phelps ME, Huang SC, Henze E, Selin CE, Schelbert HR. Positron tomography with deoxyglucose for estimating local myocardial glucose metabolism. J Nucl Med 1982;23:577-86.
4.   Phelps ME, Schelbert HR, Mazziotta JC. Positron computed tomography for studies of myocardial and cerebral function. Ann Intern Med 1983;98:339-59.
5.   Halama JR, Gratley J, DeGrado TR, Bernstein DR, Ng CK, Holden JE. Validation of 3-deoxy-3-fluoro-D-glucose as a glucose transport analogue in rat heart. Am J Physiol 1984;246:H777-87.
6.   Gambhir SS, Schwaiger M, Huang SC et al. Simple noninvasive quantification method for measuring myocardial glucose utilization in humans employing positron emission tomography and fluorine-18 deoxyglucose. J Nucl Med 1989;30:359-66.
7.   Schwaiger M, Schelbert HR, Ellison D et al. Sustained regional abnormalities in cardiac metabolism after transient ischemia in the chronic dog model. J Am Coll Cardiol 1985;6:336-47.
8.   Choi Y, Hawkins RA, Huang SC et al. Parametric images of myocardial metabolic rate of glucose generated from dynamic cardiac PET and 2-[18F]fluoro-2-deoxy-d-glucose studies. J Nucl Med 1991;32:733-8.
9.   Camici P, Ferrannini E, Opie L. Myocardial metabolism in ischemic heart disease: basic principles and application to imaging by positron emission tomography. Prog Cardiovasc Dis 1989;32:217-38.
10. Gropler RJ, Siegel BA, Lee KJ et al. Nonuniformity in myocardial accumulation of fluorine-18-fluorodeoxyglucose in normal fasted humans. J Nucl Med 1990;31:1749-56.
11. Choi Y, Brunken RC, Hawkins RA et al. Factors affecting myocardial 2-[F-18]fluoro-2-deoxy-D-glucose uptake in positron emission tomography studies of normal humans. Eur J Nucl Med 1993;20:308-18.
12. vom Dahl J, Herman WH, Hicks RJ et al. Myocardial glucose uptake in patients with insulin-dependent diabetes mellitus assessed quantitatively by dynamic positron emission tomography. Circulation 1993;88:395-404.
13. Knuuti MJ, Nuutila P, Ruotsilaanen U et al. Euglycemic hyperinsulinemic clamp and oral glucose load in stimulating myocardial glucose utilization during positron emission tomography. J Nucl Med 1991;32:565-78.
14. Schwaiger M, Brunken R, Grover-McKay M et al. Regional myocardial metabolism in patients with acute myocardial infarction assessed by positron emission tomography. J Am Coll Cardiol 1986;8:800-8.
15. Niemeyer MG, Kuijper AF, Gerhards LJ, D'Haene EG, van der Wall EE. Nitrogen-13 ammonia perfusion imaging: relation to metabolic imaging. Am Heart J 1993;125:848-54.
16. Marshall RC, Tillisch JH, Phelps ME et al. Identification and differentiation of resting myocardial ischemia and infarction in man with positron computed tomography, 18F-labeled fluorodeoxyglucose and N-13 ammonia. Circulation 1983;67:766-78.
17. Tillisch J, Brunken R, Marshall R et al. Reversibility of cardiac wall-motion abnormalities predicted by positron tomography. N Engl J Med 1986;314:884-8.
18. Schelbert HR, Schwaiger M. Positron emission tomography in human myocardial

ischemia. Herz 1987;12:22-40.
19. Tamaki N, Yonekura Y, Yamashita K et al. Positron emission tomography using fluorine-18 deoxyglucose in evaluation of coronary artery bypass grafting. Am J Cardiol 1989;64:860-5.
20. Al-Aouar ZR, Eitzman D, Hepner A et al. PET assessment of myocardial tissue viability: University of Michigan experience. J Nucl Med 1990;31:801 (Abstract).
21. Tamaki N, Yonekura Y, Yamashita K et al. Prediction of reversible ischemia after coronary artery bypass grafting by positron emission tomography. J Cardiol 1991;21:193-201.
22. Marwick TH, MacIntyre WJ, Lafont A, Nemec JJ, Salcedo EE. Metabolic responses of hibernating and infarcted myocardium to revascularization. A follow-up study of regional perfusion, function, and metabolism. Circulation 1992;85:1347-53.
23. Lucignani G, Paolini G, Landoni C et al. Presurgical identification of hibernating myocardium by combined use of technetium-99m hexakis 2-methoxyisobutylisonitrile single photon emission tomography and fluorine-18 fluoro-2-deoxy-D-glucose positron emission tomography in patients with coronary artery disease. Eur J Nucl Med 1992;19:874-81.
24. Tamaki N. Current status of viability assessment with positron emission tomography. J Nucl Cardiol 1994;1:S40-7.
25. Gropler RJ, Geltman EM, Sampathkumaran K et al. Comparison of carbon-11-acetate with fluorine-18-deoxyglucose for delineating viable myocardium by positron emission tomography. J Am Coll Cardiol 1993;22:1587-97.
26. Vom Dahl J, Eitzman DT, Al-Aouar ZR et al. Relation to regional function, perfusion, and metabolism in patients with advanced coronary artery disease undergoing surgical revascularization. Circulation 1994;90:2356-66.
27. Eitzman D, al-Aouar Z, Kanter HL et al. Clinical outcome of patients with advanced coronary artery disease after viability studies with positron emission tomography. J Am Coll Cardiol 1992;20:559-65.
28. Tamaki N, Kawamoto M, Takahashi N et al. Prognostic value of an increase in fluorine-18 deoxyglycose uptake in patients with myocardial infarction: comparison with stress thallium imaging. J Am Coll Cardiol 1993;22:1621-7.
29. Yoshida K, Gould KL. Quantitative relation of myocardial infarct size and myocardial viability by positron emission tomography to left ventricular ejection fraction and 3-year mortality with and without revascularization. J Am Coll Cardiol 1993;22:984-97.
30. DiCarli MF, Davidson M, Little R et al. Value of metabolic imaging with positron emission tomography for evaluating prognosis in patients with coronary artery disease and left ventricular dysfunction. Am J Cardiol 1994;73:527-33.
31. Lee KS, Marwick TH, Cook SA et al. Prognosis of patients with left ventricular dysfunction, with and without viable myocardium after myocardial infarction. Relative efficacy of medical therapy and revascularization. Circulation 1994;90:2687-94.
32. Zaret BL, Wackers FJ. Nuclear cardiology (first of two parts). N Engl J Med 1993;329:775-83.
33. Takahashi N, Tamaki N, Kawamoto M et al. Glucose metabolism in relation to perfusion in patients with ischaemic heart disease. Eur J Nucl Med 1994;21:292-6.
34. Sebree L, Bianco JA, Subramanian R et al. Discordance between accumulation of C-14 deoxyglucose and Tl-201 in reperfused myocardium. J Mol Cell Cardiol 1991;23:603-16.
35. Gropler RJ, Bergmann SR. Flow and metabolic determinants of myocardial viability assessed by positron-emission tomography. Coronary Artery Dis 1993;4:495-504.
36. Phelps ME, Mazziotta JC, Schelbert HR, eds. Positron emission tomography and autoradiography: principles and applications for the brain and heart. New York: Raven

Press, 1986:690.

37.   van Lingen A, Huijgens PC, Visser FC et al. Performance characteristics of a 511-keV collimator for imaging positron emitters with a standard gamma-camera. Eur J Nucl Med 1992;19:315-21.

38.   Williams KA, Taillon LA, Stark VJ. Quantitative planar imaging of glucose metabolic activity in myocardial segments with exercise thallium-201 perfusion defects in patients with myocardial infarction: comparison with late (24-hour) redistribution thallium imaging for detection of reversible ischemia. Am Heart J 1992;124:294-304.

39.   Bax JJ, Visser FC, van Lingen A et al. Detection of viable myocardium by FDG SPECT during hyperinsulinemic glucose clamping. J Nucl Med 1993;34:147P (Abstract).

40.   Bax JJ, Visser FC, van Lingen A et al. Feasibility of assessing regional myocardial uptake of 18F-fluorodeoxyglucose using single photon emision tomography. Eur Heart J 1993;14:1675-82.

41.   Bax JJ, Visser FC, van Lingen A et al. Relation between myocardial uptake of thallium-201 chloride and fluorine-18 fluorodeoxyglucose imaged with single-photon emission tomography in normal individuals. Eur J Nucl Med 1995;22:56-60.

42.   Walsh MN. Myocardial metabolic imaging with carbon-11-acetate. In: van der Wall EE, Sochor H, Righetti A, Niemeyer MN, ed. What's new in cardiac imaging? SPECT, PET, and MRI. Dordrecht, The Netherlands: Kluwer Academic Publishers, 1992:277-86.

43.   Brown MA, Marshall DR, Sobel BE, Bergmann SR. Deliniation of myocardial oxygen utilization with carbon-11-labeled acetate. Circulation 1987;76:687-96.

44.   Armbrecht JJ, Buxton DB, Brunken RC, Phelps ME, Schelbert HR. Regional myocardial oxygen consumption determined noninvasively in humans with [1-11C]acetate and dynamic positron tomography. Circulation 1989;80:863-72.

45.   Brown MA, Myears DW, Bergmann SR. Validity of estimates of myocardial oxidative metabolism with carbon-11 acetate and positron emission tomography despite altered patterns of substrate utilization. J Nucl Med 1989;30:187-93.

46.   Buxton DB, Nienaber CA, Luxen A et al. Noninvasive quantitation of regional myocardial oxygen consumption in vivo with [1-11C]acetate and dynamic positron emission tomography. Circulation 1989;79:134-42.

47.   Weinheimer CJ, Brown MA, Nohara R, Perez JE, Bergmann SR. Functional recovery after reperfusion is predicated on recovery of myocardial oxidative metabolism. Am Heart J 1993;125:939-49.

48.   Heyndrickx GR, Wijns W, Vogelaers D et al. Recovery of regional contractile function and oxidative metabolism in stunned myocardium induced by 1-hour circumflex coronary artery stenosis in chronically instrumented dogs. Circ Res 1993;72:901-13.

49.   Gropler RJ, Geltman EM, Sampathkumaran K et al. Functional recovery after coronary revascularization for chronic coronary artery disease is dependent on maintenance of oxidative metabolism. J Am Coll Cardiol 1992;20:569-77.

50.   Walsh MN, Geltman EM, Brown MA et al. Noninvasive estimation of regional myocardial oxygen consumption by positron emission tomography with carbon-11 acetate in patients with myocardial infarction. J Nucl Med 1989;30:1798-808.

51.   Henes CG, Bergmann SR, Perez JE, Sobel BE, Geltman EM. The time course of restoration of nutritive perfusion, myocardial oxygen consumption, and regional function after coronary thrombolysis. Coronary Artery Dis 1990;1:687-96.

52.   Poe ND, Robinson GD Jr, Graham LS, MacDonald NS. Experimental basis for myocardial imaging with I-123-labeled hexadecanoic acid. J Nucl Med 1976;17:1077-82.

53.   Machulla H-J, Stöcklin G, Kupfernagel C et al. Comparative evaluation of fatty acids labeled with C-11, Cl-34m, Br-77 and I-123 for metabolic studies of the myocardium: concise communication. J Nucl Med 1978;19:298-302.

54. Sobel BE, Weiss E, Welch M et al. Detection of remote myocardial infarction in patients with positron emission transaxial tomography and intravenous C-11 palmitate. Circulation 1977;55:853-7.
55. Sobel BE. Positron tomography and myocardial metabolism: an overview. Circulation 1985;72:IV22-30.
56. Schelbert HR, Henze E, Schön HR et al. C-11 palmitic acid for the noninvasive evaluation of regional myocardial fatty acid metabolism with positron emission tomography: IV: in vivo demonstration of impaired fatty acid oxidation in acute myocardial ischemia. Am Heart J 1983;106:736-50.
57. Liedtke AJ. Alterations of carbohydrate and lipid metabolism in the acutely ischemic heart. Prog Cardiovasc Dis 1981;23:321-36.
58. Lerch R. Assessment of myocardial fatty acid metabolism with carbon-11 palmitate. In: van der Wall EE, Sochor H, Righetti A, Niemeyer MG, eds. What's new in cardiac imaging? SPECT, PET, and MRI. Dordrecht, The Netherlands: Kluwer Academic Publishers, 1992:249-61.
59. Lerch RA, Ambos HD, Bergmann SR, Welch MJ, Ter-Pogossian MM, Sobel BE. Localization of viable, ischemic myocardium by positron-emission tomography with 11C-palmitate. Circulation 1981;64:689-99.
60. Schön HR, Schelbert HR, Robinson G et al. C-11 palmitic acid for the noninvasive evaluation of regional myocardial fatty acid metabolism with positron emission tomography: I: kinetics of C-11 palmitic acid in normal myocardium. Am Heart J 1981;103:532-47.
61. Rosamond TL, Abendschein DR, Sobel BE, Bergmann SR, Fox KA. Metabolic fate of radiolabeled palmitate in ischemic canine myocardium: implications for positron emission tomography. J Nucl Med 1987;28:1322-9.
62. Grover-McKay M, Schelbert HR, Schwaiger M et al. Identification of impaired metabolic reserve by atrial pacing in patients with significant coronary artery stenosis. Circulation 1986;74:281-92.
63. Schelbert HR, Henze E, Sochor H et al. Effects of substrate availability on myocardial C-11 palmitate kinetics by positron emission tomography in normal subjects and patients with ventricular dysfunction. Am Heart J 1986;111:1055-64.
64. Fox KAA, Abendschein D, Amos HD, Sobel BE, Bergmann SE. Efflux of metabolized and nonmetabolized fatty acid from canine myocardium. Implications for quantifying myocardial metabolism tomographically. Circ Res 1985;57:232-43.
65. Evans JR, Phil D, Gunton RW, Baker RG, Spears JC, Beanlands DS. Use of radioiodinated fatty acid for photoscans of the heart. Circ Res 1965;16:1-10.
66. Poe ND, Robinson GD Jr, MacDonald NS. Myocardial extraction of labeled long-chain fatty acid analogs. Proc Soc Exp Biol Med 1975;148:215-8.
67. Westera G, van der Wall EE, Heidendal GAK, van den Bos GC. A comparison between terminally radioiodinated hexadecanoic acid (I-HA) and Tl-201-thallium chloride in the dog heart. Implications for the use of I-HA for myocardial imaging. Eur J Nucl Med 1980;5:339-43.
68. van der Wall EE, den Hollander W, Heidendal GA, Westera G, Majid PA, Roos JP. Dynamic myocardial scintigraphy with 123I-labeled free fatty acids in patients with myocardial infarction. Eur J Nucl Med 1981;6:383-9.
69. van der Wall EE, Heidendal GA, den Hollander W, Westera G, Roos JP. Myocardial scintigraphy with 123I-labelled heptadecanoic acid in patients with unstable angina pectoris. Postgrad Med J 1983;59:38-40.
70. van der Wall EE, Heidendal GA, den Hollander W, Westera G, Roos JP. I-123 labeled hexadecenoic acid in comparison with Thallium-201 for myocardial imaging in coronary

heart disease. A preliminary study. Eur J Nucl Med 1980;5:401-5.

71.   van der Wall EE, Westera G, Heidendal GA, den Hollander W. A comparison between terminally radioiodinated hexadecenoic acid (125I-HA) and heptadecanoic acid (131I-HOA) in the dog heart. Eur J Nucl Med 1981;6:581-4.

72.   Visser FC, van Eenige MJ, Westera G et al. Metabolic fate of radioiodinated heptadecanoic acid in the normal canine heart. Circulation 1985;72:565-71.

73.   Van Eenige MJ, Visser FC, Duwel CMB, Karreman AJP, Van Lingen A, Roos JP. Comparison of 17-iodine-131 heptadecanoic acid kinetics from externally measured time-activity curves and from serial myocardial biopsies in an open-chest canine model. J Nucl Med 1988;29:1934-42.

74.   Chappuis F, Meier B, Belenger et al. Early assessment of tissue viability with radioiodinated heptadecanoic acid in reperfused canine myocardium: comparison with thallium-201. Am Heart J 1990;119:833-41.

75.   Machulla HJ, Marsmann M, Dutschka K. Biochemical concept and synthesis of a radioiodinated phenylfatty acid for in vivo metabolic studies of the myocardium. Eur J Nucl Med 1980;5:171-3.

76.   Dudczak R, Schmolinger R, Kletter K, Frischauf H, Angelberger P. Clinical evaluation of 123I-labeled-p-phenylpentadecanoic acid (p-IPPA) for myocardial scintigraphy. J Nucl Med Allied Sci 1983;27:267-79.

77.   Reske SN, Knapp FF, Winkler C. Experimental basis of metabolic imaging of the myocardium with radioiodinated aromatic free fatty acids. Am J Physiol Imaging 1986;1:214-29.

78.   Reske SN, Sauer W, Machulla H-J, Winkler. 15(p-[123I]-iodophenyl)pentadecanoic acid as a tracer of lipid metabolism:comparison with [1-14C]palmitic acid in murine tissues. J Nucl Med 1984;25:1335-42.

79.   Beckurts TE, Shreeve WW, Schieren R, Feinendegen LE. Kinetics of different 123I- and 14C-labelled fatty acids in normal and diabetic rat myocardium in vivo. Nucl Med Comm 1985;6:415-24.

80.   Antar MA, Spohr G, Herzog HH et al. 15-(ortho-123I-phenyl)-pentadecanoic acid, a new myocardial imaging agent for clinical use. Nucl Med Commun 1986;7:683-96.

81.   Kaiser KP, Geuting B, Grossmann K et al. Tracer kinetics of 15-(ortho-123/131I-phenyl)-pentadecanoic acid (oPPA) and 15-(para-123/131I-phenyl)-pentadecanoic acid (pPPA) in animals and man. J Nucl Med 1990;31:1608-16.

82.   Reske SN. Experimental and clinical experience with iodine 123-labeled iodophenylpentadecanoic acid in cardiology. J Nucl Cardiol 1994;1:S58-S64.

83.   Ambrose KR, Owen BA, Goodman MM, Knapp FF Jr. Evaluation of the metabolism in rat hearts of two new radioiodinated 3-methyl-branched fatty acid myocardial imaging agents. Eur J Nucl Med 1987;12:486-91.

84.   Knapp FF Jr, Goodman MM, Ambrose KR et al. The development of radioiodinated 3-methyl-branched fatty acids for evaluation of myocardial disease by single photon techniques. In: van der Wall EE, ed. Noninvasive imaging of cardiac metabolism. Dordrecht: Martinus Nijhoff, 1987:159-201.

85.   Yamamichi Y, Shirakami Y, Morishita K, Kurami M, Kusuoka H, Nishimura T. Intramyocardial metabolism of β-methyl-p-iodophenyl pentadecanoic acid (BMIPP). J Nucl Med 1994;35:97P (Abstract).

86.   Suzuki N, Kurami M, Kusuoka H, Nishimura T. Myocardial intracellular kinetics of branched-chained free fatty acid, I-123 BMIPP. J Nucl Med 1994;35:97P (Abstract).

87.   Knapp FF Jr., Goodman MM, Callahan AP, Kirsch G. Radioiodinated 15-(p-iodophenyl)-3,3-dimethylpentadecanoic acid: a useful new agent to evaluate myocardial fatty acid uptake. J Nucl Med 1986;27:521-31.

88. Sloof GW, Visser FC, Eenige van MJ et al. Comparison of uptake, oxidation and lipid distribution of 17-iodoheptadecanoic acid, 15-(p-iodophenyl)pentadecanoic acid and 15-(p-iodophenyl)-3,3-dimethylpentadecanoic acid in normal canine myocardium. J Nucl Med 1993;34:649-57.

89. Miller DD, Gill JB, Livni E et al. Fatty acid analogue accumulation:a marker of myocyte viability in ischemic-perfused myocardium. Circ Res 1988;63:681-92.

90. Nishimura T, Sago M, Kihara K et al. Fatty acid myocardial imaging using 123I-ß-methyl-iodophenyl pentadecanoic acid (BMIPP):comparison of myocardial perfusion and fatty acid utilization in canine myocardial infarction (occlusion and reperfusion model). Eur J Nucl Med 1989;15:314-5.

91. Reske SN. 123I-phenylpentadecanoic acid as a tracer of cardiac free fatty acid metabolism. Experimental and clinical results. Eur Heart J 1985;6:39-47.

92. Railton R, Rodger JC, Small DR, Harrower AD. Myocardial scintigraphy with I-123 heptadecanoic acid as a test for coronary heart disease. Eur J Nucl Med 1987;13:63-6.

93. Dudczak R, Schmoliner R, Angelberger P, Knapp FF, Goodman MM. Structurally modified fatty acids: clinical potential as tracers of metabolism. Eur J Nucl Med 1986;12:S45-8.

94. van der Wall EE, Heidendal GA, den Hollander W, Westera G, Roos JP. Metabolic myocardial imaging with 123I-labeled heptadecanoic acid in patients with angina pectoris. Eur J Nucl Med 1981;6:391-6.

95. Kennedy PL, Corbett JR, Kulkarni PV et al. Iodine-123-phenylpentadecanoic acid myocardial scintigraphy:usefulness in the identification of myocardial ischemia. Circulation 1986;74:1007-15.

96. Tamaki N, Kawamoto M. The use of iodinated free fatty acids for assessing fatty acid metabolism. J Nucl Cardiol 1994;1:S72-S8.

97. Nishimura T, Uehara T, Shimonagata T, Nagata S, Haze K. Clinical results with ß-methyl-p-(^{123}I) iodophenylpentadecanoic acid, single-photon emission computed .tomography in cardiac disease. J Nucl Cardiol 1994;1:S65-S71.

98. Corbett J. Clinical experience with iodine-123-iodophenylpentadecanoic acid. J Nucl Med 1994;35:32S-37S.

99. Hansen CL, Corbett JR, Pippin JJ et al. Iodine-123-phenylpentadecanoic acid and single photon emission computed tomography in identifying left ventricular regional metabolic abnormalities in patients with coronary artery disease; comparison with thallium-201 tomography. J Am Coll Cardiol 1988;12:78-87.

100. Chouraqui P, Maddahi J, Henkin R. Comparison of myocardial imaging with iodine-123-iodophenyl-9-methyl pentadecanoic acid and thalllium-201-chloride for asessment of patients with exercise-induced ischemia. J Nucl med 1991;32:447-52.

101. Pippin J, Corbett J, Jansen D et al. Comparison of I-123-phenylpentadecanoic acid and thallium-201 tomographic imaging for the detection of coronary artery stenoses. Circulation 1987;76:IV-508 (Abstract).

102. Tamaki N, Kawamoto M, Yonekura Y et al. Regional metabolic abnormality in relation to perfusion and wall motion in patients with myocardial infarction: assessment with emission tomography using an iodinated branches fatty acid analog. J Nucl Med 1992;33:659-67.

103. Matsunari I, Saga T, Taki J et al. Kinetics of iodine-123-BMIPP in patients with prior myocardial infarction: assessment with dynamic rest and stress images compared with thallium-201 SPECT. J Nucl Med 1994;35:1279-85.

104. Reske SN. Viability as seen with radiolabelled fatty acids - a new approach to a challenging problem. Eur J Nucl Med 1994;21:279-82.

105. Murray G, Schad N, Ladd W, et al. Metabolic cardiac imaging in severe coronary disease: assessment of viability with iodine-123-iodophenylpentadecanoic acid and multicrystal

gamma camera, and correlation with biopsy. J Nucl Med 1992;33:1269-77.

106. Murray GL, Schad NC, Magill HL, Van der Zwaag R. Myocardial viability assessment with dynamic low-dose iodine-123-iodophenylpentadecanoic acid metabolic imaging: comparison with myocardial biopsy and reinjection SPECT thallium after myocardial infarction. J Nucl Med 1994;35:43S-48S.

107. Kuikka JT, Mussalo H, Hietakorpi S, Vanninen E, Lansimies E. Evaluation of myocardial viability with technetium-99m hexakis-2-methoxyisobutyl isonitrile and iodine-123 phenylpentadecanoic acid and single photon emission tomography. Eur J Nucl Med 1992;19:882-9.

108. Henrich MM, Vester E, von-der-Lohe E et al. The comparison of 2-18F-2-deoxyglucose and 15-(ortho-123I-phenyl)-pentadecanoic acid uptake in persisting defects on thallium-201 tomography in myocardial infarction. J Nucl Med 1991;32:1353-7.

109. Visser FC, Westera G, Van Eenige MJ, van der Wall EE, Heidendal GAK, Roos JP. Free fatty acid scintigraphy in patients with successful thrombolysis after myocardial infarction. Clin Nucl Med 1985;10:35-9.

110. Franken PR, De Geeter F, Dendale P, Block P, Bossuyt A. Regional distribution of 123I-(ortho-iodophenyl)-pentadecanoic acid and 99Tcm-MIBI in relation to wall motion after thrombolysis for acute myocardial infarction. Nucl Med Commun 1993;14:310-7.

111. De Geeter F, Franken PR, Knapp FF, Bossuyt A. Relationship between blood flow and fatty acid metabolism in subacute myocardial infarction: a study by means of 99mTc-Sestamibi and 123I-β-methyl-iodo-phenyl pentadecanoic acid. Eur J Nucl Med 1994;21:283-91.

112. Dilsizian V, Rocco TP, Freedman NM, Leon MB, Bonow RO. Enhanced detection of ischemic but viable myocardium by the reinjection of thallium after stress-redistribution imaging. N Engl J Med 1990;323:141-6.

113. Dilsizian V, Bonow RO. Current diagnostic techniques of assessing myocardial viability in hibernating and stunned myocardium. Circulation 1993;87:1-20.

114. Bonow RO, Dilsizian V, Cuocolo A, Bacharach SL. Identification of viable myocardium in patients with chronic coronary artery disease and left ventricular dysfunction. Comparison of thallium scintigraphy with reinjection and PET imaging with 18F-fluorodeoxyglucose. Circulation 1991;83:26-37.

115. van Eck-Smit BLF, van der Wall EE, Kuijper AFM, Zwinderman AH, Pauwels EKJ. Immediate TI-201 reinjection following stress imaging: a novel time-saving aproach for detection of myocardial viability. J Nucl Med 1993;34:737-43.

116. Kuijper AFM, Niemeyer MG, D'Haene EGM, van der Wall EE, Pauwels EKJ. Stress-reinjection Thallium-201 scintigraphy: prediction of effect of coronary artery bypass grafting on regional myocardial perfusion. J Am Coll Cardiol 1993;21:389A (Abstract).

117. Ohtani H, Tamaki N, Yonekura Y et al. Value of thallium-201 reinjection after delayed SPECT imaging for predicting reversible ischemia after coronary artery bypass grafting. Am J Cardiol 1990;66:394-9.

118. Tamaki N, Ohtani H, Yamashita K et al. Metabolic activity in the areas of new fill-in after thallium-201 reinjection: comparison with positron emission tomography using fluorine-18-deoxyglucose. J Nucl Med 1991;32:673-8.

119. Kuijper AFM, Vliegen HW, van der Wall EE et al. The clinical impact of thallium-201 reinjection for detection of myocardial viability. Eur J Nucl Med 1992;19:783-9.

120. Beanlands RS, Dawood F, Wen WH et al. Are the kinetics of technetium-99m methoxyisobutyl isonitrile affected by cell metabolism and viability? Circulation 1990;82:1802-14.

121. Carvalho PA, Chiu ML, Kronarige JF et al. Subcellular distribution and analysis of Tc99m-MIBI in isolated perfused rat hearts. J Nucl Med 1992;33:1516-21.

122. Crane P, Laliberte R, Heminway S, Thoolen M, Orlandi C. Effect of mitochondrial viability and metabolism on technetium-99m-sestamibi myocardial retention. Eur J Nucl Med 1993;20:20-5.
123. Altehoefer C, Kaiser HJ, Dörr R, et al. Fluorine-18 deoxyglucose PET for asessment of viable myocardium in perfusion defects in 99mTc-MIBI SPET: a comparative study in patients with coronary artery disease. Eur J Nucl Med 1992;19:334-42.
124. Sawada SG, Allman KC, Muzik O et al. Positron emission tomography detects evidence of viability in rest technetium-99m sestamibi defects. J Am Coll Cardiol 1994;23:92-8.
125. Cuoculo A, Pace L, Ricciardelli B, Chiaririello M, Trimarco B, Salvatore M. Identification of viable myocardium in patients with chronic coronary artery disease. Comparison of thallium-201 scintigraphy with reinjection and technetium 99m methoxyisobutyl isonitrile. J Nucl Med 1992;33:505-11.
126. Marzullo P, Sambuceti G. 99mTc-sestamibi: its clinical role as a viability agent. J Nucl Biol Med 1992;36:259-66.
127. Piwnica-Worms D, Kronauge JF, Chiu ML. Uptake and retention of hexakis (2-methoxyisobutyl isonitrile) technetium(I) in cultured chick myocardial cells. Mitochondrial and plasma membrane potential dependence. Circulation 1990;82:1826-88.
128. Schoeder H, Friedrich M, Topp H. Myocardial viability: What do we need? Eur J Nucl Med 1993;20:792-803.
129. Valkema R, van Eck-Smit BLF, van der Wall EE. Cardiac metabolism: a technical spectrum of modalities including positron emission tomography, single-photon emission computed tomography, and magnetic resonance spectroscopy. J Nucl Cardiol 1994;1:546-60.

5   THE ROLE OF FLUORINE-18-DEOXYGLUCOSE SINGLE PHOTON EMISSION COMPUTED TOMOGRAPHY IN PREDICTING REVERSIBILITY OF REGIONAL WALL MOTION ABNORMALITIES AFTER REVASCULARIZATION

Jeroen J. Bax, Jan H. Cornel, Frans C. Visser,
Paolo M. Fioretti, Arthur van Lingen, Johannes M. Huitink,
Otto Kamp, Gerrit J.J. Teule, and Cees A. Visser

Introduction

Patients with severe coronary artery disease and left ventricular (LV) dysfunction, may improve in regional and global LV function after revascularization.[1] However, these patients have an increased risk for perioperative events.[2] Therefore, a careful selection of these patients who are likely to benefit from a revascularization procedure is necessary. Although regional contractile dysfunction is frequently due to the presence of scarred myocardium following myocardial infarction, segments can be viable as shown by positron emission tomography (PET) using F18-fluorodeoxyglucose (^{18}FDG).[3] These asynergic but viable segments are likely to improve in contractile function after revascularization, whereas the scarred segments will not improve. ^{18}FDG PET has demonstrated good predictive accuracy for improvement of viable myocardium and absence of improvement in scarred myocardium.[4]

Because PET centers are not widely available the routine clinical use of ^{18}FDG is limited. Recently, the possibility of imaging 511 keV photons with planar scintigraphy was explored in our institution.[5,6] Thereafter, we have reported on the feasibility of imaging myocardial ^{18}FDG uptake with single photon emission computed tomography (SPECT).[7,8] The initial results in 9 patients with a previous infarction showed that in 43% of the perfusion defects ^{18}FDG uptake was relatively preserved,[7] suggesting the presence of viable tissue. The remaining perfusion defects showed concomitant reduction of ^{18}FDG uptake suggesting scar tissue. To determine the value of ^{18}FDG SPECT for clinical use, the predictive value of ^{18}FDG SPECT for functional recovery after revascularization needs to determined. In the present chapter we present a study on the use of ^{18}FDG SPECT to detect viable myocardium and to predict functional improvement after revascularization.

E. E. van der Wall et al. (eds.), Cardiac Positron Emission Tomography, 75–85.
© 1995 *Kluwer Academic Publishers.*

Patients

Twenty patients that were scheduled for revascularization were enrolled in the study. All patients had coronary angiography before the SPECT study. Each individual underwent resting thallium-201 (^{201}Tl) SPECT to evaluate regional perfusion, followed by ^{18}FDG SPECT. All medication was continued during the SPECT study. To evaluate regional wall motion abnormalities, two-dimensional echocardiography was performed before revascularization and repeated 1 to 8 months after revascularization (1.5 ± 0.4 months after PTCA, 3.6 ± 2.3 months after CABG). All patients gave informed consent to the study protocol that was approved by the Ethical Committee of The Free University Hospital Amsterdam.

Acquisition of SPECT images

SPECT was performed with a dual head rotating gamma camera system (ADAC Laboratories, Milpitas, CA, USA). The method has been previously described in detail.[7] Resting perfusion was evaluated with ^{201}Tl chloride (111 MBq) and imaging was performed within 15 min after tracer injection. For ^{18}FDG SPECT the camera system was equipped with special collimators (van Mullekom, Nuclear Fields, Boxmeer, The Netherlands) to detect 511 keV photons. The characteristics have been described elsewhere.[5] ^{18}FDG was performed during hyperinsulinemic euglycemic glucose clamping, to optimize and standardize metabolic conditions during the study.[9] Imaging was performed 45 minutes after administration of 185 MBq ^{18}FDG.

Reconstruction and analysis of SPECT images

From the raw scintigraphic data 6 mm-thick (1 pixel) transaxial slices were reconstructed by filtered back projection using a Hanning filter (f_c = 0.63 cycle/cm). Slices were not corrected for attenuation. Further reconstruction yielded long- and short-axis projections. Corresponding series of ^{201}Tl and ^{18}FDG images (long- and short-axis) were displayed side by side on a videoscreen. For each study the left ventricular myocardium was divided into 5 segments (apex, anterior, lateral, inferior, and septum). Two experienced observers visually interpreted the uptake of ^{201}Tl in each of the segments. In ^{201}Tl perfusion defects the ^{18}FDG uptake was considered; hypoperfused segments with relatively increased ^{18}FDG uptake (^{18}FDG-perfusion mismatch) were defined as viable tissue, according to PET criteria for viable myocardium.[10] The hypoperfused segments with similarly decreased ^{18}FDG uptake (^{18}FDG-perfusion match) were defined as necrotic tissue.[10]
^{201}Tl and ^{18}FDG have different photon energies that may cause differences in attenuation, especially in the inferior and septal regions of the myocardium. For this reason, the predictive value of ^{18}FDG SPECT in the inferior and septal wall was compared with the predictive value in the other segments (anterior, lateral and apical).

Regional wall motion analysis

Two-dimensional echocardiography was performed with the patient in the left lateral decubitus position using a 2.5 MHz transducer and a commercially available scanner (Hewlett-Packard, Sonos 1000). Four standard views of the left ventricle (parasternal long- and short-axis, apical 2- and 4-chamber views) were recorded. All images were recorded on 0.5 inch-VHS videotape. Off-line analysis was performed by digitizing the videotaped images in a computer system (Prevue III, Nova-Microsonics, USA) using an ECG R-wave triggered mechanism. The stored images were displayed side by side in a cine-loop format on a quad-screen; thus, the baseline and post-revascularization images were displayed simultaneously in either one of 4 standard views. To evaluate regional wall motion, the left ventricle was divided into 13 segments as described previously.[11] To compare the SPECT data with the echo data, the 13 segments were combined into 5 segments: apex, anterior, lateral, inferior and septal. Each segment was scored semiquantitatively by 2 experienced observers (without knowledge of the SPECT data) as: 0) normal (normal endocardial excursion and systolic wall thickening), 1) hypokinesia (reduced excursion and wall thickening), 2) akinesia (absence of excursion and wall thickening) or 3) dyskinesia (paradoxic outward movement in systole). Baseline segmental scores were used to evaluate left ventricular dysfunction prior to revascularization. A segment was considered functionally improved if systolic thickening (either hypokinetic or normokinetic) became apparent in a segment that was akinetic or dyskinetic before revascularization, or if a hypokinetic segment returned to normal contraction after the intervention. Post-operative paradoxical motion has been described in the septal region;[12] for this reason special attention was paid to the endocardial thickening in these regions to study improvement after the revascularization. Only segments that were revascularized were included in the analysis.

Cardiac catheterization

All patients underwent coronary arteriography and left ventriculography. Lesions with >50% reduction in luminal cross-section diameter in 1 or more of the major coronary arteries were considered significant. The left ventricular ejection fraction was calculated from the right anterior oblique view of the left ventricular angiogram by the responsible angiographer.

Statistical analysis

Patient data were compared using the Student's t-test for paired data. Comparison of proportions was performed using chi-square analysis. A P-value <0.05 was considered significant. All results are expressed as mean ± 1 SD.

Results

Clinical data
The clinical details of the study population are presented in Table 1. Nineteen patients had a previous infarction; in 16 patients the infarction was more than 1 month ago (mean time-interval of infarction to the SPECT study 50 ± 68 months). Three patients had diabetes mellitus type II, which was well-regulated on oral hypoglycemics; furthermore, using the clamping technique good image quality of cardiac [18]FDG SPECT studies can be obtained in this subset of patients.[13] A PTCA procedure was performed in 8 patients, and 12 patients underwent CABG. The mean time interval of the SPECT study to revascularization was 2.3 ± 2.5 months (range 1 week to 9 months, 90% of patients ≤ 5 months).

Table 1. Clinical Characteristics of the Study Population

Sex (male/female)	19/1
Age (years)	62 ± 9
Previous infarction	19
Q wave on ECG	
*Anterior	7
*Inferior	7
Coronary anatomy	
*1-vessel disease	5
*2-vessel disease	3
*3-vessel disease	12
LVEF (%)	46.8 ± 15.3
Cardiac medication	
*Beta-blocking agents	12
*Nitrates	11
*Calcium antagonists	10
*Diuretics	1
*ACE inhibitors	6
*Aspirin	17
Revascularization	
*PTCA	8
*CABG	12

LVEF: left ventricular ejection fraction

SPECT data
In the 20 patients a total of 45 perfusion defects was identified on the ^{201}Tl images. In general, the location of the infarction correlated well with the location of perfusion defects. In 17 (38%) ^{201}Tl perfusion defects, the [18]FDG uptake was relatively increased, whereas in 28 (62%) ^{201}Tl defects the [18]FDG uptake was decreased concordantly. Thus, the pre-revascularization SPECT findings identified 17 segments as viable regions ([18]FDG-perfusion mismatch), whereas 28 segments

were identified as necrotic, scarred tissue (^{18}FDG-perfusion match). Examples of an ^{18}FDG-perfusion match and mismatch are shown in Figures 1 and 2.

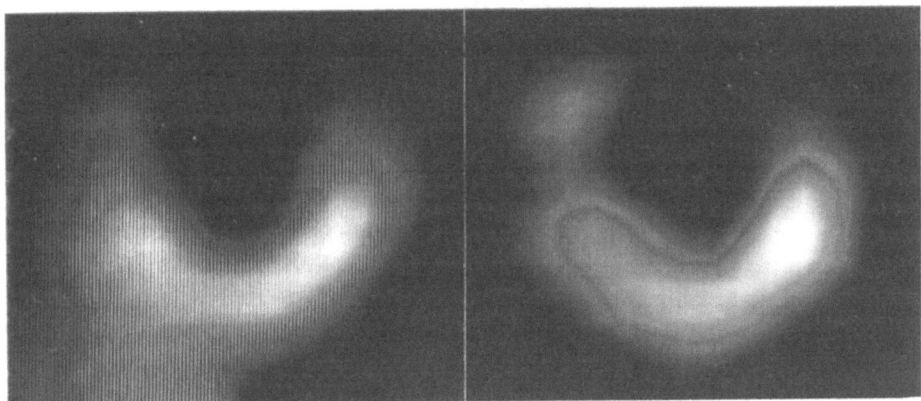

Figure 1. Two midventricular short-axis slices of a patient with an ^{18}FDG-perfusion match. Both ^{201}Tl (left) and ^{18}FDG (right) uptake are absent in the anterior wall, indicating the presence of necrotic tissue. (see for colourplate of this figure page 241).

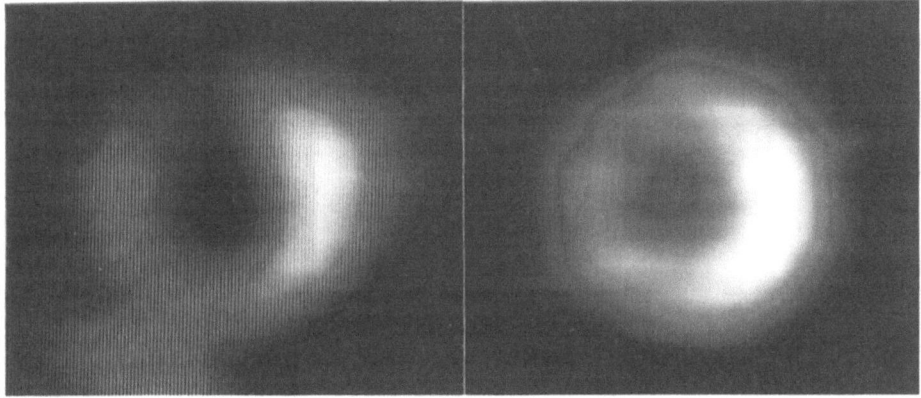

Figure 2. Two midventricular ^{201}Tl (left) and ^{18}FDG (right) short-axis slices, showing an ^{18}FDG-perfusion mismatch pattern. A ^{201}Tl perfusion defect is visible in the antero-septal wall, whereas the ^{18}FDG uptake is preserved in this region. (see for colourplate of this figure page 242).

Relation of SPECT and pre-interventional wall motion

Two segments with a perfusion defect showed normal wall motion on echocardiography. Of the remaining 43 segments, 15 (35%) were hypokinetic and 28 (62%) were a- or dyskinetic. A mismatch pattern was seen in 5 (33%) of 15 hypokinetic segments and in 10 (36%) of 28 a- or dyskinetic segments. The mean severity of pre-interventional wall motion abnormalities was not statistically different in the segments with an ^{18}FDG-perfusion match and with an ^{18}FDG-perfusion mismatch: 1.7 ± 0.6 versus 1.5 ± 0.7 (NS).

Recovery of wall motion versus SPECT data
Two segments with a perfusion defect had normal wall motion before the intervention and remained normal after the procedure; both showed a mismatch pattern. These segments were considered as mismatches that recovered in wall motion. The relation of the SPECT findings versus the mean segmental wall motion score before and after revascularization is demonstrated in Figure 3. In the segments with a mismatch on the SPECT images the mean segmental wall motion score decreased significantly after revascularization; before the intervention the score was 1.5 ± 0.7 and decreased to 0.7 ± 0.7 (P < 0.01). In the segments with a match the wall motion score remained unchanged: 1.7 ± 0.6 versus 1.7 ± 0.5 (NS). Regional wall motion abnormalities improved after the revascularization in 14 (82%) of 17 segments with a mismatch (Figure 4). In contrast, of 28 regions with a match, recovery of wall motion was seen in only 3 (11%) segments (P < 0.01 versus mismatches). Thus, the positive predictive value for recovery of wall motion in segments with a mismatch was 82%, whereas the negative predictive value for no improvement in segments with a match was 89%. The positive and negative predictive values of [18]FDG SPECT in the inferior and septal regions were not different from those in the anterior, lateral and apical regions: 71% and 88% vs 82% and 89%.

SEGMENTAL WMS

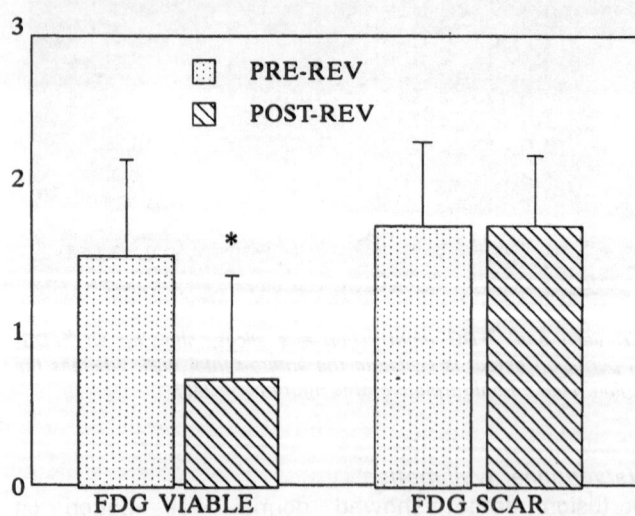

Figure 3. The relation of the SPECT data versus the mean segmental wall motion score (WMS) pre- and post-revascularization (REV) is demonstrated. Segmental wall motion score in mismatches decreased significantly (* P < 0.01), whereas in the matches the wall motion score remained unchanged.

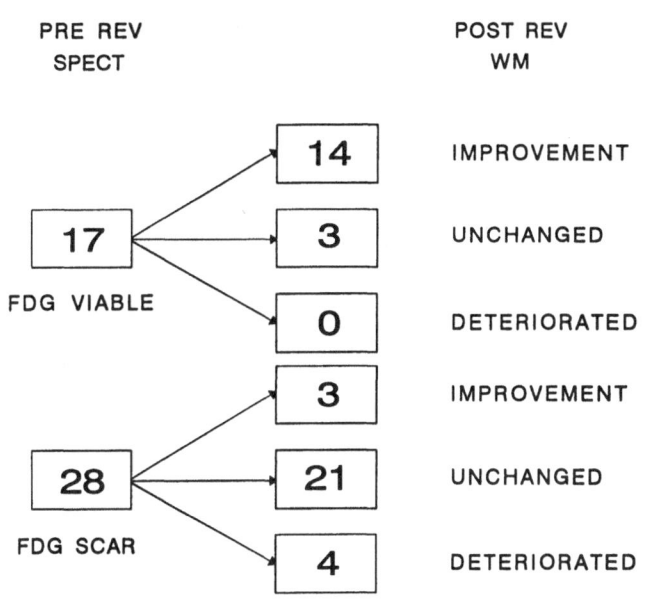

PRE REV
SPECT

POST REV
WM

Figure 4. *Changes in regional wall motion (WM) after revascularization (REV) in asynergic segments in relation to SPECT findings. Wall motion improved or remained normal after the revascularization in 14 of 17 (82%) segments with a mismatch. In contrast, of 28 regions with a match, recovery of wall motion was seen in only 3 (11%) segments (* P < 0.01 versus mismatches).*

17 → 14 IMPROVEMENT *
17 → 3 UNCHANGED
17 → 0 DETERIORATED
FDG VIABLE

28 → 3 IMPROVEMENT
28 → 21 UNCHANGED
28 → 4 DETERIORATED
FDG SCAR

Discussion

This study validates the use of ^{18}FDG SPECT imaging to predict functional recovery after revascularization. A- or hypokinesia improved after revascularization in 82% of segments with hypoperfusion and increased ^{18}FDG uptake. In contrast, no improvement in contractile dysfunction was found in 89% of segments with both decreased perfusion and ^{18}FDG uptake. These findings confirm that the presence of an ^{18}FDG-perfusion mismatch on SPECT imaging is associated with viable tissue. Our results are in agreement with those reported in ^{18}FDG PET studies, showing an average positive predictive accuracy of 83% (range 72-95%) and a negative predictive accuracy of 84% (range 75-100%).[14]

The ^{18}FDG-^{201}Tl SPECT approach
To evaluate viability ^{18}FDG uptake needs to be compared with perfusion. To evaluate perfusion an early resting ^{201}Tl SPECT was used. Melin and coworkers[15] showed that initial myocardial uptake of ^{201}Tl was directly related to perfusion as measured with microspheres. ^{201}Tl and ^{18}FDG have different photon energies that may lead to differences in attenuation especially in the inferoseptal region of the myocardium. In a study performed in normal individuals however, it was shown that no differences between tracer activities occurred in the different regions of the myocardium.[8] In the present study we demonstrated similar positive and negative predictive values in the inferior and septal regions as compared to those in the apical, anterior and lateral regions. Thus, these findings suggest that attenuation

differences between ^{201}Tl and [18]FDG play a minor role for the clinical application of the SPECT approach.

Functional improvement as the "gold standard" of myocardial viability

We have used improvement in contractile function (assessed with echocardiography) as the "gold standard" of viable myocardium. Although no patient suffered a peri-operative infarction, some myocardial necrosis may have occurred during surgery, thereby affecting post-intervention recovery. Furthermore, vessel or graft patency was not determined after the procedure. Reocclusion may partly account for the failure of some mismatches to recover. In addition, the alignment of echocardiographic and SPECT segments may be difficult. Echocardiography uses landmarks as the papillary muscles and the insertion of the right ventricle into the septum for the assignment of myocardial segments. SPECT divides the short-axis slices into 4 equidistant segments. Therefore misalignment may affect the predictive values for functional recovery. However, this limitation is present in all comparable studies that have used echocardiography for comparison with scintigraphic data.[16-18]

[18]FDG uptake occurs in viable cells. Some of these cells may be damaged to a greater extent than others. It has been demonstrated that morphological degeneration occurs at cellular level before actual cell death occurs.[19-21] Marwick et al.[17] suggested that despite the increased [18]FDG uptake, some segments may contain cells that are too severely injured to recover in function after revascularization.

Limitations of the present study

In the present study scintigrams were analyzed qualitatively. However, in a previous report, we showed that visual analysis correlated well with semiquantitative analysis.[7]

Although the predictive value of [18]FDG SPECT for reversibility of regional wall motion abnormalities has been demonstrated, recovery of global left ventricular function was not studied. Other studies have demonstrated that improvement of global function was associated with the number of segments containing viable tissue.[4,22] In the present study, the entire left ventricular myocardium was divided into only 5 segments. Several patients had one or more segments with hypoperfused but viable myocardium. In these patients ejection fraction may have improved after revascularization.

Although resolution of SPECT is inferior to PET, it showed good predictive value for the recovery of wall motion. In addition, Tillisch et al.[4] showed that a substantial amount of viable myocardium needs to be present for improvement of global ventricular function. Thus, the resolution of [18]FDG SPECT may be sufficient for routine purposes.

Clinical implications

The finding that [18]FDG SPECT can predict reversibility of wall motion abnormalities after a revascularization procedure has important clinical implications. Nesto et al.[23] showed favourable survival in patients with viable myocardium and increased ejection fraction after revascularization. Therefore, the detection of asynergic but viable myocardium (which is likely to recover after revascularization) with [18]FDG SPECT may help in the identification of patients who will benefit most from a revascularization. Cardiac [18]FDG imaging has been used for several years with PET. At present, PET is not widely available for routine clinical use. For this reason [18]FDG SPECT may contribute to a more widespread use of [18]FDG imaging for viability studies.

Conclusion

The present study reveals a positive predictive accuracy of a mismatch to recover in contractile function of 82%. Similarly, a negative predictive value of 89% was demonstrated. We conclude from the present study that [18]FDG SPECT can identify viable tissue and predict improvement of regional function after revascularization. [18]FDG SPECT may contribute to the identification of patients who may benefit from revascularization procedures.

References

1. Brundage BH, Massie BM, Botvinick EH. Improved regional ventricular function after successful surgical revascularization. J Am Coll Cardiol 1984;3:902-8.
2. Kennedy JW, Kaiser GC, Fisher LD et al. Clinical and angiographic predictors of operative mortality from the collaborative study in coronary artery surgery (CASS). Circulation 1981;63:793-802.
3. Brunken R, Tillish J, Schwaiger M et al. Regional perfusion, glucose metabolism, and wall motion in patients with chronic electrocardiographic Q wave infarctions: evidence for persistence of viable tissue in some infarct regions by positron emission tomography. Circulation 1986;73:951-63.
4. Tillisch J, Brunken R, Marshall R et al. Reversibility of cardiac wall motion abnormalities predicted by positron tomography. N Engl J Med 1986;314:884-8.
5. Van Lingen A, Huijgens PC, Visser FC et al. Performance characteristics of a 511-keV collimator for imaging positron emitters with a standard gamma-camera. Eur J Nucl Med 1992;19:315-21.
6. Huitink JM, Visser FC, van Lingen A et al. Feasibility of planar 18F-fluoro-deoxyglucose imaging after recent myocardial infarction to assess myocardial viability. J Nucl Med 1995, in press.
7. Bax JJ, Visser FC, van Lingen A et al. Feasibility of assessing regional myocardial uptake of ^{18}F-fluorodeoxyglucose using single photon emission computed tomography. Eur Heart J 1993; 14:1675-82.
8. Bax JJ, Visser FC, van Lingen A et al. Relation between myocardial uptake of thallium-201 chloride and F18-fluorodeoxyglucose imaged with SPECT in normal volunteers. Eur J Nucl Med 1994;22:56-60.
9. Knuuti MJ, Nuutila P, Ruotsalainen U et al. Euglycemic hyperinsulinemic clamp and oral glucose load in stimulating myocardial glucose utilization during positron emission tomography. J Nucl Med 1992;33:1255-62.
10. Schwaiger M, Hicks R. The clinical role of metabolic imaging of the heart by positron emission tomography. J Nucl Med 1991;32:565-78.
11. Jaarsma W, Visser CA, Eenige van MJ et al. Prognostic implications of regional hyperkinesia and remote asynergy of noninfarcted myocardium. Am J Cardiol 1986;58:394-8.
12. Righetti A, Crawford MH, O'Rourke RA et al. Interventricular septal motion and left ventricular function after coronary bypass surgery: evaluation with echocardiography and radionuclide ventriculography. Am J Cardiol 1977;39:372-7.
13. Bax JJ, Visser FC, van Lingen A et al. Image quality of F18-fluorodeoxyglucose SPECT studies in patients with coronary artery disease and diabetes mellitus type II. Eur J Nucl Med 1994;21:824 (Abstract).
14. Maddahi J, Schelbert H, Brunken R, Di Carli M. Role of thallium-201 and PET imaging in evaluation of myocardial viability and management of patients with coronary artery disease and left ventricular function. J Nucl Med 1994;35:707-15.
15. Melin JA, Becker LC. Quantitative relationship between global left ventricular thallium uptake and blood flow: effects of propranolol, ouabain, dipyridamole and coronary artery occlusion. J Nucl Med 1986;27:641-52.
16. Knuuti MJ, Nuutila P, Ruotsalainen U et al. The value of quantitative analysis of glucose utilization in detection of myocardial viability by PET. J Nucl Med 1993;34:2068-75.
17. Marwick TH, MacIntyre WJ, Lafont A, Nemec JJ, Salcedo EE. Metabolic responses of hibernating and infarcted myocardium to revascularization. Circulation 1992;85:1347-

53.

18. Nienaber CA, Brunken RC, Sherman CT et al. Metabolic and functional recovery of ischemic human myocardium after coronary angioplasty. J Am Coll Cardiol 1991;18:966-78.

19. Flameng W, Vanhaeke J, Van Belle H et al. Relation between coronary artery stenosis and myocardial purine metabolism, histology and regional function in humans. J Am Coll Cardiol 1987;9:1235-42.

20. Flameng W, Suy R, Schwartz F, Borgers M. Ultrastructural correlates of left ventricular contraction abnormalities in patients with chronic ischemic heart disease: determinants of reversible segmental asynergy post revascularization surgery. Am Heart J 1981;102:846-57.

21. Maes A, Flameng W, Nuyts J et al. Histological alterations in chronically hypoperfused myocardium. Correlation with PET findings. Circulation 1994;90:735-45.

22. Ragosta M, Beller GA, Watson DD, Kaul S, Gimple LW. Quantitative planar rest-redistribution ^{201}Tl imaging in detection of myocardial viability and prediction of improvement in left ventricular function after coronary bypass surgery in patients with severely depressed left ventricular function. Circulation 1993;87:1630-41.

23. Nesto RW, Cohn LH, Collins JH et al. Inotropic contractile reserve: a useful predictor of increased 5 year survival and improved postoperative left ventricular function in patients with coronary artery disease and reduced ejection fraction. Am J Cardiol 1982;50:39-44.

6   PARAMETRIC POSITRON EMISSION TOMOGRAPHY IMAGING OF MYOCARDIAL PERFUSION AND METABOLISM

Antoon T.M. Willemsen, Paul K. Blanksma,
and Anne M.J. Paans

Introduction

In clinical cardiology, knowledge of the characteristics of both the normal and abnormal heart is of paramount importance in the diagnosis and treatment of cardiological patients. The characteristics can be obtained using many different techniques such as biochemical analysis and the electrocardiogram (ECG), or the various imaging techniques [coronary angiography, ultrasound, magnetic resonance imaging (MRI), single photon emission computed tomography (SPECT), positron emission tomography (PET)]. Of course, each technique has its own advantages and disadvantages which should be known in order to be able to select the appropriate technique for a given patient. In this chapter, an overview of cardiac PET will be presented showing which parameters can be obtained, how the measurements are performed and how the data can be analyzed (for an extensive and detailed introduction see e.g. [1]). Emphasis will be placed on the determination of the myocardial blood flow and metabolism. It will be shown how the data can be represented in polarmaps and how a statistical analysis can be performed by comparing the data with a database obtained in healthy volunteers. These procedures are performed semi-automatically requiring little effort and attention.

Positron emission tomography

In PET, a molecule is labeled with a positron emitting radionuclide. The radionuclides mostly used are ^{11}C, ^{13}N, ^{15}O and ^{18}F with half-lives ranging from 2 minutes up to 2 hours. When a nucleus disintegrates a positron is emitted which will annihilate with an electron to form two 511 keV photons moving in opposite direction. With a ring of detectors the photons can be detected in coincidence and the so called line of response (LOR) is established. By filtered backprojection the data thus obtained can be transformed to calculate the underlying radioactivity distribution. The two photons

E. E. van der Wall et al. (eds.), Cardiac Positron Emission Tomography, 87–96.

are detected in coincidence, i.e. the disintegration will only be accepted when both photons are detected within 8 ns of each other. This reduces background noise substantially resulting in an increased signal to noise ratio. The chance that either photon is absorbed is given by the total amount of absorption on the LOR, irrespective of the original position of the disintegration. This enables the measurement of the attenuation for each LOR with an external source, and thus the subsequent correction for this attenuation. Thus the radioactivity distribution can be measured quantitatively and as a function of time.

Parameters

For a number of radiopharmaceuticals a model has been proposed and validated, describing the relation between the input i.e. the radioactivity in arterial plasma and the output i.e. the radioactivity distribution in tissue as a function of time as measured with the PET camera. Combining both, often model parameters can be obtained which are related to some physiological or functional parameter. This enables the measurement of various parameters as shown in Table 1.

Table 1. Overview of some of the parameters which can be measured with positron emission tomography and the corresponding tracers

Parameter	Tracer
Blood flow	$^{13}NH_3$, $H_2^{15}O$, $C^{15}O_2$
Blood volume	$C^{15}O$
Metabolism	
Glucose metabolism	^{18}FDG
Protein synthesis rate	L[1-^{11}C]tyrosine, L-[1-^{11}C]leucine
DNA synthesis rate	^{11}C-thymidine
Fatty acids	^{11}C-palmitate
Oxidative	^{11}C-acetate
Receptors	(a)
Wall thickness	^{18}FDG
Wall movement	^{18}FDG
Ejection fraction	$C^{15}O$

(a): For an overview see A. van Waarde et al.[14]

To obtain accurate estimations of the wall thickness, wall movement and the ejection fraction it is essential that the PET system supports gated acquisition. With gating the acquisition is synchronized to the R-peak of the ECG and each heartbeat is dynamically divided into 16 or 32 gates, automatically compensating for changes in heart rate. For a heart rate of 60 bpm this results in gates of either 60 or 30 ms.

Here, we will focus on the determination of myocardial blood-flow and glucose metabolism using the tracers $^{13}NH_3$ and ^{18}FDG respectively. Ammonia extraction by the myocardium is flow-dependent. Thus the amount of activity in the myocardium is a measure of the blood flow to that region.[2,3] Two potential problems must be considered. First, the extraction fraction is dependent on the flow itself. This is corrected for, using data obtained from animal experiments. Second, ammonia is rapidly metabolized and a redistribution of activity can be observed which obscures the flow-dependent activity accumulation. This can be solved by extending the model to incorporate these processes. However, we apply a simpler model which requires only data over the first 2 minutes when metabolism is still negligible.[4,5] The effectiveness of the method was demonstrated by comparing the flow-distribution with the activity distribution in healthy volunteers.[6] It was shown that whereas the flow distribution was homogeneous, the activity distribution was not with reduced values in the posterolateral region indicating a redistribution of activity after 2 minutes post injection.

^{18}FDG is metabolized to ^{18}FDG-6-phosphate which, on the time scale of the experiment, is irreversibly trapped in the cell as it is not metabolized further nor reduced to ^{18}FDG. As the relationship between ^{18}FDG and glucose has been established the accumulation of activity in the myocardium can be used to calculate the corresponding glucose metabolism. This can be performed using the graphical Patlak analysis[7] which requires the plasma activity to be known over the total duration of the experiment, whereas the tissue data is mainly of importance between 20 and 50 minutes. The model requires both a constant glucose plasma level and a constant glucose metabolism. This requires dietary precautions while in the case of diabetic subjects a glucose clamp technique may be required in which the glucose level is stabilized.

Measurements

After positioning the subject in the camera a rectilinear transmission scan is made. This gives an image of the absorption over an axial length of typically 30 cm and takes 6 minutes. On these images the exact position of the heart is established and the final positioning is then performed. A transmission scan is performed (20 minutes) using the same external ring source for subsequent correction of photon attenuation. The radiopharmacon is injected intravenously and the radioactivity distribution is measured as a function of time. The length of the individual time-frames and the total study duration are determined by the radiopharmaceutical used and can range from 2 to 50 minutes for a single study. For $^{13}NH_3$ the frames are 12*10s, 1*2, 4 and 6 minutes and for ^{18}FDG the frames are 8*15 s, 4*30s, and 1*1, 5, 10, 15 and 20 minutes. Generally several consecutive studies are performed e.g. flow-metabolism and flow(rest)-flow(stress)-metabolism, where the stress is induced by infusion of dipyridamole. Using the flow-tracer $^{13}NH_3$ and applying the standard of 5 half-lives between two injections total study time could be longer than 2 hours exclusive transmission and rectilinear scan. To reduce total scan time we developed a program to automatically compensate for remaining activity of the previous scan. This program uses the finding that the ^{13}N-activity in the myocardium is virtually constant (< 4%)

in the period from 5 to 40 minutes post injection. Because the injection times are known, the remaining activity of the previous scan can easily be corrected for. In case of a second flow study, the error is further reduced as the flow is determined by the first 2 minutes of data when the activity is high. In case of a [18]FDG study the error is further reduced by the difference in half-life and because the [18]FDG model requires predominantly data obtained between 20 and 50 minutes post injection. This compensation was tested in healthy volunteers. Comparing the flow values of three consecutive [13]NH$_3$ studies with 20 minutes between the scans, significant statistical differences could not be observed. As a result scan time for the three emission scans is reduced from 2 to 1 hour.[8]

To determine the input function, i.e. the radioactivity of the free compound in arterial plasma, one generally requires arterial sampling. In the case of cardiac studies however, a blood-pool value can be obtained by measuring the whole blood activity in the cavity of the left ventricle or left atrium directly from the PET images. Whether or not these blood-pool values are representative of the arterial plasma values must be checked for each radiopharmaceutical. For [18]FDG this was found to be correct whereas for [13]NH$_3$ studies this is correct for the first few minutes only.

For longer living isotopes, a gated study can be performed after the dynamic scan. Using a homogeneous phantom and a ECG simulator the correction for dead-time and decay was investigated. The effect of missed and skipped beats, due to unacceptable RR interval times, was investigated also. It was found that this gated acquisition gave reliable activity distributions irrespective of the above mentioned factors. The resulting gated study can indeed be averaged to obtain a single frame of data, identical to a conventional non-gated study of the same duration. Thus the last frame of the dynamic study is now changed into a gated acquisition of 20 minutes. Afterwards, this frame is reconstructed from the gated study. In effect, for the [18]FDG study, a gated study is obtained at little additional costs.

Analysis

After reconstruction, attenuation correction and the correction for remaining activity, the data can be analyzed. Therefore, the data is re-oriented to short axis images.[9] First the image of the last time frame is displayed and the long axis of the heart is drawn manually, Figure 1. A new image perpendicular to the previous one is now displayed and the long axis is drawn again. This defines the myocardial long axis in three dimensions. The apex and base are defined and the data is then resliced to 10 short axis images perpendicular to the long axis. When possible, identical reslice parameters, which can be saved and restored, are used for all studies of a single subject, although movement of the subject can cause problems. Using the appropriate model the parameter of interest can be calculated by supplying the activity as measured in the blood-pool and the activity as measured in a segment of the myocardium. The blood-pool data is calculated using a circular region of interest in three slices near the base and calculating the average value. The tissue activity can be measured for each single pixel, effectively resulting in a functional image, or by selecting a group of pixels. We use a wedge-shaped region of interest dividing the short axis image into 48 segments of 7.5° each. Each segment is defined by two circles which describe the

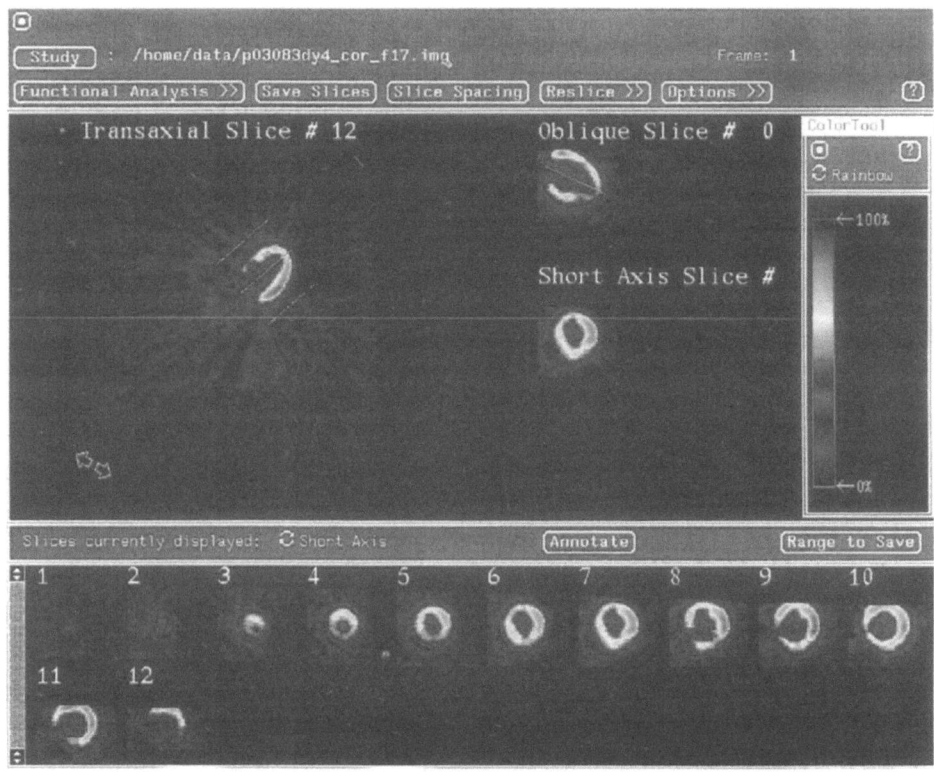

Figure 1 Construction of the short axis images. First the long axis is drawn and the boundaries of the myocardium are given, top left. The data is resampled and the vertical long axis is drawn again, top right. This defines the long axis in three dimensions. Finally the data is resampled perpendicular to the long axis and the resulting short axis images can be saved, bottom right and bottom.(see for colourplate of this figure page 242).

inner and outer dimension of the myocardium. Both the origin and their radii can be changed manually, Figure 2. In each segment thus defined, the average of all pixels and the average of nine pixels around the maximum activity is calculated. If one's primary interest is in obtaining the maximum value than the difference between the inner and outer circles can be taken rather large to insure that all the myocardium is analyzed. Contrary, for the average value the inner and outer dimensions must be close together to insure that only myocardium is analyzed. For ^{18}FDG and ^{13}NH$_3$ studies we generally apply the maximum segment activity. These setting can be saved and restored to use identical setting for different consecutive measurements. With 10 short axis images this results in 480 time-activity curves for both the average and the maximum activity, which must be transformed to 480 values for the physiological parameter. Therefore the time-activity curves are saved on disk and further processing is performed using dedicated software written within the framework of MATLAB (The MathWorks Inc, Natick, Mass. USA). This results in an ASCII data file representing the

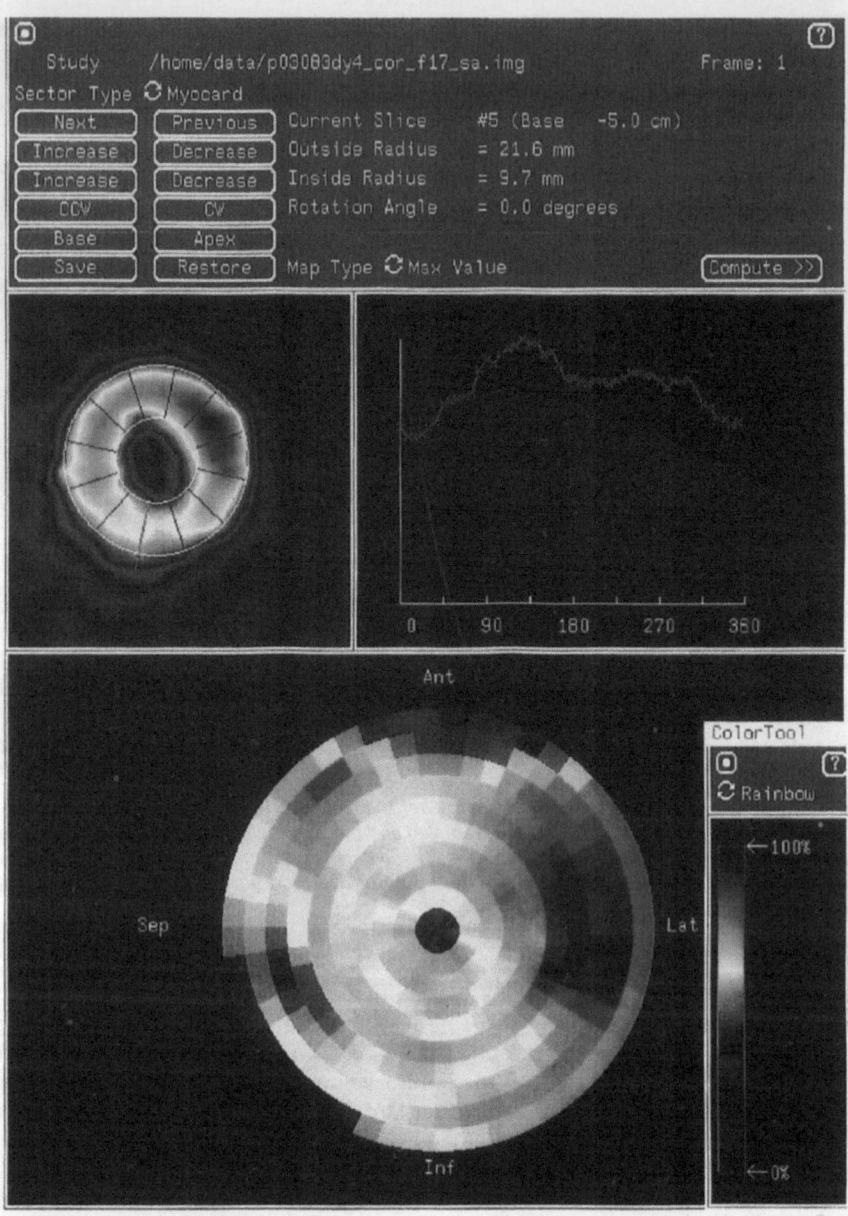

Figure 2 Construction of a single activity polarmap. For each of the slices from base to apex, which can be defined manually, the inner and outer dimensions of the myocardium are set, top left. Then the average and maximum activity in 48 segments along the circles are calculated and presented in a polarmap, bottom. The polarmaps constitutes of the apex at the center to the base at the rim. The activity profile for the 48 segments of a single slice are given also, top right.   (see for colourplate of this figure page 243).

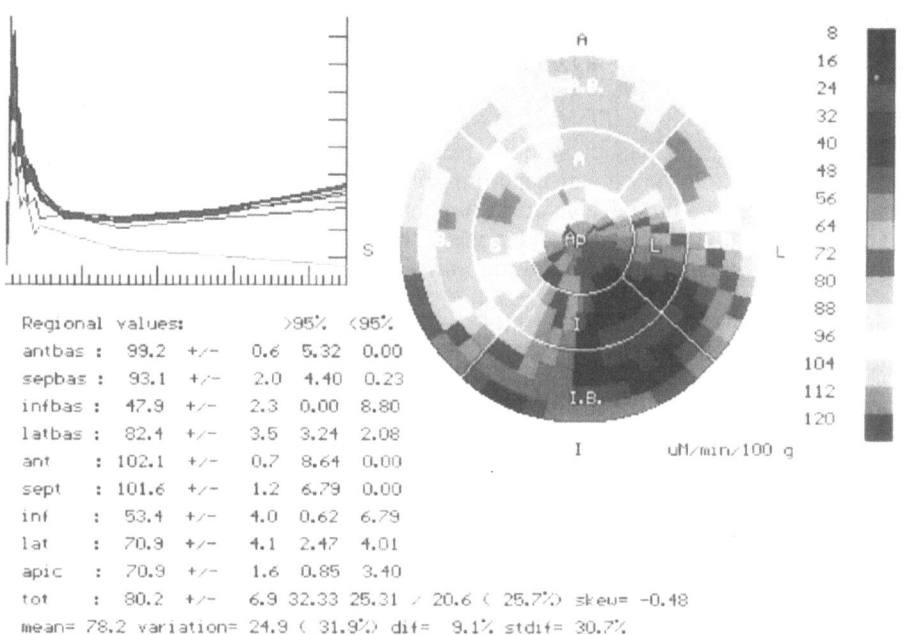

Regional values: >95%   <95%
antbas : 99.2 +/- 0.6 5.32 0.00
sepbas : 93.1 +/- 2.0 4.40 0.23
infbas : 47.9 +/- 2.3 0.00 8.80
latbas : 82.4 +/- 3.5 3.24 2.08
ant   : 102.1 +/- 0.7 8.64 0.00
sept   : 101.6 +/- 1.2 6.79 0.00
inf   : 53.4 +/- 4.0 0.62 6.79
lat   : 70.9 +/- 4.1 2.47 4.01
apic   : 70.9 +/- 1.6 0.85 3.40
tot   : 80.2 +/- 6.9 32.33 25.31 / 20.6 (25.7%) skew= -0.48
mean= 78.2 variation= 24.9 (31.9%) dif= 9.1% stdif= 30.7%

Figure 3 Functional polarmap of a patient studied with FDG. The blood-pool time activity curve together with the average time activity curves for the 9 regions are shown at the top left. Below it the mean and standard deviations for each region are given together with some statistical parameters. At the right the glucose metabolism is given in μmol/min/100g tissue as a functional polarmap. (see for colourplate of this figure page 244).

flow or metabolism data for all 480 segments together with information on the original file and the processing applied. This file is used for further statistical analysis as described below. Additionally, a polarmap data file is made with the apex at the center and the base at the rim, Figure 3, which can be displayed and manipulated using a polarmap calculator (pmcalc, CTI/Siemens, Knoxville, USA). The same procedure can be followed to calculate e.g. the receptor density[10] or the activity distribution at a given time point. Because the generation of the short axis images and the time-activity curves for each segment is independent of the tracer used, the only difference is in the model selected where the transformation of time-activity data to physiological parameter is performed. This also enables the investigation of alternative models or the effect of various forms of data (pre-)processing without recalculation of the time-activity curves.

Another advantage of this approach is the possible combination with automatic contour detection of inner and outer myocardium boundaries. This way, wallthickness and wall movement can be obtained and represented in a similar polarmap. Knowledge of wall thickness also enables the estimation of the partial volume effect, i.e. the smoothing of activity due to the limited resolution (FWHM 6mm) of the system and thus its compensation.

The data files are transported to a personal computer where they are compared with a data base of polarmaps obtained in healthy volunteers. From this database 95% confidence intervals are obtained (mean +/- two standard deviations).[8] Combining the data of the three consecutive scans a classification can be made as shown in Table 2.

Again, the analysis is based on data from healthy volunteers. This data can be represented in a truly functional polarmap indicating normal, infarcted and ischemic myocardium.[10-12] The data is also combined in nine regions where for each region the percentages are given. The final diagnosis is based on all the above mentioned data including the original activity distribution images.

Table 2. Discrimination of normal, infarcted and ischemic myocardium using PET

Flow rest	Flow stress	Glucose Metabolism	Diagnosis
Normal	Normal	Normal	Normal myocardium
Reduced	Reduced	Reduced	Infarcted myocardium
Normal	Normal	Reduced	Infarcted myocardium (luxury perfusion)
Reduced	Reduced	Normal/Increased	Ischemic myocardium (rest)
Normal	Reduced	Normal/Increased	Ischemic myocardium (provocable)

Discussion

Quantitation of myocardial flow and metabolism is of great importance as it enables the detection of absolute changes in addition to relative distribution differences. Furthermore, this also enables the comparison of the data of a single subject with a database obtained from healthy volunteers. The subsequent statistical analysis which has thus become available, offers the opportunity to assess myocardial infarction and ischemia in a until now unprecedented rigour.

Considering the relative good resolution of present PET scanners to base such a statistical analysis on manually drawn regions of interest is impractical as this discards the majority of the data. Furthermore in some studies we found the coefficient of variation to be a most important parameter which requires a relative large amount of regions. However, an analysis of the total myocardium must be highly automated to prevent excessive work load. The calculation of a functional image where the flow and metabolism are calculated on a pixel by pixel basis was not attempted. Although the construction of such these images may actually be rather fast,[13] the results require further processing unless the analysis is to be performed visually only. A statistical analysis combining the data of the (three) consecutive scans and the pooled data of a group of healthy subjects would be impractical if not impossible on a pixel by pixel basis. In the presented method the myocardium is divided into 480 segments (assuming 10 slices of 48 segments) and processed. Due to the reslicing and interpolating steps the correlation between neighboring segments is high which minimizes the effect of small displacements. Although various steps are not particularly fast, the actual user interaction is dominated by the manual determination of the long axis of the left ventricle and the setting of the inner and outer dimensions of the resulting short axis images. Using the multi-tasking capabilities of present workstations these two steps can be performed almost in parallel. As a result, the total analysis time of 1 hour for three consecutive PET studies requires only 15 to 20 minutes of user interaction.

Because different parameters are represented in identical polarmap format the assessment of various correlations can easily be obtained. Also, analysis methods developed for a specific topic can easily be transformed to be applied for all measurements. The main improvement is expected from the automatic detection of the inner and outer myocardium. This will have three advantages. First, user interaction can be further reduced although visual quality inspection may be required. This should also enable the analysis of gated acquisition which was impractical until now. Second, this will give an estimate of wall thickness. Consequently a proper correction for partial volume effect may become feasible. Third, the combination of wall thickness assessment and gated studies should enable the assessment of wall movement. Thus wall motion and wall thickness measurements can be combined with the functional parameters flow and glucose metabolism. The potential of such a combination in the assessment of myocardial function is evident.

References

1. Positron Emission Tomography of the Heart. S.R. Bergmann and B.E. Sobel, editors. Mount Kisco, New York: Futura Publishing Company, 1992.
2. Bellina CR, Parodi O, Camici P et al. Simultaneous in vitro and in vivo validation of nitrogen-13-ammonia for the assessment of regional myocardial blood flow. J Nucl Med 1990;31:1335-43.
3. Shah A, Schelbert HR, Schwaiger M et al. Measurement of regional myocardial blood flow with N-13 ammonia and positron emission tomography in intact dogs. J Am Coll Cardial 1985;5:92-100.
4. Yoshida K, Endo M, Hime T et al. Measurement of regional myocardial blood flow in hypertrophic cardiomyopathy: application of the first-pass flow model using [13N]ammonia and PET. Am J Physiol Imaging 1989;4:97-104.
5. Weinberg LN, Huang SC, Hoffmann EJ et al. Validation of PET-acquired input functions for cardiac studies. J Nucl Med 1988;9:241-7.
6. De Jong RM, Blanksma PK, Willemsen ATM et al. The "posterolateral defect" of the mormal human heart investigated with nitrogen-13 ammonia and dynamic positron emission tomography. J Nucl Med (In press).
7. Patlak CS, Blasberg RG, Fenstermacher JD. Graphical evaluation of blood-to-brain transfer constants from mulitple-time uptake data. J Cereb Blood Flow Metab 1983;3:1-7.
8. Blanksma PK, Willemsen ATM, De Jong RM et al. Quantitative myocardial mapping of perfusion and metabolism using parametric polar map displays in cardiac PET. J Nucl Med 1995;36:1-6.
9. Laubenbacher C, Rothley J, Sitomer J et al. An automated analysis program for the evaluation of cardiac PET studies: initial results in the detection and localization of coronary artery disease using nitrogen-13 ammonia. J Nucl Med 1993;34:968-78.
10. Anthonio RL, Van Waarde A, Willemsen ATM et al. Experimental and clinical beta receptor studies. In: Cardiac PET, Blanksma P.K., Niemeyer M.G., Paans A.M.J., van der Wall E.E. (eds). Kluwer Academic Publishers, Dordrecht/Boston/London, 1995.
11. Tan ES. Positron emission tomography assessment of myocardial viability. In: Cardiac PET, Blanksma P.K., Niemeyer M.G., Paans A.M.J., van der Wall E.E. (eds). Kluwer Academic Publishers, Dordrecht/Boston/London, 1995.
12. Blanksma PK, Posma JI, De Jong RM et al. PET characterization of the myocardium in Hypertrophic cardiomyopathy. in Cardiac PET, Blanksma P.K., Niemeyer M.G., Paans A.M.J., van der Wall E.E. (eds). Kluwer Academic Publishers, Dordrecht/Boston/London, 1995.
13. Choi Y, Huang SC, Hawkins RA et al. A simplified method for quantification of myocardial blood flow using nitrogen-13-ammonia and dynamic PET. J Nucl Med 1993;34:488-97.
14. van Waarde A, Elsinga PH, Anthonio RL et al. Study of Cardiac Receptor Ligands. In: Cardiac PET, Blanksma P.K., Niemeyer M.G., Paans A.M.J., van der Wall E.E. (eds). Kluwer Academic Publishers, Dordrecht/Boston/London, 1995.

7   POSITRON EMISSION TOMOGRAPHY COMPARED TO SINGLE PHOTON EMISSION COMPUTED TOMOGRAPHY IN THE EVALUATION OF MYOCARDIAL VIABILITY: A PRELIMINARY COST-EFFECTIVENESS ANALYSIS

Maria G.M. Hunink

Introduction

Using positron emission tomography (PET) in determining a revascularization strategy reduces the number of "events" after revascularization. This yields a benefit in terms of event-free survival and reduced (downstream) treatment costs because events are averted. However, PET is more expensive than single photon emission computed tomography (SPECT) and could result in an increase in the number of revascularization procedures.

To evaluate two diagnostic strategies with respect to costs and effectiveness one could perform a randomized controlled trial. However, such a trial may not always be feasible or ethical and the potential for confounding by treatment variables raises the question whether such a study design is applicable to diagnostic tests. Decision analysis provides an analytical method to compare diagnostic strategies. Using mathematical modeling, it weighs and integrates risks, benefits, and costs.[1-3]

This chapter addresses the question which health benefit and additional costs are associated with the use of PET versus SPECT in deciding on a revascularization strategy in patients with possible residual ischemia after a myocardial infarction, and how the costs are related to the benefit gained. We address this question using decision and cost-effectiveness analysis.

The model

Based on the available data from the literature and a number of assumptions we can structure the problem as in Figure 1. The two strategies considered are:

1. Revascularization strategy based on the PET result, i.e. if PET is positive perform revascularization (REV+), if PET is negative do not perform revascularization (REV-).

E. E. van der Wall et al. (eds.), Cardiac Positron Emission Tomography, 97–102.
© 1995 Kluwer Academic Publishers.

2. Revascularization strategy based on the SPECT result, i.e. if SPECT is positive perform revascularization (REV+), if SPECT is negative do not perform revascularization (REV-).

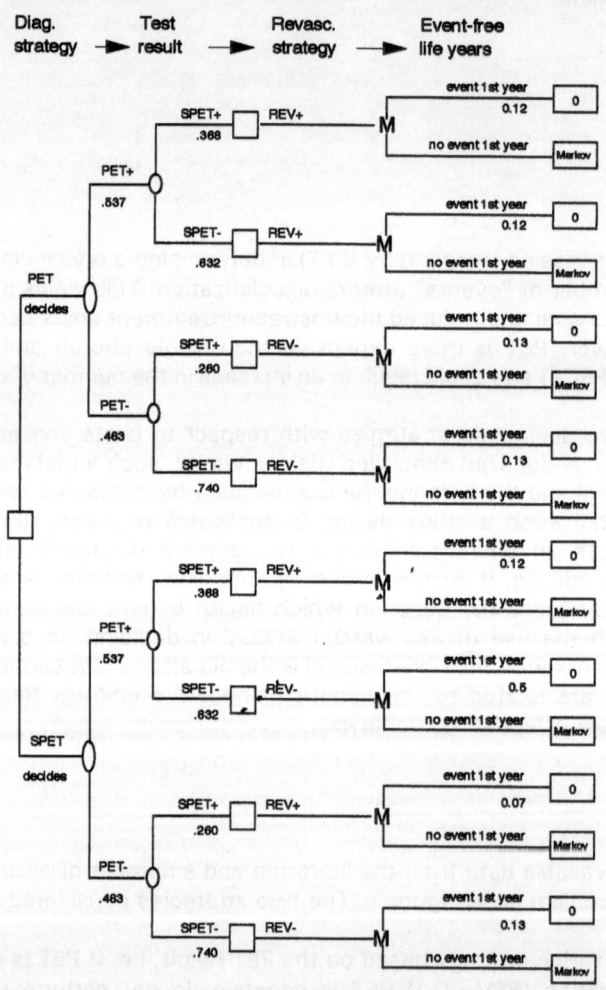

Figure 1. The decision model for the choice between PET and SPECT in deciding whether revascularization is required in patients with myocardial ischemia.

Moving from left to right we have modeled consecutively the two possible diagnostic strategies, the possible test results if both tests are performed, the revascularization strategy (based on only one of the two tests), and the outcome in terms of survival or event-free life expectancy. The model consists of a decision tree incorporating the initial diagnostic procedure and the revascularization strategy, and a Markov model to model the follow-up (Figure 1). Only the first year of follow-up (and of the Markov model) is shown in the figure. The follow-up period models downstream events, which include mortality, recurrent myocardial infarction, recurrent angina pectoris, heart failure, ventricular tachycardia, atrium fibrillation requiring hospitalization, and/or the need for revascularization during follow-up.

Although in daily practice only one test would be used, both test results have been included in the analytical model to enable a fair comparison of the two strategies. Thus, the diagnostic cost estimates for each strategy included only the costs of the test determining the revascularization strategy. Other costs included were those of the revascularization procedure and of downstream events.

Cost-effectiveness (CE) ratios were calculated using the following equation:

$$CEratio = \frac{C_{pet} - C_{spect}}{E_{pet} - E_{spect}}$$

With:

C_{PET} = costs of the PET strategy, i.e. costs of PET + costs of the revascularization procedure + costs of downstream events

C_{SPECT} = costs of the SPECT strategy, i.e. costs of SPECT + costs of the revascularization procedure + costs of downstream events

E_{PET} = effectiveness expressed in terms of event-free life years with the PET strategy

E_{SPECT} = effectiveness expressed in terms of event-free life years with the SPECT strategy

The analysis was performed from the perspective of the health care system. Calculations were performed with a 1-, 2-, and 5-year time frame.

Data and assumptions

The analysis was based on the following data and simplifying assumptions:

Eitzman et al.[4] demonstrated that in a group of patients with a poor ejection fraction (mean 35%) and an average of two affected coronary arteries, the PET result was positive in 54% of the examined patients (i.e. a mismatch). This data was used to calculate the distribution of the test results (Figure 1).

Brunken et al.[5] demonstrated how SPECT and PET test results are correlated. Using their data we calculated the following conditional probabilities (Figure 1).

Probability of SPECT + given PET + = 0.368
Probability of SPECT - given PET + = 0.632
Probability of SPECT + given PET - = 0.260
Probability of SPECT - given PET - = 0.740

Eitzman et al.[4] demonstrated that event rates after one year of follow-up depend on the result of the PET test and the revascularization strategy (REV). They found the following one-year event rates:

PET+ REV+   PET+ REV-   PET- REV+   PET- REV-
0.12   0.50   0.07   0.13

The estimated costs of the tests were (in 1994 Dutch guilders, one guilder = 1.75 US dollar):

cost of SPECT test = f 1000 (570 US $)
cost of PET test   = f 2000 (1140 US $)

The cost of revascularization and an event are based on Wong et al.[6] We assume that half of the revascularizations will be balloon angioplasty (PTCA) and the other half coronary artery bypass surgery (CABG) yielding an average cost of f 25470 (14550 US $)for a revascularization procedure. The cost of an event was estimated to be equal to that of a myocardial infarction, i.e. f 14400.-- (8225 US $).[6]

Results

Event-free survival, the total costs, and the incremental cost-effectiveness ratio depend on the time frame considered (Table 1).

Table 1. Event-free survival, costs, and incremental cost-effectiveness ratios of PET and SPECT for different time frames

| Time frame | Event-free survival | | Costs | | Incremental cost/effect |
	PET	SPECT	PET	SPECT	PET vs SPECT
1 year	0.88	0.75	,17472 (9985 US $)	12647 (7725 US $)	39632 (22645 US $)
2 years	0.77	0.61	19054 (10890 US $)	14709 (8405 US $)	15690 (8965 US $)
5 years	0.51	0.38	22750 (13000 US $)	18048 (10315 US $)	6637 (3795 US $)

Event-free survival is always higher for the PET strategy. However, the total cost is also always higher for PET. The incremental cost-effectiveness ratio of PET vs SPECT decreases as the time frame is extended. The reason for this is that the longer observations are continued, the more events will be prevented by the improved revascularization strategy.

Discussion

This preliminary decision analysis suggests that using PET to determine the revascularization strategy can reduce the number of events after revascularization. Although the PET strategy is associated with higher costs than SPECT, the incremental cost-effectiveness ratio of PET vs SPECT is favorable (from the first year less than *f* 40,000 (22855 US $)/event-free life year gained), with a low ratio after five years. The annual long-term costs after an event were not considered (only the short-term costs of the event itself). However, taking long-term costs into account would strengthen the conclusion because events which are prevented by PET, would induce more costs.

References

1. Weinstein MC, Feinberg HV. Clinical decision analysis. Philadelphia: W.B. Saunders & Co., 1980.
2. Drummond MF, Stoddart GL, Torrance GW. Methods for the economic evaluation of health care programmes. Oxford: Oxford Medical Publications, 1988.
3. Weinstein MC, Stason WB. Foundations of cost-effectiveness analysis for health and medical practices. N Engl J Med 1977;296:716-21.
4. Eitzman D, Al-Aouar Z, Kanter HL et al. Clinical outcome of patients with advanced coronary artery disease after viability studies with positron emission tomography. J Am Coll Cardiol 1992;20:559-65.
5. Brunken RC, Kottou S, Nienaber CA et al. PET detection of viable tissue in myocardial segments with persistent defects at T1-201 SPECT. Radiology 1989;172:65-73.
6. Wong JB, Sonnenberg FA, Salem DN, Pauker SG. Myocardial revascularization for chronic stable angina. Analysis of the role of percutaneous transluminal coronary angioplasty based on data available in 1989. Ann Intern Med 1990; 113:852-71.

8

ASSESSMENT OF MYOCARDIAL VIABILITY BY PHARMACOLOGICAL STRESS ECHOCARDIOGRAPHY

Jan H. Cornel, and Paolo M. Fioretti

Introduction

The assessment of myocardial viability is an issue of considerable clinical relevance in the current era of thrombolytic therapy and coronary revascularization[1,2] in selected cases (Figure 1). The awareness of the potential of even severe regional and global dyssynergic myocardium to improve its functional state, has resulted in a search for the optimal diagnostic approach for its noninvasive assessment. The identification of myocardial regions with high and low probability of functional improvement after myocardial infarction or revascularization is of vital importance since this can be crucial for the decision of performing revascularization procedures in individual patients with (multiple) severe wall motion abnormalities.

Myocardial viability, defined as a potentially reversible depression of myocardial contractility, may be caused by ischemia, stunning, hibernation or even sepsis.

Myocardial stunning is defined as transient prolonged postischemic dysfunction that may occur after the restoration of normal flow.[1] Despite the absence of irreversible damage, mechanical dysfunction may persist after coronary reperfusion in different clinical situations, like after coronary angioplasty,[3] coronary artery bypass surgery, unstable angina[3,4] or acute myocardial infarction with early reperfusion.[5-12] Spontaneous recovery may occur within weeks after the event and is dependent on the "area at risk", the duration of coronary occlusion, the amount and location of myocardial necrosis and the presence and extent of collateral vessels.[13]

In chronically ischemic and hibernating myocardium, chronic reduction in myocardial blood flow is thought to be matched by downregulation of the contractile cellular function.[14,15] Successful coronary revascularization may lead to a recovery of wall motion. In clinically apparently stable patients with chronic coronary artery disease, repetitive stunning may also lead to hypocontractile myocardial segments, which recover after revascularization.[16] In contrast, myocardial necrosis and scar tissue formation do not lead to reversibility of contractile dysfunction. In individual patients, all types of reversible and irreversible

E. E. van der Wall et al. (eds.), Cardiac Positron Emission Tomography, 103–115.
© 1995 Kluwer Academic Publishers.

contractile dysfunction may coexist and in them it is not possible to distinguish myocardial stunning from hibernation.

The use of stress echocardiography to detect viable myocardium has recently gained increasing attention. The echocardiographic hallmark for viability is the improvement of contractility of a dyssynergic segment after a stress stimulus since the degree of dyssynergy at rest cannot predict viability. The concept of metabolically viable myocardium must be distinguished from recovery of regional function. Viable myocardium not necessarily results in improvement of function since a substantial portion of the myocardium can still be viable and not show recovery of contractility. Still the clinical goal is to improve the functional state of severe dyssynergic myocardium.

In this chapter we will discuss the role of pharmacological stress echocardiography for the assessment of myocardial viability resulting in improvement of function in different clinical settings.

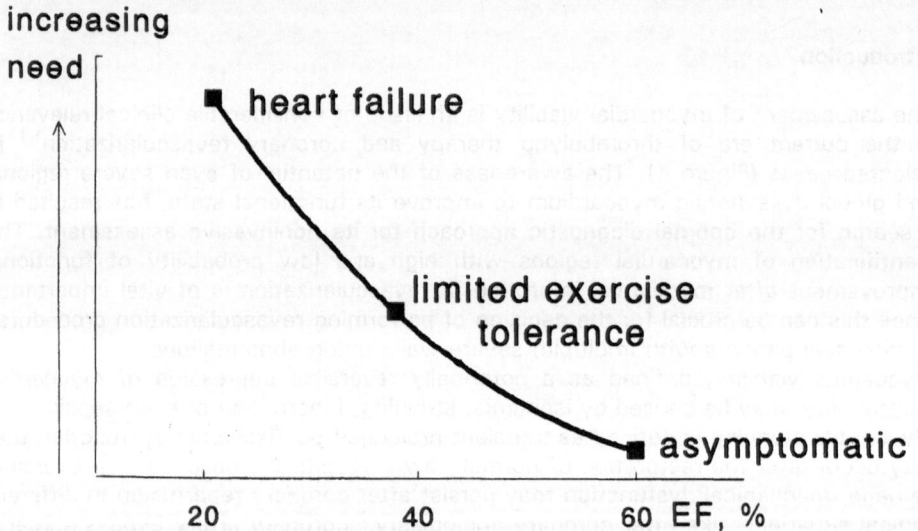

Figure 1.   The assessment of myocardial viability is an important clinical tool, which should be addressed in limited conditions, and not necessary applied on a routine basis

Rationale for pharmacologic stress echocardiography

Although positron emission tomography (PET), because of its ability to demonstrate metabolic activity in dysfunctional myocardial cells, is considered the gold standard for myocardial viability, its limited availability and high costs have led to search for a more cost-effective and simpler alternative. During the last decade particularly thallium-201 scintigraphy has received much attention and is now considered to be a reliable tool for the identification of viable myocardium.[17,18]

Most recently, the inotropic challenge of dyssynergic regions with a "low dose" dobutamine infusion in conjunction with echocardiography has been proposed as a simpler alternative method for the assessment of residual myocardial viability both in patients early after acute myocardial infarction[19-23] and in patients with stable chronic ischemic heart disease.[24-27] The rationale is based upon the fact that "low-dose" dobutamine increases myocardial contractility without changing heart rate.[28] The inotropic effect of dobutamine is already nearly maximal at doses that do not increase heart rate, and augmented myocardial contractility is associated with a concomitant increase in myocardial blood flow.[29]

Wall thickening rather than wall motion has been advocated as echocardiographic marker of myocardial contractility. Experimental data suggest that wall thickening diminishes linearly with reduction in coronary flow, whereas a selective increase in flow results in some enhancement of wall thickening.[30] In the non-infarcted myocardium wall thickening predominantly occurs in the endocardium and not in the epicardium.[31] This implies that necrosis or ischemia of just the endocardium significantly affect wall thickening at rest.[32] Thus, loss of wall thickening at rest does not preclude the presence of viable myocardium. On the other hand, wall motion analysis is affected not only by the tethering effect of adjacent areas and translational effects but also by changes in the loading conditions. Therefore it seems preferable to assess thickening rather than motion.

Moreover, experimental studies have shown that the functional reserve of dyssynergic but viable segments can be recruited after moderate inotropic stimulation.[33,34] Thus, in the absence of myocardial ischemia, myocardial contractility in dyssynergic but viable segments will enhance and lead to appearance or improvement of myocardial thickening. If dobutamine causes ischemia at higher doses, it can result in worsening of regional contractility. Since non-viable myocardium cannot lead to ischemia, even detoriation of function implies the presence of myocardial viability.

An increase in contractility of dyssynergic segments has also been observed early during dipyridamole infusion.[35] Dipyridamole induces coronary arterial vasodilatation leading to an increase of blood flow. Possibly through the "inotropic" effect of an increased flow (Gregg phenomenon), the presence of myocardial viability can be demonstrated. However, severe coronary stenoses may preclude coronary blood flow to increase and thus to improve regional myocardial thickening of dyssynergic segments.

Two-dimensional echocardiography is a simple technique to explore regional left ventricular wall motion and thickening which can be easily repeated over time. Although the image quality of echocardiography depends on several factors, patient related or related to the skills of the echocardiographer, a reasonable quality can be acquired in the majority of patients. But by using stimuli to influence the contractility of the heart, it is of paramount importance that the same classical views are recorded over time. Conditional to these circumstances, a reliable judgement can be made of the segmental changes in wall motion and thickening during the test.

Low-dose dobutamine echocardiography

Most institutions have chosen dobutamine as pharmacon to detect viability in dysfunctional myocardium. The test should be performed after stopping betablockers for at least 24 hours. Since no standard protocol exist, dobutamine is infused through an antecubital vein at doses ranging between 4 to 15 µg/kg/min. In our institution we currently start with a dose of 5 µg/kg/min for 5 minutes, continuing with 10 and 15 µg/kg/min respectively. Continuous monitoring of the echocardiogram is obtained during the test, and recorded on videotape. The echocardiographic images are also digitized and displayed side by side in quad-screen format to facilitate the comparison of rest and dobutamine images.

What is the optimal dose of dobutamine needed to show functional improvement? A recently published experimental study shows that, in a model of acute myocardial infarction, the dose of dobutamine needed to show improvement of wall thickening was related to infarct size.[36] However, in this study the infarct-related artery was not flow-limiting. Since furthermore recovery in regional function is the clinical goal, it is probably best to interpretate the test at the lower stages of 5 and 10 µg/kg/min of dobutamine. Based on experimental[36] and clinical data,[21] the sensitivity to predict reversible dysfunction is highest at low doses when hemodynamics are not altered and the endocardium increases its thickening.

The interpretation of the echocardiograms is based on both the digitized images displayed in a quad-screen format and by reviewing the images recorded on the video. The assessment is semi-quantitative. Wall motion, including wall thickening, of every segment is scored preferably with a 4-point scoring system: 1 = normal wall motion and thickening, 2 = moderately hypokinetic, 3 = severely hypokinetic, 4 = akinetic or dyskinetic. We define a segment as severely hypokinetic in the presence of minimal wall thickening with a limited inward motion of ≥ 2 mm; as akinetic in the absence of systolic wall thickening, whenever possible confirmed by M-mode tracing; as dyskinetic in the presence of systolic outward wall motion with thinning. To circumvent the confounding effect of tethering, segmental wall thickening is analyzed mainly during the first half of systole.

Myocardial viability is judged to be present in a dyssynergic segment when wall thickening improves during the infusion of low-dose dobutamine by at least one point of the scoring system. Thus, a severe hypokinesis becoming moderately hypokinetic or systolic myocardial thickening becoming apparent in a previously akinetic segment are considered as markers of viability. An example of a positive low-dose dobutamine echocardiogram is shown in Figure 2. In order to get an impression of the global left ventricular function, a wall motion score index can be calculated by dividing the sum of the scores of each segment by the total number of segments analyzed. The wall motion score index is only affected by abnormally contracting segments since hyperdynamic segments during dobutamine infusion are scored as normal.

Recovery of function after myocardial infarction

Transient prolonged postischemic dysfunction has been observed in several clinical conditions, including in patients after acute myocardial infarction treated with thrombolysis.[5-12] But even in the presence of a persistently occluded infarct-related artery, experimental data show that regional ventricular dysfunction recovers in

Rest

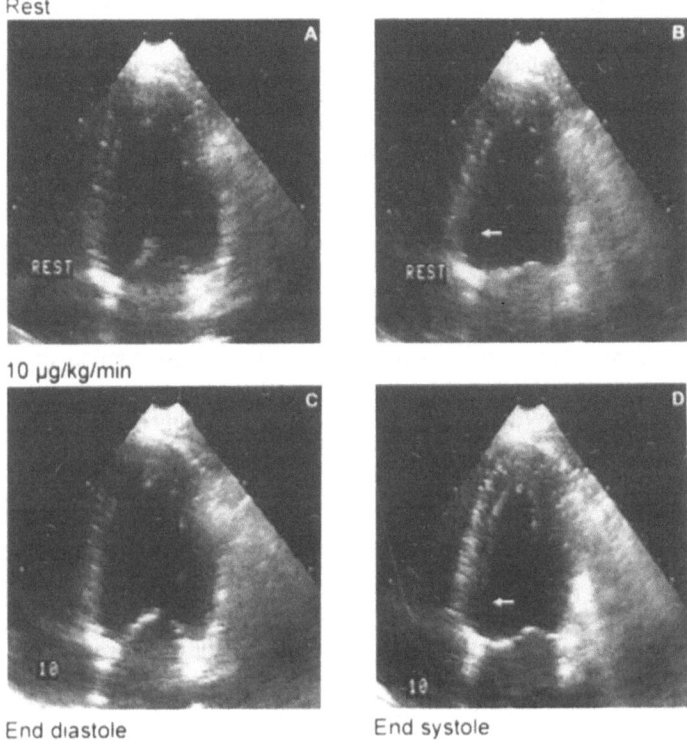

10 µg/kg/min

End diastole   End systole

Figure 2. Representative example of myocardial viability as demonstrated by low-dose dobutamine stress echocardiography. Top panels show resting apical four-chamber views at end diastole (A) and end systole (B). Marked dyssynergy is present in the posteroseptal segment (arrow). Bottom panels show the same views during dobutamine infusion (10µg/kg/min). At end systole a clear improvement in wall thickening has occurred after the inotropic stimulus (arrow in panel D).

some degree within several weeks.[37] Spontaneous recovery of wall motion after a Q-wave myocardial infarction, especially in patients with inferior infarction and normal ventricular size, has been frequently demonstrated with echocardiography.[38] Although most improvement takes places within the first 2 weeks,[39] recovery of perfusion and wall motion may continue for up to 7 months.[40] This implies that independent of the patency of the infarct-related artery, in all patients early after myocardial infarction, the specific evaluation of myocardial viability is desirable, when clinically required (particularly in view of revascularization of dyssynergic segments). The outcome of this evaluation can possibly influence the choice between medical treatment or coronary revascularization in selected patients.

The recovery of regional dysfunction may occur within weeks after the event and its degree is not only dependent on the "area at risk", the duration of coronary occlusion, the amount of myocardial necrosis and the presence and extent of collateral vessels[13] but also on the presence of an open infarct-related artery.[10] However, an open infarct-related artery does not result in functional recovery of all patients. But this does not mean that there is no viable myocardium left. It is possible that despite irreversible damage of the endocardium still viable myocardium is present in the sub-epicardial layers. In these cases, regional wall thickening will not improve, but left ventricular dilatation can be prevented.[12]

Studies about the usefulness of low-dose dobutamine stress echocardiography for the prediction of recovery of left ventricular function after acute myocardial infarction have recently been published.[19-23]

In a comparative study with PET, Pierard et al.[19] demonstrated in 17 patients with acute anterior myocardial infarction that improved wall thickening of the infarcted area during low-dose dobutamine infusion (10 µg/kg/min) identifies reversible dysfunction after a follow-up of 9 months. PET revealed the presence of viable myocardium in 11 patients (62% of infarct-related segments). All 5 patients with normal perfusion by PET showed improvement of wall thickening with dobutamine infusion and all showed functional recovery at follow-up. The 6 patients with viable but jeopardized myocardium, as shown by an abnormally high glucose to perfusion ratio, showed in 15/21 segments at follow up signs of necrosis, despite additional revascularization in 4 (PTCA in 2 and CABG in 2). Not surprisingly, although initially 3 patients showed improvement of wall thickening with dobutamine, functional recovery was found at follow-up in only 1 of the 6. All patients in whom no viable myocardium was found either with PET or dobutamine echocardiography showed no improvement of regional function at follow-up.

Barillà and coworkers[20] assessed the sensitivity of low-dose (5-10 µg/kg/min) dobutamine echocardiography for the identification of viable myocardium and the prediction of the extent of improvement after acute anterior infarction treated with coronary revascularization (either with PTCA or CABG). The study group consisted of 21 patients with either a documented non-Q wave myocardial infarction (n = 16) or post-thrombolytic therapy (n = 15) and all had a significant residual stenosis in the infarct-related artery. Wall motion improved during dobutamine infusion in all but one patient, as indicated by a reduction of wall motion score index. At follow up of 40 ± 15 days, all patients showed an improvement in contractility, although the magnitude was greater in the 13 patients who underwent revascularization. Interestingly, already 5 days after revascularization recovery had occurred almost to the level of dobutamine infusion.

In order to explore the optimal dose of dobutamine to achieve the highest sensitivity and specificity for the prediction of functional recovery in patients after thrombolytic therapy who are not always further revascularized, Smart and coworkers[21] performed an interesting study. They investigated the role of different the role of different indicators of reversible postischemic dysfunction (multistage dobutamine stress echocardiography (4 and 12 µg/kg/min), non-Q wave infarction and peak CK). They reported in 22 (41%) of the 51 patients an improvement of wall motion 2 months after thrombolytic therapy of acute myocardial infarction. Reversible dysfunction was defined as improved wall thickening in at least two contiguous segments at follow-up. The lowest dose of dobutamine infusion, which did not alter hemodynamics, had the highest sensitivity (86%) with a specificity of 90% for the prediction of reversible dysfunction and was sensitive and specific in all infarct locations (Table 1). The test was more accurate than clinical data for the identification of patients with functional recovery. Apart from the low-dose dobutamine echocardiography, non-Q wave infarction was the only independent predictor of reversible dysfunction. In this study, 22 patients were revascularized before hospital discharge on the basis of angiographic findings alone, and this could have affected the recovery of hypoperfused myocardium.

Table 1. Low-dose dobutamine echocardiography to predict recovery of left ventricular function

	pts	indication	therapy	sensitivity (%)	specificity (%)
Smart[21]	51	acute MI	thrombolysis (100%) additional revascularization (43%)	86	90
Salustri[23]	57	acute MI	thrombolysis (47%) no further revascularization	64	91
Marzullo[24]	14	chronic CAD	revascularization	82	92
Cigarroa[26]	25	chronic CAD	revascularization	82	86
La Canna[27]	33	chronic CAD	CABG	92	75

CABG = coronary artery bypass grafting; CAD = coronary artery disease; MI = myocardial infarction

Watada et al.[22] further explored the optimal dose of dobutamine to achieve the highest sensitivity and specificity for the detection of post-ischemic reversible dysfunction. They studied 21 patients after mechanical reperfusion of anterior myocardial infarction (acute PTCA) using 2 stages of 5 and 10 μg/kg/min dobutamine infusion for 6 minutes each. All infarct-related coronary arteries were patent and not significantly narrowed at the time of the dobutamine infusion, 3 days after the acute event. Follow-up echocardiography was performed at 25 days. In 57% (66/116) of the segments wall thickening improved at follow-up. In this study although the specificity was similar (92% vs 86%), at the higher dobutamine dose of 10 ug/kg/min sensitivity to predict functional recovery was better (62% vs 83%). These results are at first glance in contrast with the report by Smart et al.[21] But in the latter study myocardial ischemia may have been evoked by the intermediate dose of dobutamine stress (12 μg/kg/min) since the majority of patients had residual coronary lesions. This fact may account for the lower sensitivity of the test at intermediate stage as shown. Watada and coworkers[22] also demonstrated that low-dose dobutamine echocardiography can be used to quantitate the extent of the irreversible dysfunction since the extent of dyssynergy during dobutamine infusion correlated well with that at follow-up.
Our group[23] recently described the natural history and dobutamine responsiveness

of dyssynergic segments independent of treatment with thrombolytic agents. At this aim 57 patients after a first uncomplicated myocardial infarction (thrombolysis n = 27, Q-wave n = 49) not undergoing additional revascularization procedures were studied. In this study, one fourth of myocardial segments showed recovery of function after three months. The incidence of spontaneous recovery was higher in hypokinetic than in akinetic segments (35% vs 19%). Viability at low-dose dobutamine echocardiography (5-10 μg/kg/min) was considered to be present in case of an improvement of ≥ 1 grade in dyssynergic segments from rest to low dose dobutamine. Using this definition, low-dose dobutamine echocardiography seems a very specific method to predict the lack of late recovery of regional left ventricular dysfunction (94%). But, although the sensitivity is high in hypokinetic segments, in akinetic segments our initial data show a rather low sensitivity (87% vs 35%). Since the target population for the proper identification of myocardial viability is based mainly on those with severe multiple dyssynergic regions, it remains unclear what the ideal diagnostic and therapeutic approach is in this patient group. The low number of akinetic segments showing improved wall thickening and the high percentage of false positive tests possibly due to incomplete reperfusion are arguments to explain the low sensitivity as reported. We recently found that T-wave normalization during low-dose dobutamine infusion is a promising ancillary sign of viable myocardium after acute myocardial infarction and increases the sensitivity of echocardiography for the prediction of late spontaneous recovery of function.[41]

Recovery of function after revascularization in chronic ischemic heart disease

Although normal contractile myocardium is obviously viable, a mixture of normal myocardium with scar or stunned/hibernating myocardium can both be present in a hypokinetic myocardial region, but only that segment which contains a "critical mass" of stunned/hibernating myocardium may potentially improve after coronary revascularization. Several studies in patients with coronary artery disease indicate that coronary revascularization may lead to improvement of left ventricular function.[42-45] Recently it has been demonstrated that even in severe left ventricular dysfunction, ejection fraction can improve in selected patients.[46] These results implicate the potential to prolong survival as well as the quality of life in patients with left ventricular dysfunction.[47,48] Thus patients with chronic advanced ischemic left ventricular dysfunction, even when eligible for heart transplantation, may improve after successful revascularization. Several factors may affect the outcome of such approach however. It is conceivable that in patients with hibernating myocardium, repetitive episodes of superimposed stunning exist due to transient ischemia. Since by definition stunning represents transient dysfunction and the amount and severity of dyssynergic myocardium involved may be variable, myocardial stunning may influence functional recovery. A predominance of myocardial stunning may also influence the timing of recovery. Furthermore, not only the presence but more importantly the amount of jeopardized myocardium by hibernation and the degree of myocardial scarring affect the outcome of revascularization. Other factors important to keep in mind are the success of revascularization, concomitant cardiomyopathy and the preoperative left ventricular dimensions. Patients with severe left ventricular dilatation may be less likely to recover. Anyway, recovery of ventricular function may underestimate the real extent of myocardial viability due to several factors like inadequate restoration of regional myocardial blood flow. In Figure 3 an example of positive low-dose dobutamine echocardiogram followed by an improvement of wall motion after successful PTCA is represented.

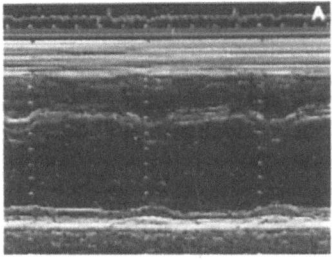

Rest

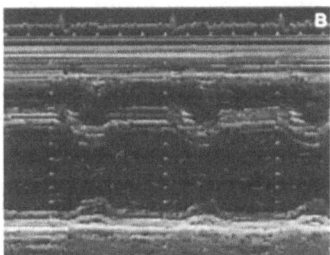

Low-dose Dobutamine

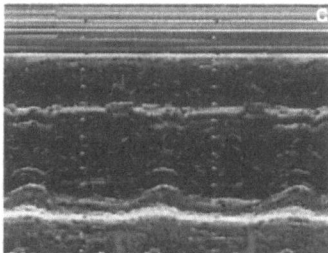

Post-Revascularization

Figure 3. Example of post-revascularization improvement of posterior wall thickening as predicted by low-dose dobutamine stress echocardiography. M-mode tracings of the parasternal long axis view demonstrate at rest severe hypokinesia of the posterior wall (panel A). At low-dose dobutamine infusion wall thickening improved (panel B), after successful revascularization wall thickening at rest recovered to the level as predicted by low-dose dobutamine infusion.

A few studies about the usefulness of low-dose dobutamine stress echocardiography for the prediction of recovery of left ventricular function after successful revascularization have been recently published.[24-27] In a small study comprising 14 patients, Marzullo et al.[24] explored this issue. They studied patients with moderate left ventricular dysfunction (ejection fraction 39 ± 7%) who were at least > 9 weeks after myocardial infarction. After a follow-up of 11 weeks 65% of the dyssynergic segments improved. In this study, low-dose dobutamine echocardiography (10 µg/kg/min) revealed both a high specificity (92%) as well as a high sensitivity (82%) for the prediction of reversible dysfunction (Table 1). Cigarroa and coworkers[25] used in their study not a fixed "low-dose" but various doses of dobutamine (5-20 µg/kg/min) to assess the contractile reserve of dyssynergies. Even after a postoperative follow-up of only 4 weeks, dobutamine stress echocardiography predicted postoperative recovery. Interestingly, the presence of totally occluded coronary arteries did not preclude the identification of contractile reserve by dobutamine infusion. Arnese et al.,[26] from our group, further explored the predictive accuracy of the test in severely hypokinetic as well as in akinetic segments of 20 patients with severe chronic left ventricular dysfunction. Wall thickening during low-dose dobutamine infusion (5-10 µg/kg/min) improved more frequent in severely hypokinetic (7/26) than in akinetic (3/54) segments (27% vs 6%, p=0.01). An example of a positive dobutamine echocardiogram with subsequent post-revascularization improvement is shown in Figure 2. Marzullo et al.[24] and Cigarroa et al.[25] reported a higher incidence of dobutamine responsive wall thickening in akinetic regions (47% and 39%). This discrepancy may relate to different methodologies (due to the subjective criterion also severely hypokinetic segments possibly were classified as akinetic) and patient selection. Postoperative improvement of regional function after 3 months was found in only 10/80 segments. Nevertheless low-dose dobutamine infusion resulted in a positive predictive value of 90% and a negative predictive value of 99%.

To clarify the time course of postoperative functional recovery, La Canna et al.[27] selected 33 patients with chronic coronary artery disease without extensive left ventricular scar/aneurysm. At baseline they reported a remarkably high number of akinetic segments (314/528) although the mean ejection fraction was not severely reduced (0.33 ± 0.08). This discrepancy may relate to previously mentioned subjective interpretation of echocardiograms. In this study 179 of the 314 akinetic segments improved at 3 months follow-up and recovery predominantly occurred immediately after surgical revascularization. The akinetic segments that recovered after revascularization showed greater end-diastolic wall thickness at baseline (10 ± 4 vs 6 ± 3 mm, p<0.001). In contrast to other studies, La Canna et al.[27] reported a rather low specificity (74%) of low-dose dobutamine echocardiography to predict late follow-up (Table 1). Due to strict exclusion criteria adopted in this study, the results cannot be considered representative of the value of the test in a general population of patients with chronic coronary artery disease.

Although these reports are encouraging, still many questions have to be answered and further studies are needed on larger series and with longer follow-up before a definite conclusion about the predictive value of this technique can be drawn.

Also, it can be foreseen that quantification methods will increasingly be applied to echocardiographic images and that contrast echocardiography will be used in conjunction with wall motion analysis.[49]

References

1. Bolli R. Myocardial "stunning" in man. Circulation 1992;86:1671-91.
2. Dilsizian V, Bonow RO. Current diagnostic techniques of assessing myocardial viability in patients with hibernating and stunned myocardium. Circulation 1993;87:1-20.
3. Marzullo P, Parodi O, Sambuceti G et al. Does the myocardium become 'stunned' after episodes of angina at rest, angina on effort, and coronary angioplasty? Am J Cardiol 1993;71:1045-51.
4. Nixon JV, Brown CN, Smitherman TC. Identification of transient and persistent segmental wall motion abnormalities in patients with unstable angina by two-dimensional echocardiography. Circulation 1982;65:1497-503.
5. Patel B, Kloner RA, Przyklenk K, Braunwald E. Postischemic myocardial "stunning": a clinically relevant phenomenon. Ann Intern Med 1988;108:626-8.
6. Bourdillon PDV, Broderick TM, Williams ES et al. Early recovery of regional left ventricular function after reperfusion in acute myocardial infarction assessed by serial two-dimensional echocardiography. Am J Cardiol 1989;63:641-6.
7. Serruys PW, Simoons ML, Suryapranata H et al. Preservation of global and regional left ventricular function after early thrombolysis in acute myocardial infarction. J Am Coll Cardiol 1986;7:729-42.
8. Charuzi Y, Beeder C, Marshall LA et al. Improvement in re.   .l and global left ventricular function after intracoronary thrombolysis: assessment with two-dimensional echocardiography. Am J Cardiol 1984;53:662-5.
9. Widimsky P, Cervenka V, Gregor P et al. First month course of left ventricular asynergy after intracoronary thrombolysis in acute myocardial infarction. A longitudinal echocardiographic study. Eur Heart J 1985;6:759-65.
10. Touchstone DA, Beller GA, Nygaard TW, Tedesco C, Kaul S. Effects of successful intravenous reperfusion therapy on myocardial function and geometry in humans: a tomographic assessment using two-dimensional echocardiography. J Am Coll Cardiol 1989;13:1506-13.
11. Penco M, Romano S, Agati L et al. Influence of reperfusion induced by thrombolytic treatment on natural history of left ventricular regional wall motion abnormality in acute myocardial infarction. Am J Cardiol 1993;71:1015-20.
12. Marino P, Zanolla L, Zardini P, on behalf of the GISSI study. Effect of streptokinase on left ventricular modeling and function after myocardial infarction: the GISSI trial. J Am Coll Cardiol 1989;14:1149-58.
13. Sabia P, Powers ER, Ragosta M, Sarenbock IJ, Burwell LR, Kaul S. An association between collateral blood flow and myocardial viability in patients with recent myocardial infarction. N Engl J Med 1992;327:1825-31.
14. Rahimtoola SH. A perspective on the three large multicenter randomized clinical trails of coronary bypass surgery for chronic stable angina. Circulation 1985;72(Suppl V):123-35.
15. Braunwald E, Rutherford JD. Reversible ischemic left ventricular dysfunction: evidence for the hibernating myocardium. J Am Coll Cardiol 1986;8:1467-70.
16. Vanoverschelde J-LJ, Wijns W, Depré C et al. Mechanisms of chronic regional postischemic dysfunction in humans: New insights from the study of noninfarcted collateral-dependent myocardium. Circulation 1993;87:1513-23.
17. Zaret BL, Wackers FJ. Nuclear cardiology (first of two parts). N Engl J Med 1993;329:775-83.
18. Zaret BL, Wackers FJ. Nuclear cardiology (second of two parts). N Engl J Med 1993;329:855-63.
19. Piérard LA, De Landsheere CM, Berthe C, Rigo P, Kulbertus HE. Identification of viable myocardium by echocardiography during dobutamine infusion in patients with

myocardial infarction after thrombolytic therapy: comparison with positron emission tomography. J Am Coll Cardiol 1990;15:1021-31.
20. Barilla F, Gheorghiade M, Alam M, Khaja F, Goldstein S. Low-dose dobutamine in patients with acute myocardial infarction identifies viable but not contractile myocardium and predicts the magnitude of improvement in wall motion abnormalities in response to coronary revascularization. Am Heart J 1991;122:1522-31.
21. Smart SC, Sawada S, Ryan T et al. Low-dose dobutamine echocardiography detects reversible dysfunction after thrombolytic therapy of acute myocardial infarction. Circulation 1993;88:405-15.
22. Watada H, Ito H, Oh H et al. Dobutamine stress echocardiography predicts reversible dysfunction and quantitates the extent of irreversibly damaged myocardium after reperfusion of anterior myocardial infarction. J Am Coll Cardiol 1994;24:624-30.
23. Salustri A, Elhendy A, Garyfallydis P et al. Prediction of improvement of ventricular function after first acute myocardial infarction using low-dose dobutamine stress echocardiography. Am J Cardiol 1994;74:853-6.
24. Marzullo P, Parodi O, Reisenhofer B et al. Value of rest thallium-201 / technetium-99m sestamibi scans and dobutamine echocardiography for detecting myocardial viability. Am J Cardiol 1993;71:166-72.
25. Cigarroa CG, de Filippi CR, Brickner ME, Alvarez LG, Wait MA, Grayburn PA. Dobutamine stress echocardiography identifies hibernating myocardium and predicts recovery of left ventricular function after coronary revascularization. Circulation 1993;88:430-6.
26. Arnese M, Cornel JH, Maat APWM, Reijs AEM, Fioretti PM. Prediction of recovery of severe left ventricular dyssynergies after bypass surgery: dobutamine echocardiography vs thallium scintigraphy (abstract). Circulation 1994;90:I-117.
27. La Canna G, Alfieri O, Giubbini R, Gargano M, Ferrari R, Visioli O. Echocardiography during infusion of dobutamine for identification of reversible dysfunction in patients with chronic coronary artery disease. J Am Coll Cardiol 1994;23:617-26.
28. Meyer SL, Curry GC, Donsky MS, Twieg DB, Parkey RW, Willerson JT. Influence of dobutamine on hemodynamics and coronary blood flow in patients with and without coronary artery disease. Am J Cardiol 1976;38:103-8.
29. Sonnenblick EH, Frishman WH, LeJemtel TH. Dobutamine: A new synthetic cardioactive sympathetic amine. N Engl J Med 1979;300:17-22.
30. Kaul S. Echocardiography in coronary artery disease. Curr Probl Cardiol 1990;15:233-98.
31. Myers JH, Stirling MC, Choy M, Buda AJ, Gallagher KP. Direct measurement of inner and outer wall thickening dynamics with epicardial echocardiography. Circulation 1986;74:164-72.
32. Weintraub WS, Hattori S, Aggarwal JB, Bodenheimer MM, Banks VS, Helfant RH. The relationship between myocardial blood flow and contraction by myocardial layer in the canine left ventricle during ischemia. Circ Res 1981;48:430-8.
33. Bolli R, Zhu WX, Myers ML, Hartley CJ, Roberts R. Beta-adrenergic stimulation reverses postischemic myocardial dysfunction without producing subsequent functional deterioration. Am J Cardiol 1985;56:964-8.
34. Becker LC, Levine LH, Di Paula AF, Guarnieri T, Aversano T. Reversal of dysfunction in postischemic stunned myocardium by epinephrine and postextrasystolic potentiation. J Am Coll Cardiol 1986;7:580-9.
35. Picano E, Marzullo P, Gigli G et al. Identification of viable myocardium by dipyridamole-induced improvement in regional left ventricular function assessed by echocardiography in myocardial infarction and comparison with thallium scintigraphy in rest. Am J Cardiol 1992;70:703-10.
36. Sklenar J, Ismail S, Villanueva FS, Goodman NC, Glasheen WP, Kaul S. Dobutamine

echocardiography for determining the extent of myocardial salvage after reperfusion. An experimental evaluation. Circulation 1994;90:1502-12.

37. Gibbons EF, Hogan RD, Franklin TD, Nolting M, Weyman AE. The natural history of regional dysfunction in a canine preparation of chronic infarction. Circulation 1985;71:394-402.

38. Picard MH, Wilkins GT, Ray PA, Weyman AE. Natural history of left ventricular size and function. Assessment and prediction by echocardiographic endocardial surface mapping. Circulation 1990;82:484-94.

39. Ito H, Tomooka T, Sakai N et al. Time course of functional improvement in stunned myocardium in risk area in patients with reperfused anterior infarction. Circulation 1993;87:355-62.

40. Galli M, Marcassa C, Bolli R et al. Spontaneous delayed recovery of perfusion and contraction after the first 5 weeks after anterior infarction. Evidence for the presence of hibernating myocardium in the infarcted area. Circulation 1994;90:1386-97.

41. Salustri A, Garyfallidis P, Elhendy A et al. T wave normalization during dobutamine echocardiography for the diagnosis of viable myocardium. Am J Cardiol 1995, in press.

42. Rees G, Bristow JD, Kremkau KLE et al. Influence of aortocoronary bypass on left ventricular performance. N Engl J Med 1971;284:1116-20.

43. Brundage BH, Massie BM, Botvinick EH. Improved regional ventricular function after successful surgical revascularization. J Am Coll Cardiol 1984;3;902-8.

44. Topol EJ, Weiss JL, Guzman PA et al. Immediate improvement of dysfunctional myocardial segments after coronary revascularization: detection by intraoperative transesophageal echocardiography. J Am Coll Cardiol 1984;4:1123-34.

45. De Feyter PJ, Suryapranata H, Serruys PW, Beatt K, Van Den Brand M, Hugenholtz PG. Effects of successful percutaneous transluminal coronary angioplasty on global and regional left ventricular function in unstable angina pectoris. Am J Cardiol 1987;60:993-7.

46. Elefteriades JA, Tolis G, Levi E, Mills LK, Zaret BL. Coronary artery bypass grafting in severe left ventricular dysfunction: excellent survival with improved ejection fraction and functional state. J Am Coll Cardiol 1993;22:1411-7.

47. Alderman EL, Bourassa MG, Cohen LS et al. Ten-year follow-up of survival and myocardial infarction in the randomized coronary artery surgery study. Circulation 1990;82:1629-46.

48. Nesto RW, Cohn LH, Collins JJ, Wynne J, Holman L, Cohn PF. Inotropic contractile reserve: a useful predictor of increased 5-year survival and improved postoperative left ventricular function in patients with coronary artery disease and reduced ejection fraction. Am J Cardiol 1982;50:39-44.

49. Rovai D, Zanchi M, Lombardi M et al. Contractile reserve of reversibly damaged myocardium is linked to a residual coronary flow reserve. Eur Heart J 1994;15:331 (Abstract).

9   ASSESSMENT OF MYOCARDIAL VIABILITY BY MAGNETIC RESONANCE IMAGING TECHNIQUES

Christian A. Schneider, Frank Baer, Eberhard Voth,
Peter Theissen, and Udo Sechtem

Introduction

In contrast to the well established scintigraphic methods such as single photon emission computed tomography (SPECT) and positron emission tomography (PET), which are routinely used in the assessment of myocardial viability, magnetic resonance (MR) imaging and MR spectroscopy techniques have only recently been applied to address these questions. Due to its excellent spatial resolution MR imaging is well suited for the exact assessment of morphological and functional changes after myocardial infarction.[1-5] A chronic, transmural myocardial infarct, e.g. a myocardial infarct which is older than 16 weeks, is in general characterized by a significant reduction in wall thickness.[6-8] In contrast, a chronic myocardial infarct with hibernating myocardium will show less wall thinning, although wall motion may be severely impaired in both conditions. Therefore, measurement of wall thickness alone may provide important information about the presence of clinically relevant amounts of residual viable myocardium. An acute transmural myocardial infarct without residual viability may or may not yet exhibit a significant reduction in wall thickness. Assessment of myocardial wall thickness in acute myocardial infarcts will therefore not be helpful to distinguish between viable and scarred myocardium. This problem may be overcome by MR spectroscopy techniques, which detect key molecules (ATP, phosphocreatine) of the metabolic pathways, in an area of acute or subacute myocardial infarcts.[9]

The purpose of this chapter is to review the features of viable and scarred myocardium as characterized by MR imaging and to compare MR imaging to other methods currently used for the identification of viable myocardium. In addition, the potential of MR spectroscopy for the diagnosis of viability will be discussed.

Pathophysiological characterization of acute and chronic myocardial infarcts

In general, there are different possible outcomes for the myocardial cell after an

117

E. E. van der Wall et al. (eds.), Cardiac Positron Emission Tomography, 117–128.
© 1995 Kluwer Academic Publishers.

ischemic event, depending on the time to restoration of blood flow. If the blood flow is restored within minutes, either no changes in contractile or metabolic function can be detected or the contractile and metabolic function are transiently depressed for a certain time ("stunned").[10-12] If blood flow is not restored within a critical time window (minutes), the myocardial cell will either die and loose functional and metabolic properties, or will remain in a basal metabolic state without contractile function, kept alive by a minimal "rescue" blood flow (chronic ischemia, "hibernation").[13,14] Another possible fate of the myocardium is restoration of blood flow after only a short time period of occlusion but a lack of recovery of function because repetitive episodes of ischemic injury in the presence of a residual high grade coronary artery stenosis maintain the state of severely impaired contractility (repetitive stunning). For each of these conditions magnetic resonance techniques compete with scintigraphic and echocardiographic techniques to answer the clinically important question whether myocardium is viable or not.

MR techniques and viability in acute and subacute myocardial infarcts

Wall motion abnormalities

Although wall motion abnormalities can be easily depicted by MR imaging -especially by the gradient-echo technique[15]- measurement of this parameter is not very helpful in making the distinction between stunned and necrotic myocardium in the acute phase of myocardial infarct, because both conditions can lead to severe wall motion abnormalities. Consequently, quantification of the region of severe hypokinesia from MR images is not reliable to determine the infarct size, even though these measurements correlate well with the extent of wall motion abnormalities on left ventriculography.[16]

However, residual wall thickening is an unequivocal indicator of residual viability which cannot be influenced in the same way as wall motion by traction of surrounding hypercontractile myocardium. Johnston et al.[17] studied 24 patients 6 days after an acute infarct by using adenosine thallium-201 (^{201}Tl) scintigraphy and redistribution scintigraphy after 4 hours. To analyze wall thickening all patients had magnetic resonance imaging. Ten of 11 patients with ^{201}Tl signs of viability (redistribution) showed wall thickening in the area of the infarct. In addition, MR imaging was more sensitive in detecting viable myocardium, because 6/13 patients with fixed ^{201}Tl defects had also preserved wall thickening, the remaining 7 patients with fixed ^{201}Tl defects had absent wall thickening by MR imaging. This paper demonstrates, that the analysis of wall thickening after acute myocardial infarct can detect residual viability in areas with persistent ^{201}Tl defects, which is in good concordance with papers demonstrating preserved glucose metabolism in areas with persistent ^{201}Tl defects.[18] The use of ^{201}Tl reinjection techniques[19] would possibly have reduced the number of patients with fixed ^{201}Tl defects and wall thickening of the infarct areas.

Inotropic stimulation by various pharmacological agents, which results in improved contractile function of hibernating myocardium, can be employed with MR imaging.[20] Preliminary data indicate that an increase of systolic myocardial wall thickening after dobutamine of more than 20% as compared to the resting value can serve as an index of myocardial viability early after the event. Further experience using recently developed fast imaging sequences[21] is necessary before the clinical value of dobutamine MR imaging in the detection of viability in patients with acute myocardial infarct can be assessed.

Signal intensity changes on spin-echo images
An increase in signal intensity of freshly infarcted myocardium, which appears on T2 weighted spin-echo MR images only a few hours after occlusion of a coronary artery can be used to determine the extent of irreversible myocardial damage.[22,23] However, it is unclear, whether this area of increased signal intensity that is seen within the first week after the event only represents necrotic myocardium or incorporates some edematous viable myocardium.[24,25] After three weeks, true infarct size may be more closely approximated by the area of increased signal intensity, because the edema surrounding the infarct has presumably regressed and signal abnormalities are restricted to the pathophysiologically determined infarct area.[26]
When measuring the area of increased „myocardial" signal intensity, one has to consider that slow blood flow adjacent to a region with severe hypokinesia also results in high signal intensity of the blood. This signal from blood may blend with the signal of the myocardium and may lead to the false impression of increased signal intensity within the myocardium.[27] The use of signal intensity changes for making a diagnosis of complete myocardial necrosis is further complicated by the fact that in vivo MR imaging sometimes results in artifacts caused by breathing or cardiac arrhythmias. Thus spurious increases in signal intensity may also be found in normal persons.[28]
Only one paper directly addresses the question, whether reversibly and irreversibly injured myocardium can be distinguished on the basis of signal intensity measurements.[29] In a canine model transient occlusion of a coronary artery was used to produce stunned or infarcted myocardium. In contrast to infarcted myocardium, stunned myocardium did not show increases in signal intensity despite regional systolic dysfunction.

MR contrast agents
T1-enhancing contrast agents like gadolinium and manganese chelats have been employed in animal models to distinguish between reversible and irreversible injury on the basis of MR signal enhancement.[30,31] Reperfused, reversibly injured myocardium and normal myocardium enhance in a similar way. Irreversibly injured myocardium, however, shows increased signal enhancement.[30,31]
T2-enhancing agents cause a decrease in signal intensity in normal myocardium by dephasing water molecules, which diffuse through local magnetic field gradients induced by heterogenous distribution of the contrast agent at the microscopical level. The heterogenous distribution in normal myocardium occurs because the cell membrane is a barrier, which limits effectively the access of the contrast agent to the intracellular space. If cell death has occurred cell membranes become leaky and the contrast agent is distributed homogenously throughout the cells and the interstitium leading to an increase in signal intensity. This was recently confirmed in an animal model of reperfused myocardial infarcts, which showed less signal loss after administration of dysprosium-DTPA-bis(methylamide) than normal myocardium on T2-weighted spin-echo images.[32] However, these interesting results must be confirmed in humans.

MR-spectroscopy

MR spectroscopy is an exciting tool for the direct measurement of ischemia induced changes of high-energy phosphates and the intracellular pH in in-vivo animal models using coils directly applied to the surface of the heart. During ischemia ATP and phosphocreatine (PCr) levels decrease, whereas the level of inorganic phophate increases.[9] After brief periods of ischemia PCr levels recover during reperfusion.[33,34] Based on these findings, PCr was proposed as an indicator for the balance of myocardial perfusion and actual energy requirement.[33] After the onset of ischemia, the concentration of PCr decreases much faster than that of ATP resulting in a rapid increase of the PCr/ATP ratio.[33,34] In contrast to these changes, chronically hypoperfused myocardium should be characterized by a balanced reduction of ATP and PCr, because the PCr pool can be replenished under these circumstances after a certain recovery time.[35-37] However, no spectroscopy data are currently available which apply these experimental data to patients with evidence of hibernation (e.g. severe wall motion abnormality with increased glucose metabolism and decreased myocardial blood flow in the region of wall motion abnormality). Unfortunately, the quantification of metabolism by MR spectroscopy in humans is not without problems because volumes of interest are relatively large as compared to myocardial wall thickness. Further technical progress is necessary in order to correctly quantify the amount of viable myocardium contained within a small volume of interest.[38]

Recently, new pulse sequences and high field magnets have permitted separate observation of the endocardial and epicardial portion of the left ventricle in animal models.[39] The ability to selectively gather information from both of these layers may further improve the detection of residual viable cells, which are preferentially located near the epicardium.[40]

Viability in chronic myocardial infarcts

Chronic transmural infarcts are characterized by a significant reduction in wall thickness. Approximately 16 weeks after the ischemic event the formation of scar tissue is complete.[1-5] This consistent finding of wall thinning (Figure 1) in large chronic Q-wave infarcts on MR images[41] and data from animal and pathology studies led to the hypothesis that scarred myocardium could be distinguished from viable myocardium on the basis of diastolic wall thickness. Transmural infarcts in rats, known to have only very little collateral circulation, led to a reduction of wall thickness of about one third, whereas the wall thickness of non-transmural infarcts remained normal.[42] In contrast, infarcts in dogs remain usually non-transmural due to their extensive collateral network and have only minor reduction in wall thickness.[43]

In humans there is confusion of terms as what should be regarded as transmural or non-transmural.[44] Pathologists define transmural scars as infarcts which span the full wall from the epicardium at least at one point of the left ventricular circumference.[45] The infarct may extend through the full wall thickness of the myocardium over most of the left ventricular region supplied by the infarct artery or it may be transmural only at one point of this territory. This was confirmed in a histopathologic study, which examined thickness of viable myocardium in more than 200 patients who came to autopsy with a single myocardial infarct.[46] In the majority of the infarcts, the thickness

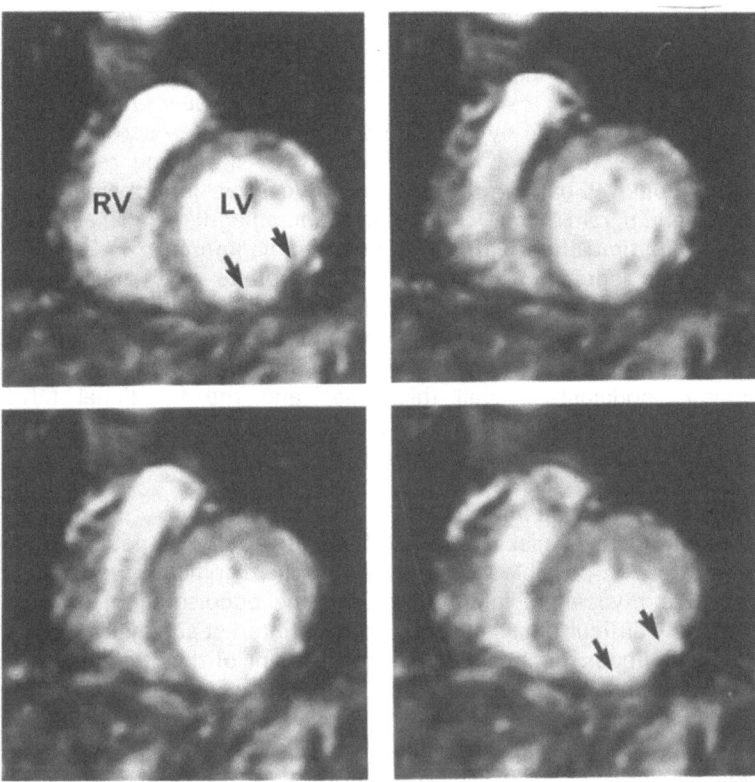

Figure 1A. Four phases of the cardiac cycle in patient with a remote inferior-lateral Q-wave myocardial infarct. Short axis gradient-echo MR images of the heart (upper left: end-diastole;upper right: early systole; lower left: mid-systole; lower right: end-systole) are shown. Severe thinning of the inferior lateral wall (two arrows, upper left) is evident at end-diastole. There is no thickening of the area with severely reduced enddiastolic wall thickness, whereas the posterior septum and the anterior wall thicken normally during systole.(Reproduced from Baer FM et al: Magnetic resonance imaging techniques for the assessment of residual myocardial viability. Herz 1994; 1: 51-64, with permission)

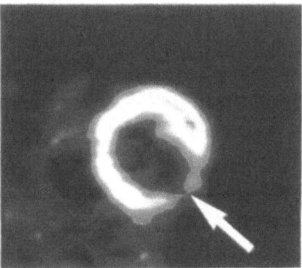

Figure 1B. ¹⁸FDG-PET image on a midventricular level of the same patient. The region without ¹⁸FDG-uptake (small arrow) matches exactly the region with severe wall thinning on the diastolic gradient echo MR image. The remaining myocardial regions have normal ¹⁸FDG-uptake and normal enddiastolic wall thickness and systolic wall thickening. (see for colourplate of this figure page 244).

Dobutamine-MR imaging for the assessment of contractile reserve in chronic infarcts
In animal models it was shown that contractile dysfunction can be reversed by the infusion of dobutamine,[52] indicating that underperfused and akinetic regions can preserve their contractile response to positive inotropic stimulation. Low dose dobutamine can be employed by in patients with chronic myocardial infarct and wall motion abnormalities to detect residual viability by improving regional contractile function. We studied 35 patients with chronic myocardial infarcts and akinesia in the left ventricular angiogram by [18]FDG-PET and MR imaging (Figure 2) at rest and during positive inotropic stimulation with 10 μg dobutamine/kg/min.[49] In 31 of 35 patients (89%) there was agreement between [18]FDG-uptake and dobutamine induced contraction reserve as documented by MR imaging. Of 251 initially akinetic myocardial regions, which showed wall thickening of > 1 mm after dobutamine stimulation, 242 (96%) had [18]FDG-uptake > 50% on PET images. The combination of the morphologic MR parameter „enddiastolic wall thickness" and the functional MR-parameter „dobutamine induced systolic wall thickening" gave the best result for sensitivity (88%) and positive predictive accuracy (92%).

MR spectroscopy in chronic infarcts
Currently no data are available about MR-spectroscopy in patients with *chronic* myocardial infarcts. A possible reason might be the significant wall thinning usually found in chronic myocardial infarcts, making the acquisition of interpretable MR spectra extremely difficult: the smallest volume of interest achievable with any spatial localization technique is much larger than the amount of thinned myocardium within the measurement volume.

Conclusions

MR imaging can reliably identify viable myocardium in patients with chronic myocardial infarction and left ventricular dysfunction on the basis of wall thickness, systolic wall thickening and the response to positive inotropic stimulation. In contrast to [18]FDG-PET, MR imaging does not provide any biochemical or metabolic insights into the infarcted myocardium. Although initial data show that MR imaging detects viability in patients with chronic myocardial infarcts as well as [18]FDG-PET, no data have yet been published about the ability of MR imaging to predict functional recovery of akinetic areas after revascularization which is the ultimate verification of all viability tests. These data are needed to make a final judgement about the precision of MR diagnoses of viability. In combination with MR spectroscopy, magnetic resonance techniques may in the future provide an unique approach to assess viability at the morphological, functional and metabolic level.

of the surviving myocardium formed a continuous range from less than 10% to more than 80% of neighbouring wall thickness. The relationship between enddiastolic wall thickness and viability was addressed by a study of Dubnow et al.[47] demonstrating that the total wall thickness of chronic transmural myocardial infarcts was usually less than 6 mm. In addition, intraoperative biopsies from asynergic left ventricular regions showed < 10% muscle loss if regional function was postoperatively improved whereas muscle loss was more than 50% in regions without recovery.[14] Thus non-contractile myocardium thinner than 6 mm is very likely to be so severely damaged that recovery of regional function after revascularization is unlikely.

Comparison of wall thickness and wall thickening at rest by MR imaging with [18]*F-Fluorodeoxyglucose (*[18]*FDG)-uptake by PET*
The hypothesis that thinned and akinetic regions represent chronic scar has been tested by comparing MR imaging data to PET and SPECT findings in identical myocardial regions.[48,49] This comparison is facilitated by the fact that MR imaging provides a three-dimensional set of sections through the left ventricle, which is very similar to reconstructed PET and SPECT sections.

In a recent study from our institution[49] wall thickness measurements were made from short axis MR tomograms in 35 patients with chronic infarcts (infarct age older than 4 months) and regional akinesia on left ventricular angiograms. An akinetic segment was considered viable if enddiastolic wall thickness on gradient-echo MR images was > 5,5mm (2,5 standard deviations below the mean of a control group). Segments were graded viable by PET if [18]FDG-uptake was > 50% of the maximum [18]FDG uptake in a region with normal wall motion. Viability of the infarct region was diagnosed by [18]FDG-PET in 23/35 patients (66%) and gradings based on [18]FDG-uptake and myocardial morphology were identical in 29/35 (83%) patients. There was a total of 2200 segments, 482 (23%) of which were akinetic (Table 1). Of these akinetic segments, 234 (48%) had preserved end-diastolic wall thickness and 299 (62%) were viable by [18]FDG-PET, yielding a sensitivity of 72%, a specificity of 89% and a positive predictive accuracy of 91%. In addition, the average [18]FDG-uptake did not differ between segments with systolic wall thickening at rest or akinesia as long as wall thickness was preserved. Thus, enddiastolic left ventricular wall thickness predicted residual viability nearly as accurate as metabolic findings by [18]FDG-PET in our study.

Other authors[50] comparing PET and MR imaging findings in patients with coronary artery disease and reduced left ventricular function found that [18]FDG-uptake was largely independent of regional end-diastolic wall thickness. In this study the large overlap between the [18]FDG-uptake of akinetic/dyskinetic and hypokinetic/normokinetic regions made the wall thickness measurements not helpful in identifying viability.

Possible explanations for their finding of a lack of metabolic activity in regions with normal enddiastolic wall thickness include differences in the study population (patients with chronic and acute myocardial infarct) as well as the use of spin-echo technique with short echo-times (20 ms). Especially with short echo-times slow blood flow adjacent to regions with wall motion abnormalities can be confused with myocardium and lead to an overestimation of the wall thickness.[51]

Comparison of MRI gradings based on dobutamine induced systolic wall thickening, end-diastolic wall thickness and combined evaluation of both MRI parameters with PET defined viability

Rest-MRI (akinetic segments; n=482)

		MRI-DWT		
		viable	scar	
FDG-PET	viable	214	85	299
	scar	20	163	183
		234	248	482

Table 3 a

Dobutamine-MRI (10 µg/kg/min) (akinetic segments; n=482)

		MRI-SWT		
		viable	scar	
FDG-PET	viable	242	57	299
	scar	9	174	183
		251	231	482

Table 3 b

Rest &Dobutamine-MRI (akinetic segments; n=482)

		MRI-DWT & SWT		
		viable	scar	
FDG-PET	viable	263	36	299
	scar	24	159	183
		287	195	482

Table 3 c

Table 1. Comparison of MR imaging viability gradings in 35 patients with 482 left ventricular myocardial segments, which were akinetic at rest MR imaging, based on enddiastolic wall thickness (left), dobutamine induced systolic wall thickening (middle), and combination of both parameters (right) with viability gradings based on relative [18]FDG-uptake on PET images. DWT = enddiastolic wall thickness; [18]FDG-PET = 18F-fluorodeoxyglucose positron emission tomography; MR imaging = gradient-echo magnetic resonance imaging; SWT = systolic wall thickening during dobutamine infusion (Reproduced from F.M.Baer et al.: Dobutamine-gradient-echo MR imaging: A functional and morphologic approach to the detection of residual myocardial viability. Circulation 1995 (in press), with permission).

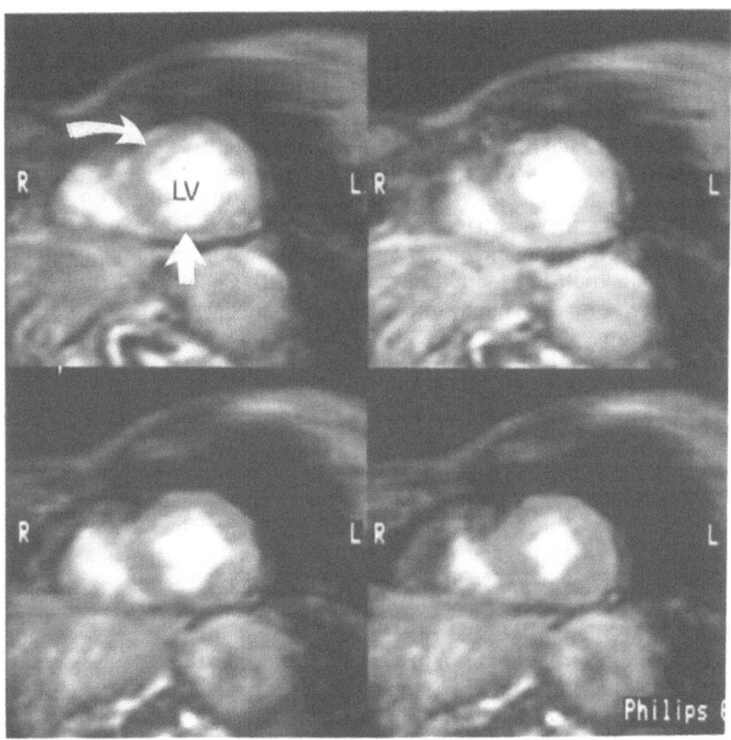

Figure 2A. Four phases short axis gradient-echo MR images (TR = 28ms, TE = 12ms) during dobutamine infusion (10 µg/kg/min) in a patient with chronic anteroseptal and inferior myocardial infarct.
Upper left: Enddiastolic image. There is some wall thinning in the anteroseptal region (curved arrow) and markedly reduced wall thickness in the inferior wall (single white arrow). Upper right: The endsystolic image demonstrates hypokinesia of the anteroseptal region, and akinesia of the inferior region.
Lower left: Enddiastolic image during dobutamine: Lower right: At endsystole, there is perfectly normal wall thickening of the inferior and anterior wall.

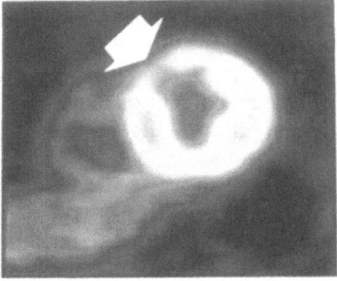

Figure 2B: The corresponding ¹⁸FDG-PET image shows reduced uptake in the anteroseptal region (arrow), but relative uptake is larger than 50%. Therefore, this region is also viable by PET-criteria. The inferior wall shows normal ¹⁸FDG-uptake (see for colourplate of this figure page 245).

References

1. Akins EW, Hill JA, Sievers KW, Conti CR. Assessment of left ventricular wall thickness in healed myocardial infarction by magnetic resonance imaging. Am J Cardiol 1987;59:24-8.
2. Higgins CB, Lanzer P, Stark D et al. Imaging by nuclear magnetic resonance in patients with chronic ischemic heart disease. Circulation 1984;69:523-31.
3. Pflugfelder PW, Sechtem UP, White RD, Higgins CB. Quantification of regional myocardial function by rapid cine MR imaging. Am J Roentgenol 1988;150:523-9.
4. White RD, Holt WW, Cheitlin MD et al. Estimation of the functional and anatomic extent of myocardial infarction using magnetic resonance imaging. Am Heart J 1988;115:740-8.
5. Sechtem U, Sommerhoff BA, Markiewicz W, White RD, Cheitlin MD, Higgins CB. Regional left ventricular wall thickening by magnetic resonance imaging: evaluation of normal persons and patients with global and regional dysfunction. Am J Cardiol 1987;59:145-51.
6. Schlichter J, Hellerstein HK, Katz LN. Aneurysm of the heart. A correlative study of 102 proven cases. Medicine 1954;33:43-86.
7. Fishbein MC, Maclean D, Maroleo PR. The histopathologic evolution of myocardial infarction. Chest 1978;73:843-9.
8. Mallory GK, White PD, Salcedo-Galger J. The speed of healing of myocardial infarction: a study of the pathologic anatomy in 72 cases. Am Heart J 1939;18:647-71.
9. Bottomley PA, Smith LS, Brazzamano S, Hedlund LW, Redington RW, Herfkens RJ. The fate of inorganic phosphate and pH in regional myocardial ischemia and infarction: a noninvasive 31P NMR study. Magn Reson Med 1987;5:129-42.
10. Braunwald E, Kloner RA. The stunned myocardium: prolonged, postischemic ventricular dysfunction. Circulation 1982;66:1146-9.
11. Kloner RA, Allen J, Cox TA, Zheng Y, Ruiz CE. Stunned left ventricular myocardium after exercise treadmill testing in coronary artery disease. Am J Cardiol 1991;68:329-34.
12. Bolli R, Zhu WX, Thornby JI, O'Neill PG, Roberts R. Time course and determinants of recovery of function after reversible ischemia in conscious dogs. Am J Physiol 1988;254:102-14.
13. Rahimtoola S. The hibernating myocardium. Am Heart J 1989;117:211-21.
14. Bodenheimer MM, Banka VS, Hermann GA, Trout RG, Pasdar H, Helfant RH. Reversible asynergy. Histopathologic and electrographic correlations in patients with coronary artery disease. Circulation 1976;53:792-6.
15. Meese RB, Spritzer CE, Negro VR, Bashore T, Herfkens RJ. Detection, characterization and functional assessment of reperfused Q-wave acute myocardial infarction by cine magnetic resonance imaging. Am J Cardiol 1990;66:1-9.
16. Johns JA, Leavitt MB, Newell JB et al. Quantitation of acute myocardial infarct size by nuclear magnetic resonance imaging. J Am Coll Cardiol 1990;15:143-9.
17. Johnston DL, Gupta VK, Wendt RE, Mahmarian JL, Verani MS. Detection of viable myocardium in segments with fixed defects of thallium-201 scintigraphy: usefulness of magnetic resonance imaging early after acute myocardial infarction. Magn Res Imaging 1993;11:949-56.
18. Brunken R, Schwaiger M, Grover-McKay M, Phelps ME, Tillisch J, Schelbert HR. Positron emission tomography detects tissue metabolic activity in myocardial segments with persistent thallium perfusion defects. J Am Coll Cardiol 1987;10:557-67.
19. Dilsizian V, Rocco TP, Freedman MT, Leon MB, Bonow RO. Enhanced detection of ischemic but viable myocardium by the reinjection of thallium after stress-redistribution imaging. N Engl J Med 1990;323:141-6.
20. Nienaber CA, Rochau T, Chatterjee T, Nicolas V. Dobutamin-Magnetresonanztomographie und 201-Thallium-SPECT: Nachweis von vitalem Myokard in der Postinfarktphase (abstr).

Z Kardiol 1993;82(Suppl 1):17.
21. Atkinson DJ, Edelman RR. Cineangiography of the heart in a single breath hold with a segmented turbo FLASH sequence. Radiology 1991;178:357-63.
22. Tscholakoff D, Higgins CB, McNamara MT, Derugin N. Early-phase myocardial infarction: evaluation by MR imaging. Radiology 1986;159:667-72.
23. Rokey R, Verani MS, Bolli R et al. Myocardial infarct size quantification by MR imaging early after coronary occlusion in dogs. Radiology 1986;158:771-4.
24. Buda AJ, Aisen AM, Juni JE, Gallagher KP, Zotz RJ. Detection and sizing of myocardial ischemia and infarction by nuclear magnetic resonance imaging in the canine heart. Am Heart J 1985;110:1284-90.
25. Bouchard A, Reeves RC, Cranney G, Bishop SP, Pohost GM. Assessment of myocardial infarct size by means of T2-weighted magnetic resonance imaging. Am Heart J 1989;117:281-9.
26. Wisenberg G, Prato FS, Carroll SE, Turner KL, Marshall T. Serial nuclear magnetic resonance imaging of acute myocardial infarction with and without reperfusion. Am Heart J 1988;115:510-8.
27. McNamara MT, Higgins CB, Seheehtmann N et al. Detection and characterization of acute myocardial infarction in man with use of gated magnetic resonance. Circulation 1985;71:717-24.
28. Filipchuk NG, Peshock RM, Malloy CR et al. Detection and localization of recent myocardial infarction by magnetic resonance imaging. Am J Cardiol 1986;58:214-9.
29. Ryan T, Tarver RD, Duerk JL, Sawada SG, Hollenkamp NC. Distinguishing viable from infarcted myocardium after experimental ischemia and reperfusion by using nuclear magnetic resonance imaging. J Am Coll Cardiol 1990;15:1355-64.
30. McNamara MT, Tscholakoff D, Revel D et al. Differentiation of reversible and irreversible myocardial injury by MR imaging with and without gadolinium-DTPA. Radiology 1986;158:765-9.
31. Saeed M, Wendland MF, Takehara Y, Higgins CB. Reversible and irreversible injury in the reperfused myocardium: differentiation with contrast material-enhanced MR imaging. Radiology 1990;175:633-7.
32. Saeed M, Wendland MF, Masui T, Higgins CB. Myocardial infarctions on Tl- and susceptibility-enhanced MRI: evidence for loss of compartimentalization of contrast media. Magn Res Med 1994;31:31-9.
33. Guth BD, Martin JF, Heusch G, Ross JJ. Regional myocardial blood flow, function and metabolism using phosphorus-31 nuclear magnetic resonance spectroscopy during ischemia and reperfusion in dogs. J Am Coll Cardiol 1987;10:673-81.
34. Camacho SA, Lanzer P, Toy BJ et al. In vivo alterations of high-energy phosphates and intracellular pH during reversible ischemia in pigs: -a 31P magnetic resonance spectroscopy study. Am Heart J 1988;116:701-8.
35. Arai AE, Pantely GA, Anselone CG, Bristow J, Bristow JD. Active downregulation of myocardial energy requirements during prolonged moderate ischemia in swine. Circ Res 1991;69:1458-69.
36. Pantely GA, Malone SA, Rhen WS et al. Regeneration of phosphocreatine in pigs despite continued moderate ischemia. Circ Res 1990;67:1481-93.
37. Schulz R, Guth PD, Pieper K, Martin C, Heusch G. Recruitment of inotropic reserve in moderately ischemic myocardium at the expense of metabolic recovery: a model of short-term hibernation. Circ Res 1992;70:1282-95.
38. Menon RS, Hendrich K, Hu X, Ugurbil K. 31P NMR spectroscopy of the human heart at 4 T: detection of substantially uncontaminated cardiac spectra and differentiation of subepicardium and subendocardium. Magn Reson Med 1992;26:368-76.

39. Gober JR, Schaefer S, Camacho SA et al. Epicardial and endocardial localized 31P magnetic resonance spectroscopy: evidence for metabolic heterogeneity during regional ischemia. Magn Reson Med 1990;13:204-15.

40. Bottomley PA, Herfkens RJ, Smith LS, Bashore TM. Altered phosphate metabolism in myocardial infarction: P-31 MR spectroscopy. Radiology 1987;172:53-8.

41. Baer FM, Smolarz K, Theissen P, Voth E, Schicha H, Sechtem U: Assessment of myocardial viability by quantification of 99mTc-methoxyisobutyl-isonitrile uptake at rest: comparison with parameters of myocardial viability obtained from gradient-echo magnetic resonance imaging. Eur Heart J 1994;15:97-107.

42. Roberts CS, Maclean D, Braunwald E, Maroko PR, Kloner RA. Topographic changes of the left ventricle after experimentally induced myocardial infarction in the rat. Am J Cardiol 1983;51:872-6.

43. Sasayama S, Gallagher KP, Kemper WS, Franklin D, Ross JJ. Regional left ventricular wall thickness early and late after coronary occlusion in the conscious dog. Am J Physiol 1981;240:H293-9.

44. Phibbs B. "Transmural" versus "subendocardial" myocardial infarction: An electrocardiographic myth. J Am Coll Cardiol 1983;1:561-4.

45. Preifeld AG, Schuster EH, Bukley BH. Nontransmural versus transmural myocardial infarction. A morphologic study. Am J Med 1983;75:423-32.

46. Pirolo JS, Moore GW, Hutchins GM. Continuum of the thickness of surviving myocardial wall with single myocardial infarcts. Arch Pathol Lab Med 1986;110:382-4.

47. Dubnow MH, Burchell HB, Titus JL. Postinfarction left ventricular aneurysm. A clinicomorphologic and electrocardiographic study of 80 cases. Am Heart J 1965;70:753-60.

48. Baer FM, Smolarz K, Jungehülsing M et al. Chronic myocardial infarction: assessment of morphology, function, and perfusion by gradient echo magnetic resonance imaging and 99mTc-methoxyisobutyl-isonitrile SPECT. Am Heart J 1992;123:636-45.

49. Baer FM, Voth E, Theissen P, Schneider CA, Schicha H, Sechtem U. Dobutamine-gradient-echo MRI: a functional and morphologic approach to the detection of residual myocardial viability. Circulation (In press).

50. Perrone-Filardi P, Bacharach SL, Dilsizian V et al. Metabolic evidence of viable myocardium in regions with reduced wall thickness and absent wall thickening in patients with chronic ischemic left ventricular dysfunction. J Am Coll Cardiol 1992;20:161-8.

51. Von Schulthess GK, Fisher MR, Crooks LE, Higgins CB. Gated MR imaging of the heart: intracardiac signal in patients and healthy subjects. Radiology 1985;156:125-32.

52. Horn HR, Teichholz LE, Cohn PF, Herman MV, Gorlin RG. Augmentation of left ventricular contraction pattern in coronary artery disease by an inotropic catecholamine. Circulation 1974;49:1063-71.

10   CLASSIFICATION OF HYPERTROPHIC CARDIOMYOPATHY WITH MAGNETIC RESONANCE IMAGING COMPARED WITH ECHOCARDIOGRAPHY

Jan L. Posma, Paul K. Blanksma,
and Kong I. Lie

Introduction

Hypertrophic cardiomyopathy is a myocardial disorder with an autosomal pattern of inheritance characterized by an increased wall mass of a non-dilated left ventricle with heterogeneity in wall thickness and myocyte and myofibrillar disarray. Common symptoms are dyspnea, angina, fatigue and syncope. Patients with hypertrophic cardiomyopathy vary greatly in terms of the patterns and extent of left ventricular hypertrophy, ranging from localized subaortic hypertrophy to full-length septal involvement together with anterolateral wall extension.[1] It is important to assess the degree of left ventricular hypertrophy in the individual patient since it may be a major determinant of symptoms and prognosis.[2,3] In hypertrophic cardiomyopathy regional wall thickness is directly associated with systolic[4] and diastolic[5] function. Correct anatomic classification of patients with hypertrophic cardiomyopathy is necessary for interpretation and understanding the results of studies with positron emission tomography.

Traditionally, echocardiography has been the imaging modality most widely used in the morphologic evaluation of patients with hypertrophic cardiomyopathy. Although in the majority of patients echocardiography allows diagnostic anatomic and hemodynamic evaluations, this technique is highly dependent on operator skills and expertise in case of complex heart disease. Furthermore, imaging of certain parts of the myocardium by ultrasonography may be hampered by limited windows and/or presence of adjacent lung tissue. A substantial part of patients show insufficient echogenicity to allow adequate delineation of endocardial and epicardial borders in all regions of the left ventricle. In recent years, magnetic resonance (MR) imaging has been effectively used in defining the extent of diverse myocardial abnormalities. We will discuss the potential role of MR imaging in the diagnostic procedure of patients with hypertrophic cardiomyopathy.

E. E. van der Wall et al. (eds.), Cardiac Positron Emission Tomography, 129–135.
© 1995 Kluwer Academic Publishers.

MR imaging: orientation to cardiac axis for optimal assessment of morphology

In the early years of cardiovascular MR imaging, the use of this technique in clinical practice was generally restricted to imaging in standard transaxial, sagittal and coronal views. These orthogonal body planes are oblique to the heart axes and poorly suited to the measurement of cardiac dimensions. Many of the image slices in a transaxial series are tangential to the myocardial wall and the myocardium appears thicker than it actually is. In contrast, image planes oriented to intrinsic cardiac axes can be rigorously standardized and compared from patient to patient. They can also be compared directly with other cardiac imaging techniques including two-dimensional echocardiography.[6] In order to obtain short-axis and long-axis views electronic angulation in two planes can be used.[7] In our institution a combination of patient positioning and electronic oblique angulation is used, as described in detail by Dinsmore et al.[6,8] In short, the patient's right shoulder is rotated 30 degree upward from the supine position so that a line through the long axis of the left ventricle, from aortic valve to apex, is horizontal. First the position of the left ventricle is determined by a transversal scout scan at the fourth intercostal space. A coronal image is made through the center of the left ventricular cavity in the long-axis plane parallel to the septum. This plane is analogous to the 30 degree right anterior oblique ventriculogram. From this image the horizontal long-axis view that passes through both the left ventricular apex and the aortic orifice is selected. This view is perpendicular to the septum.[7] This plane is comparable with the parasternal long-axis view in two-dimensional echocardiography. From the horizontal long-axis view, four parallel short-axis image planes (perpendicular to the long axis) are identified. Basal and apical planes are first located. The basal plane passes just below the mitral valves and cut through the muscular septum, and the apical plane passes just above the apical endocardium. The remaining two midventricular image planes are then defined to trisect equally the interval between the apical and the basal planes. The four parallel short-axis and the long-axis images are acquired at end-diastole.

MR imaging in hypertrophic cardiomyopathy

Higgins et al.[9] showed a good agreement between MR imaging and two-dimensional echocardiography in defining the distribution of abnormal wall thickness in 14 patients with hypertrophic cardiomyopathy. Because fixed orthogonal body planes were used for MR imaging, the patterns of distribution could not be directly compared with the two-dimensional echocardiographic studies. Although Boon et al.[10] used *ungated* MR imaging, which was compared with M-mode echocardiography, they obtained in 11 patients with hypertrophic cardiomyopathy a good correlation (p=0.71, p<0.001) for septal thickness measurements. The MR imaging measurements were larger than those obtained with echocardiography probably because orthogonal body planes were used. Sardanelli et al.[11] used MR imaging oriented to the cardiac axes. In 23 patients they found an excellent correlation (r=0.93) between MR imaging and echocardiography for septal wall thickness. For posterolateral wall thickness they found a good correlation (r = 0.74). In addition to the morphologic study, Sardanelli et al.[11] also performed a functional study in which they compared cine MR imaging and Doppler echocardiography. Good agreement was found for semiquantitative estimates of mitral regurgitation and dynamic obstruction. Park et al.[12] obtained good results in measuring wall thickness and semiquantitative classification of different subtypes of hypertrophic cardiomyopathy with spin-echo MR imaging, but no comparisons with echocardiography were made. Allison et al.[13] compared measurement of left ventricular mass in hypertrophic cardiomyopathy using MR imaging with echocardiography. MR imaging measurements of left ventricular mass in 6 ex-vivo hearts were within 8% of the mass determined by actually weighing the hearts. In contrast, they found a poor correlation (r = 0.17) between echocardiography and MR imaging in 12 patients with hypertrophic cardiomyopathy. This is explained by an inadequate echocardiographic technique. The used method of M-mode echocardiography in assessing left ventricular mass is not suitable in patients with hypertrophic cardiomyopathy, since in hypertrophic cardiomyopathy the left ventricle shows a very irregular pattern of hypertrophy. Dong et al.[4] determined regional wall thickness and systolic thickening in 17 patients with hypertrophic cardiomyopathy using MR imaging tagging and three-dimensional volume-element reconstruction, but no comparison with echocardiography was made.

MR imaging compared with echocardiography: own results

It has been our impression that in some patients with hypertrophic cardiomyopathy, spin-echo MR imaging provided additional clinically useful morphologic information in the primary diagnostic work-up that was not readily available by echocardiography. Therefore, we prospectively investigated the diagnostic value of spin-echo MR imaging in quantitative assessment of the severity of the hypertrophic process in 52 consecutive patients with hypertrophic cardiomyopathy and compared its diagnostic performance with those of transthoracic echocardiography. The diagnosis of hypertrophic cardiomyopathy was based on clinical, electrocardiographic, echocardiographic, and angiographic findings demonstrating a hypertrophied, nondilated left ventricle in the absence of identifiable cardiac or systemic stimuli to hypertrophy.[14] There were 35 men and 17 women. The mean age was 47 ± 15 years (range 19-82 years). All patients had regular sinus rhythm and had no contraindication for MR imaging. New York Heart Association classification was I or II in 40 patients and III or IV in 12 patients. Systolic anterior motion of the mitral valve was present in 25 patients, and a resting pressure gradient > 30 mmHg in the outflow tract was present in 9 patients (mean 55 ± 25 mmHg).

Electrocardiographically gated end-diastolic MR imaging oriented to the cardiac axes were obtained using a 1.5-T unit (Gyroscan S15, Philips, Eindhoven, The Netherlands). Spin-echo T1-weighted images were obtained with an echo time of 30 ms and pulse repetition time dependent on the R-R interval. Complete two-dimensional echocardiographic and Doppler examinations were performed in standard parasternal long-axis, short-axis and apical four chamber views and recorded on videotape. Medication remained unchanged. A commercially available phased-array echocardiograph (Toshiba 65A) with a 3.75-MHz and 2.5-MHz transducer was used. All measurements were made at end-diastole without knowledge of the results obtained by MR imaging. Magnitude of left ventricular hypertrophy was assessed primarily from the parasternal short-axis planes; however, the parasternal long-axis and apical views were also used to integrate the observations obtained from the short-axis views. The median time between MR imaging and echocardiography was 5 days (range 1-14 days). None of the patient's clinical conditions changed during the interval between MR imaging and echocardiography. For both imaging modalities the quality of obtained morphologic information was scored: non-diagnostic, anatomy not completely delineated and/or poor quality image, or anatomy completely delineated. A consensus was reached in all cases.

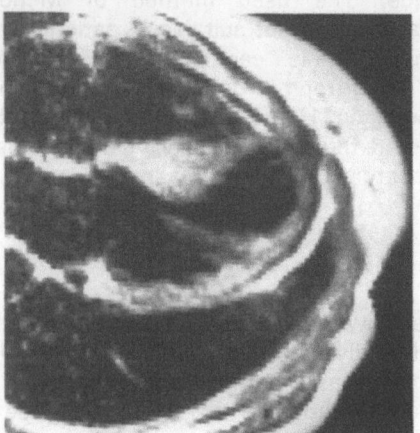 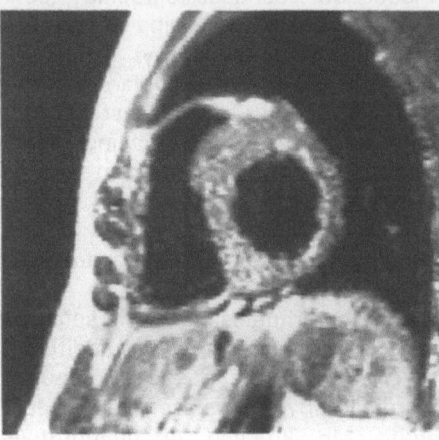

Figure 1. MR imaging of a patient with hypertrophic cardiomyopathy. Left panel: long-axis view showing localized hypertrophy of the basal part of the interventricular septum. Right panel: short-axis view showing hypertrophy of the posterior and anterior parts of the septum and of the anterior part of the left ventricular free wall.

In the 52 patients we obtained 51 spin echo MR images that showed hypertrophic cardiomyopathy in all cases (Figure 1). In 1 patient MR imaging was not possible due to claustrophobia. In 49 (94%) MR imaging studies, a sharp delineation of total endocardium and epicardium allowed complete assessment of myocardial anatomy. The apical region was not visible in 1 case; in another case the thickness of the lateral free wall could not be measured.

Also, echocardiography demonstrated hypertrophic cardiomyopathy in all patients, but only 33 (63%) patients showed sufficient echogenicity to allow reliable wall thickness measurements in all segments. In the remaining 19 patients echocardiography demonstrated asymmetric septal hypertrophy, but in 17 patients the lateral wall was not clearly visible, in 13 cases the apical region could not be visualized, and in 12 patients imaging of the posterior part of the septum was inadequate. The patients with inadequate echocardiograms did not differ in age or extent of hypertrophy from the patients with adequate echocardiograms.

For 32 patients in whom both MR imaging and echocardiography provided complete morphologic information, wall thickness measurements obtained with both imaging modalities were compared. MR imaging wall thickness measurements correlated well with those obtained by echocardiography (Table 1). However, in 18 patients with poor echogenicity and good MR images poor correlations were found especially in the posteroseptal and anterolateral regions (Table 2).

Table 1. Linear regression analysis of results with MR imaging versus echocardiography for patients with good echogenicity.

	n	MRI	Echo	r	SEE	p value
anteroseptal (mm)	32	27±7	27±7	0.93	2.5	<0.001
posteroseptal (mm)	32	19±8	19±7	0.93	2.7	<0.001
anterolateral (mm)	32	16±5	16±5	0.88	2.3	<0.001
posterior (mm)	32	12±2	12±2	0.66	1.8	<0.001

n = number of segments that could be compared, r = correlation coefficient, SEE = standard error of the estimate (mm).

Table 2. Linear regression analysis of results with MR imaging versus echocardiography for patients with poor echogenicity.

	n	MRI	Echo	r	SEE	p value
anteroseptal (mm)	18	26±7	25±6	0.86	3.0	<0.001
posteroseptal (mm)	12	19±5	18±6	0.55	4.0	ns
anterolateral (mm)	9	17±4	16±6	0.18	6.3	ns
posterior (mm)	15	15±4	14±2	0.77	1.4	<0.001

n = number of segments that could be compared, r = correlation coefficient, SEE = standard error of the estimate (mm), ns = not significant.

Discussion

Based on our experience in 51 consecutive patients, MR imaging provided additional morphologic information in 18 patients (35%), which was not available with echocardiography. We found that accurate assessment of lateral and posteroseptal wall thickness was not possible in 33% and 23% of the patients, respectively. This is probably due to the small angle between the ultrasound beam and the reflecting surface of these parts of the myocardium, causing weak echoes.[15] However, as is evident from Tables 1 and 2, in the cohort of patients with good echogenicity there was an excellent correlation between MR imaging and echocardiography for the measurements of the anteroseptal and posteroseptal regions (r=0.93). Even in patients with poor echogenicity the best correlation between the two methods was found for the anteroseptal segment (r = 0.86). In 20% of the patients, echocardiography was not conclusive in assessing the wall thickness of the apical part of the interventricular septum. Due to technical difficulties intrinsic to echocardiography this imaging modality is often less accurate in the apical region dependent of the angle of the ultrasound beam and the left ventricular wall segment.[16] Conversely, MR imaging has the characteristic capability to delineate clear margins of both the endocardium and the epicardium at the apical level of the left ventricle.[17,18]

Conclusion

In hypertrophic cardiomyopathy the heart shows a complex geometric shape and anatomic configuration. Spin-echo MR imaging has an important role in the diagnostic evaluation of these patients. MR imaging provides excellent morphologic information necessary for quantitative assessment of the extent of hypertrophy that is not available by echocardiography in a substantial part of patients. In addition to echocardiography, MR imaging provides a high-quality diagnostic information necessary for patient-care and research in patients with hypertrophic cardiomyopathy.

References

1. Maron BJ, Gottdiener JS, Epstein SE. Patterns and significance of the distribution of left ventricular hypertrophy in hypertrophic cardiomyopathy: a wide-angle, two-dimensional echocardiographic study of 125 patients. Am J Cardiol 1981;48:418-28.
2. Wigle ED, Sasson Z, Henderson MA et al. Hypertrophic cardiomyopathy: the importance of the site and the extent of hypertrophy. A review. Prog Cardiovasc Dis 1985;28:1-83.
3. Spirito P, Maron BJ. Relation between extent of left ventricular hypertrophy and occurrence of sudden cardiac death in hypertrophic cardiomyopathy. J Am Coll Cardiol 1990;15:1521-6.
4. Dong SJ, MacGregor JH, Crawley AP et al. Left ventricular wall thickness and regional systolic function in patients with hypertrophic cardiomyopathy. A three-dimensional tagged magnetic resonance imaging study. Circulation 1994;90:1200-9.
5. Hayashida W, Kumada T, Kohno F et al. Left ventricular regional relaxation and its nonuniformity in hypertrophic nonobstructive cardiomyopathy. Circulation 1991;84:1496-504.
6. Dinsmore RE. MRI determination of cardiac dimensions. In: Van der Wall EE, De Roos A, editors. Magnetic Resonance Imaging in Coronary Artery Disease. Dordrecht: Kluwer Academic Publishers, 1991:97-111.
7. AHA/ACC recommendation on tomographic imaging: standardization of cardiac tomographic imaging. An ACC/AHA policy statement. J Am Coll Cardiol 1992;20:255-6.
8. Dinsmore RE, Wismer GL, Levine RA, Okada RD, Brady TJ. Magnetic resonance imaging of the heart: position and gradient angle selection for optimal imaging planes. Am J Radiol 1984;143:1135-42.
9. Higgins CB, Byrd BF, Stark D et al. Magnetic resonance imaging in hypertrophic cardiomyopathy. Am J Cardiol 1985;55:1121-6.
10. Been M, Kean D, Smith MA, Douglas RHB, Best JJK, Muir AL. Nuclear magnetic resonance in hypertrophic cardiomyopathy. Br Heart J 1985;54:48-52.
11. Sardanelli F, Molinari G, Petillo A et al. MRI in hypertrophic cardiomyopathy: a morphofunctional study. J Comput Assist Tomogr 1993;17:862-72.
12. Park JH, Kim YM, Chung JW, Park YB, Han JK, Han MC. MR imaging of hypertrophic cardiomyopathy. Radiology 1992;185:441-6.
13. Allison JD, Flickinger FW, Wright JC et al. Measurement of left ventricular mass in hypertrophic cardiomyopathy using MRI: comparison with echocardiography. Magn Reson Imaging 1993;11:329-34.
14. Maron BJ, Epstein SE. Hypertrophic cardiomyopathy: a discussion of nomenclature. Am J Cardiol 1979;43:1242-4.
15. Hamer JPM. Practical echocardiography in the adult with Doppler and color-Doppler flow imaging. Dordrecht: Kluwer Academic Publishers, 1990:10.
16. Vacek JL, Davis WR, Bellinger RL, McKiernan TL. Apical hypertrophic cardiomyopathy in American patients. Am Heart J 1984;108:1501-6.
17. Casolo GC, Trotta F, Rostagno C et al. Detection of apical hypertrophic cardiomyopathy by magnetic resonance imaging. Am Heart J 1989;117:468-72.
18. Suzuki J, Watanabe F, Takenaka K et al. New subtype of apical hypertrophic cardiomyopathy identified with nuclear magnetic resonance imaging as an underlying cause of markedly inverted T waves. J Am Coll Cardiol 1993;22:1175-81.

11   POSITRON EMISSION TOMOGRAPHY CHARACTERIZATION OF THE MYOCARDIUM IN HYPERTROPHIC CARDIOMYOPATHY

Paul K. Blanksma, Jan L. Posma, Richard M. de Jong, Jan Pruim,
Antoon T.M. Willemsen, Rutger L. Anthonio, Evert van der Wall,
Willem Vaalburg, and Kong I. Lie

Introduction

Angina pectoris is a common symptom in patients with hypertrophic cardiomyopathy. Contrary to patients with coronary artery disease a variety of underlying pathological factors can be held responsible, such as impeded blood flow due to asymmetric hypertrophy of the left ventricle and subaortic left ventricle outflow tract obstruction, inducing myocardial ischemia and consequently left ventricle diastolic dysfunction.[1] A localized thickening in the interventricular septum is the most prominent pathologic feature, but thickening may also be present in the left ventricle free wall. In the hypertrophic left ventricle wall smaller or larger areas of myocardial fiber disarray are present, histologically featured by myocytes disorderly arranged at perpendicular and oblique angles to each other. Functionally this random fiber orientation will result in an isometric contraction pattern. This may explain the frequent lack of systolic wall thickening in these myocardial areas. Especially in older patients areas of myocardial necrosis and scarring have been found accompanied by a decreased left ventricle systolic function.

In patients with hypertrophic cardiomyopathy, myocardial ischemia has been demonstrated by thallium scintigraphy and positron emission tomography (PET), showing both reversible and irreversible myocardial perfusion defects and a reduced myocardial perfusion reserve.[1-5] These findings are suggestive of significant myocardial ischemia as a cause of the symptoms. Because PET is the most accurate non-invasive method to demonstrate regional myocardial ischemia and viability, we studied 12 patients with hypertrophic cardiomyopathy and angina pectoris while on verapamil treatment. $^{13}NH_3$ (ammonia) PET and ^{18}FDG (fluoro-deoxyglucose) PET were used for studying myocardial perfusion and myocardial glucose uptake, respectively. The results were compared to the results in a group of normal volunteers, using a new technique for the semi-automated generation of parametric polar maps recently described by our group.[6]

E. E. van der Wall et al. (eds.), Cardiac Positron Emission Tomography, 137–148.
© 1995 Kluwer Academic Publishers.

Methods

Study group
Twelve patients (7 men and 5 women; age range 16 to 70 years, mean 47.3 years, Table 1) with symptomatic hypertrophic cardiomyopathy using adequate doses of verapamil were included in this study. Myocardial perfusion was studied using dynamic $^{13}NH_3$ imaging of the heart, as described by Schelbert and colleagues[7-9] and Bellina et al.[10] A control group of 22 volunteers was studied with $^{13}NH_3$ of whom 13 also underwent a dipyridamole stress test. Furthermore, a separate group of 7 volunteers were studied with ^{18}FDG. The protocol was approved by the local Medical Ethical Committee and all subjects agreed to the study.

Table 1. Clinical characteristics of the patients with hypertrophic cardiomyopathy

patient (no)	age (yrs)	sex	echogradient (mmHg)	symptoms	therapy
1	70	female	0	heart failure	4 x 80 mg verapamil, furosemide
2	54	female	0	fatigue	3 x 40 mg verapamil
3	16	female	50	fatigue	3 x 80 mg verapamil
4	17	female	50	angina	3 x 40 mg verapamil
5	53	male	0	angina	2 x 240 mg verapamil
6	17	male	85	angina	3 x 40 mg verapamil
7	54	male	10	angina	2 x 240 mg verapamil, nitrates
8	70	female	25 - 150	angina	2 x 240 mg verapamil
9	58	male	66	angina	3 x 120 mg verapamil, metoprolol,amiodarone
10	61	male	20	angina	2 x 120 mg verapamil, metoprolol
11	57	male	50	angina	3 x 120 mg verapamil
12	41	male	107	angina	sotalol, quinidine

Study protocol (Figure 1)
None of the subjects did use vasoactive medication (ß-blocking agents, calcium antagonists, long acting nitrates) for 24 hours prior to the study. The study was approved by the local ethical committee and all volunteers and patients gave their informed consent. Subjects were positioned in a 951 Siemens positron camera with a rectilinear scan, imaging 31 planes simultaneously over 0.8 cm. Measured resolution of the system was 6 mm full width half maximum. Data was corrected automatically for accidental coincidence and dead time. Photon attenuation was measured with a transmission scan using a retractable internal ring source filled with $^{68}Ge/^{68}Ga$. Dynamic data acquisition was started at the time of $^{13}NH_3$ injection (370 MBq) and

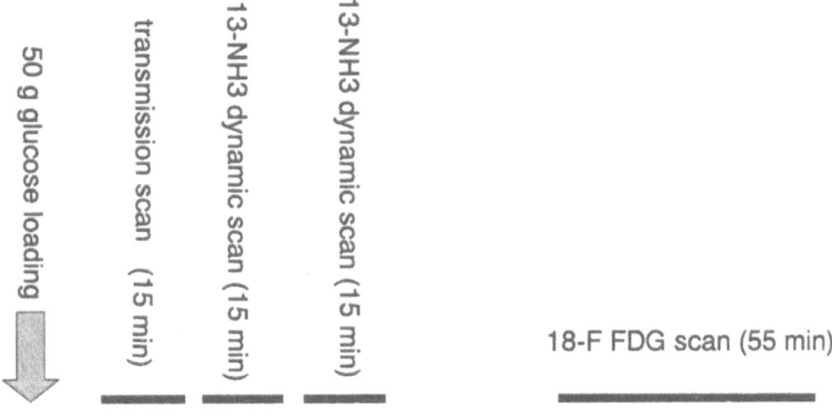

Figure 1. Scheme of the study protocol. The protocol consists of: a) transmission scan for correction of photon attenuation; b) control perfusion scan with 370 MBq $^{13}NH_3$; c) second perfusion scan with 370 MBq $^{13}NH_3$, preceded by an intravenous injection of dipyridamole in ad dose of 0.56 mg/kg body weight; d) ^{18}FDG scan for myocardial viability. Before the subject is positioned in the camera glucose loading is performed with 50 g oral glucose solution.

continued for 15 minutes (frames: 12 x 10 sec, 1 x 2 min, 1 x 4 min, 1 x 7 min). Twenty minutes after the baseline $^{13}NH_3$ injection, the study was repeated. In the repeated study injection of $^{13}NH_3$ was preceded by provocation with dipyridamole in a dose of 0.56 mg dipyridamole/kg body weight from 6 to 2 minutes before $^{13}NH_3$ injection.

The study of myocardial glucose uptake was started 50 minutes after the second injection of $^{13}NH_3$, when the count rate of the camera had decreased below 2000 counts per second. An amount of 50 g of glucose was administered orally before subjects were positioned in the camera. The study was performed with ^{18}FDG, according to the methods described by Krivokapich et al.[11] and Ratib et al.[12] A 17 frame protocol of: 8 x 15 sec, 4 x 30 sec, 1 x 1 min, 1 x 5 min, 1 x 10 min, 1 x 15 min, 1 x 20 min was used. During the whole procedure heart rate and blood pressure were monitored continuously by a Dynamap automatic blood pressure monitor, and the rate pressure product was calculated.

Data analysis
The data of the $^{13}NH_3$ provocation study was corrected for remaining activity of the baseline study by subtracting the activity in the last frame of the baseline study (correction frame). Next, data of each study consisting of 31 transversal image planes perpendicular to the long axis of the body, was reoriented by the computer to 10 short axis images perpendicular to the long axis of the left ventricle. For reorientation a manually defined long axis in the left ventricle was used. The myocardium in each of

the 10 short-axis images was divided into 48 segments i.e. 7.5° per segment. Using the maximum activity in each segment, time activity curves were established in every segment of all slices.[13] A blood pool was defined in three short-axis images near the base to avoid myocardial spillover as much as possible. The average radioactivity of the three blood pools was used to calculate a single blood pool time activity curve. Finally, the results of segmental myocardial perfusion and glucose uptake were presented as polar maps.[8] The results were displayed in concentric circles with the apical data in the centre, and the more basal data towards the periphery of the display. In contrast to usual polar map displays as described by Porenta et al.,[13] our data were quantitative. For each of the 48 segments of all 10 transversal images myocardial perfusion and myocardial glucose uptake was calculated. For perfusion calculation the model as described by Schelbert et al.[7] was used. A correction for flow mediated extraction of the tracer was applied, using an equation as described by these authors:

$$E = E_0 . (1\text{-}0.607 . \exp[\text{-}1.25/\text{Flow}])$$

For the [18]FDG studies the Patlak analysis was used,[14] as adapted for myocardial glucose uptake by Gambhir et al.[15] and Hicks et al.[16] From the perfusion maps of the control and the provoked situation, perfusion ratio polar maps were constructed by calculating the ratio for each individual myocardial segment. To demonstrate inducible ischemia a ratio polar map was calculated based on the results of the [18]FDG study and the dipyridamole stress test perfusion study. For statistical analysis the total myocardium was divided into 9 regions (Figure 2). Values per region were calculated for perfusion, dipyridamole stress test perfusion ratio and glucose consumption.

From the studies in the healthy volunteers, we defined 95% confidence intervals for the normal values for each imaging modality and for each myocardial region (mean ± two standard deviations.[13] (Table 2) The measurements in the patients were compared with these intervals. As a result, 95% confidence maps could be made in all patients, indicating which myocardial segment was within, above, or below the corresponding 95% confidence interval for control perfusion, induced perfusion and glucose consumption. In this way calculations per region could also be made of the percentage of myocardium above and below the 95% confidence interval of the inducible ischemic area. To quantify inducible ischemic myocardium, the percentage myocardium above the 95% interval was calculated from the ratio map of [18]FDG study and of dipyridamole stress test perfusion study ("mismatch defect calculation"). To quantify nonviable myocardium a map was constructed of the [18]FDG uptake ("metabolism defect calculation"). From this metabolic map the percentage myocardium below the 95% confidence interval was calculated (Figure 2). The percentage myocardium beyond the 95% normal confidence limits was considered to be significant if it exceeded 10% of the total myocardium.

Statistical analysis

The results are indicated by its mean value and standard deviation. The results in the hypertrophic cardiomyopathy patients were compared with the results obtained in the normal volunteers by a two-tailed Students-*t*-test.

Table 2. Normal values of myocardial perfusion at control situation, during a dipyridamole stress test, of the DST ratio, and of ^{18}F-FDG uptake obtained in 22 healthy volunteers

	mean	SD	number
control perfusion (ml/min/100 g)	95.8	18.6	(n = 22)
Rate-pressure product (mmHg.min^{-1})	6774	1210	(n = 22)
DST perfusion (ml/min/100 g)	191.3	60.1	(n = 13)
DST Rate-pressure product (mmHg.min^{-1})	9972	1749	(n = 13)
DST ratio (%)	196.0	33.5	(n = 13)
^{18}F-FDG uptake (μmol/min/100 g)	54.8	14.7	(n = 7)

Values are given as the mean and standard deviation (SD). DST: dipyridamole stress test. DST ratio: DST perfusion divided by control perfusion, expressed as a percentage.

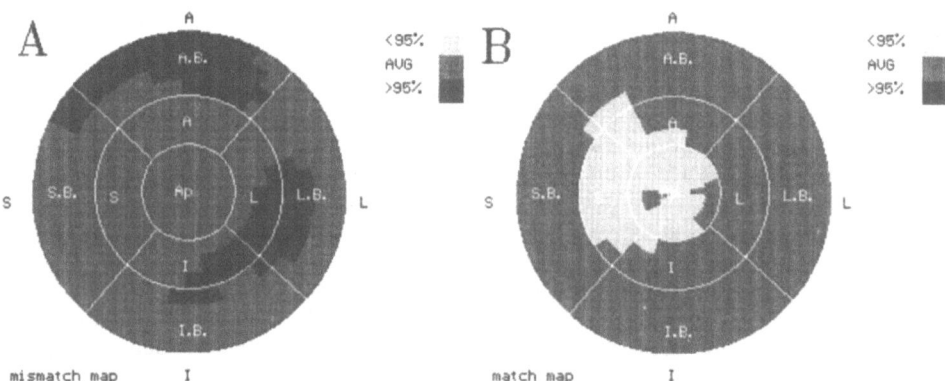

Figure 2. Mismatch polar map (A) and metabolism defect polar map (B) in a 57-year old male with extensive septal and lateral wall ischemia and anteroseptal wall fibrosis. The dark-shaded area in B is the myocardial area above the 95% normal confidence interval, derived from the normal volunteers. The light-shaded area in A is the myocardial area below the 95% confidence interval obtained from the normal volunteers. The shades of gray are indicated at right of the polar maps. A = anterior region; S = septal region; I = inferior region; L = lateral region.

Results

The percentage of myocardial tissue above and below the 95% confidence interval as obtained in the normal volunteers, was in patients calculated for baseline perfusion, dipyridamole stress test perfusion, dipyridamole stress test ratio, and the perfusion-metabolism mismatch and metabolic defects as described above. The results are given in Table 3. It may be evident that in the major part of the myocardium values of resting perfusion are above normal in all but two patients (mean 73.1 ± 36.7% of the total myocardium). However, myocardial perfusion during the dipyridamole stress test was within normal limits in the hypertrophic cardiomyopathy patients. The dipyridamole stress test ratio was below normal values in a considerable part of the myocardium in 5/10 patients (mean 29.8 ± 30.8%). Total myocardial [18]FDG uptake was within normal values. Heart rate, blood pressure, and the rate pressure product at rest and during the dipyridamole stress test were also within normal confidence limits in the hypertrophic cardiomyopathy patients. A flow - metabolism mismatch was found in eight patients (mean 18.3 ± 9.8%), and a metabolic defect in three patients (mean 7.8 ± 7.9%). The metabolic defects did not match a decreased perfusion since perfusion reserve within these defects was 159.5 ± 35.4%, which was not different from the mean value in hypertrophic cardiomyopathy patients.

Discussion

The results of our study contribute to the understanding of the myocardial pathophysiology in hypertrophic cardiomyopathy. Our method of parametric imaging of myocardial perfusion and metabolism is specifically suitable for the study of regional differences of these parameters. The following aspects of myocardial ischemia in these patients can be studied with PET:

a. Increased myocardial oxygen consumption due to myocardial fiber disarray

In all but two patients baseline perfusion was above the 95% confidence limit of normal perfusion in a significant part of the myocardium (>10%). This may be explained by the presence of an increased myocardial oxygen consumption per gram tissue at rest, apparently due to isometric fiber contractions in the areas of myocardial fiber disarray.

b. Decreased perfusion reserve

In 5 of the 12 patients studied we found a decreased dipyridamole stress test ratio, mainly caused by an already increased perfusion at rest. This finding is in line with the observations reported by Camici et al.,[2] who also found a decreased myocardial perfusion reserve, as measured with a dipyridamole stress test. A decreased perfusion reserve may be caused by the above mentioned increased baseline perfusion in combination with a normal upper limit. Another cause might be sclerosis of the microvasculature, causing a decreased dilating capacity of these vessels. At the occurrence of chronotropic stimulation as is the cause during a dipyridamole stress test, the relative duration of the systolic phase increases compared to the diastolic phase, thus restricting the increase of myocardial perfusion during the dipyridamole stress test.

Table 3. Results of positron emission tomography in 12 patients with hypertrophic cardiomyopathy

patient (no)	Control			Dypiridamole stress test				^{18}F-FDG mismatch		
	RPP (mmHg.min^{-1})	perfusion (ml/min/100g)	>95% c.l. (%)	RPP (mmHg.min^{-1})	perfusion (ml/min/100g)	ratio (%)	>95% c.l. (%)	uptake (μmol/min/100g)	<95%c.l. (%)	>95%c.l. (%)
1	7095	128.1	54.9	9514	131.5	103.4	92.7	39.4	3.3	11.4
2	8568	119.0	0.5	9417	202.1	230.6	0.0			
3		215.9	100.0		252.4	117.1		56.3		
4	5555	132.0	61.9	8346	162.6	253.0	43.1	3.2		
5	6903	92.5	1.2	10586	228.7	169.8	0.0	35.8	3.4	16.7
6	8175	170.5	94.3	12305	283.3	158.1	3.8	86.5	0.7	11.8
7	7313	199.3	97.5	10976	297.4	136.3	27.7	54.0	20.3	32.9
8	8547	175.9	97.6	10864	233.9	151.2	23.6	31.2	19.1	32.7
9	7638	154.7	96.1	8700	230.1	146.2	4.5	58.8	2.3	5.4
10	7150	144.6	83.8	8611	206.0	120.7	9.9	46.5	4.2	10.5
11	10028	160.9	91.4	8640	189.7	119.0	50.0	37.1	17.9	19.0
12	7139	204.9	97.5	7888	236.7		59.3	68.1	3.9	24.0
mean	7646	158.2	73.1	9622	221.2	155.0	29.8	50.1	7.8	18.3
SD	1160	37.3	36.7	1379	46.9	47.5	30.8	17.1	7.9	9.8

control:control condition; RPP: rate pressure product; >95% c.l. percentage of the myocardium with values exceeding the 95% confidence limits of normal; <95% c.l.: percentage of the myocardium with values below the 95 % confidence limits of normal; ratio: perfusion during the dipyridamole stress test divided by perfusion in the control condition, expressed as a percentage; SD: standard deviation.

c. Dynamic coronary artery obstruction
Another cause of myocardial ischemia, which may be operative in cases with a decreased perfusion during the dipyridamole stress test in some myocardial areas, may be a dynamic systolic obstruction of the septal branches of the left anterior descending coronary artery. In such cases during coronary angiography the "milking sign" of the septal branches can be found. An actual decrease of myocardial perfusion, indicating coronary steal, during the dipyridamole stress test was found in this study in three patients, an example of which is shown in Figure 3 (patient no 3). Here, the parametric polar maps are shown of a 16-year old female presenting with severe dyspnea at exercise associated with ST-segment depressions in the electrocardiogram. When it is considered, that in these three patients normal coronary arteries were found on angiography, this decrease of perfusion during dipyridamol infusion is particularly remarkable, since this phenomenon can otherwise only be observed in a myocardial area with exclusive blood supply from collateral circulation because of total occlusion of the nutritive coronary artery.

d. Impeded perfusion due to hypertrophy
Due to localized myocardial hypertrophy, the amount of myocardium, which has to be supplied with blood is increased. Furthermore the distance, in which intramural coronary branches are running intramyocardially is increased. This may cause a transmural gradient of myocardial blood supply. In one patients this was found both at rest and during dipyridamole stress test. Figure 4 illustrates this finding showing the horizontal long axis images of a 54-year old male, 7 years after a septal myotomy/myectomy (patient no 7). Despite a successfully relieved outflow tract obstruction, he continued to suffer from severe angina pectoris functional class III according to NYHA. Images are displayed of perfusion at rest, during a dipyridamole stress test and of ^{18}FDG uptake. It can be noticed that myocardial perfusion at rest is higher in the septal area than in the lateral free wall. However, during the dipyridamole stress test septal perfusion decreases particularly in the subendocardial region. In contrast, the ^{18}FDG image shows a high uptake in the septum also mainly in the subendocardial region. The combination of these findings points to the presence of septal ischemia predominantly in the subendocardial layer.

e. Decreased myocardial viability due to fibrosis
The results of this study also suggest an age dependent difference in ^{18}FDG uptake. In three patients over 50 years of age metabolic defects were seen on the ^{18}FDG image In Figure 5 myocardial perfusion at baseline and during dipyridamole stress test and ^{18}FDG uptake is displayed of a 57-year old patient with hypertrophic cardiomyopathy (patient no 11). ˙Also myocardial dipyridamole stress test perfusion reserve is displayed. In the septum a large area of decreased viability can be seen, indicated by a decreased ^{18}FDG uptake. Note that within the viability defect, normal baseline and dipyridamole stress test perfusion is found. Within a fibrotic area, dynamic obstruction of the coronary arteries cannot be expected, since regional contractile force is diminished. In the surrounding septal area a decreased perfusion reserve is present in which ^{18}FDG uptake is increased. Decreased viability is assumed to be caused by myocardial infarctions and areas of fibrosis due to long standing myocardial ischemia much in the same way as in occlusive coronary artery disease.

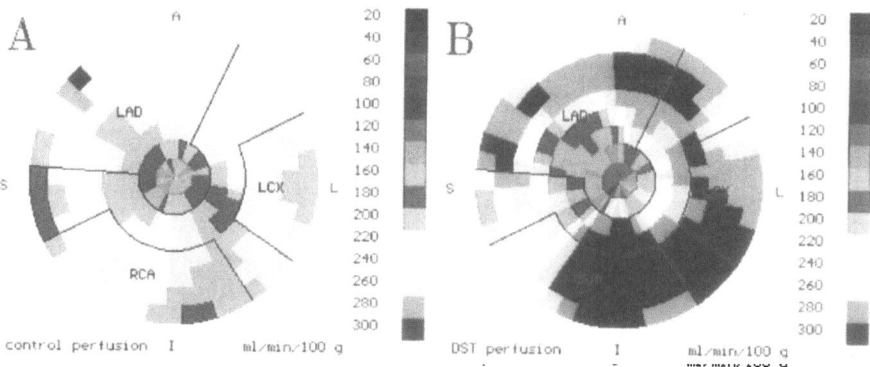

Figure 3. Functional polar maps of myocardial perfusion in the control situation (A) and during a dipyridamole stress test (B) obtained by $^{13}NH_3$ PET, from a 16 year old female with severe hypertrophic cardiomyopathy. It can be noticed that in the septal and apical region perfusion actually decreases during the dipyridamole stress test. This indicates to dynamic obstruction in the LAD or septal vessels. Note that myocardial perfusion is abnormally high during the control situation in the whole myocardium (180 - 300 ml/min/100 g). At the right side of the polar maps a color scale is given which indicates myocardial perfusion in ml/min/100 g of myocardial tissue. Regions as indicated in Figure 2. (see for colourplate of this figure page 245).

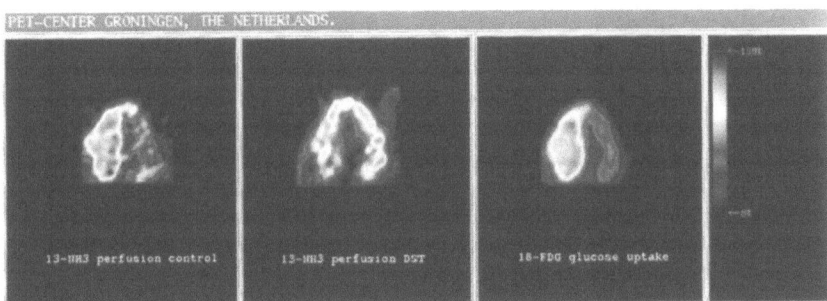

Figure 4. Horizontal long axis images of control perfusion (A), dipyridamole stress test perfusion (B) and ^{18}FDG uptake (C) from a 54-year male with old hypertrophic cardiomyopathy (patient nr 7), who underwent a successful myotomy/myectomy 7 years before, but continued to experience angina pectoris class III NYHA. Septal perfusion is increased compared to the lateral wall in the control situation. During the dipyridamole stress test, perfusion decreases especially in the subendocardial region. ^{18}FDG uptake is increased in the septum especially in the subendocardial region. The combination of these findings points to inducible ischemia in the septum, most prominently in the subendocardial region. (see for colourplate of this figure page 245).

Necropsy studies in hypertrophic cardiomyopathy have frequently shown areas of myocardial fibrosis and even transmural infarctions.[3,4] Perrone-Filardi et al.[3] recently described a relationship with left ventricular function and ^{18}FDG defects. In younger patients Kagaya et al.[4] observed a more heterogeneous uptake of ^{18}FDG than in middle aged and older patients, whereas Nienaber et al.[5] reported a prevalence of mismatch flow defects at exercise in younger patients. Probably at younger age, alterations in myocardial perfusion resulting in myocardial ischemia are more pronounced due to an increased oxygen consumption caused by myocardial fiber disarray and dynamic

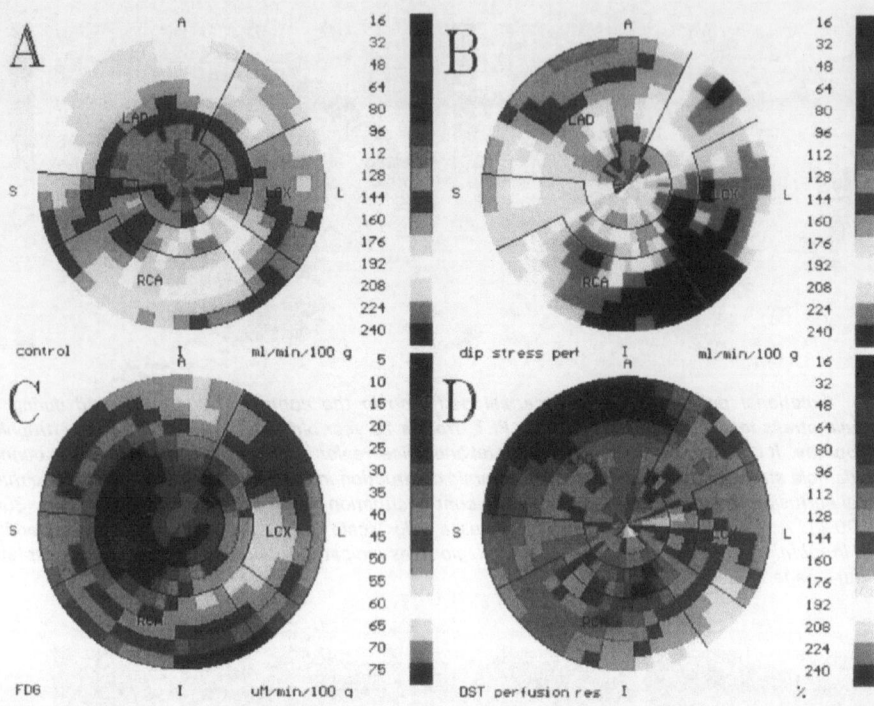

Figure 5. Parametric polar maps of myocardial perfusion (A) at rest, during a dipyridamole stress test (B), of ^{18}FDG uptake (C) and of dipyridamole stress test perfusion reserve (D) in a 57-year old male patient with symptoms of diminished exercise tolerance and angina. An inhomogeneous pattern of perfusion is present with decreased perfusion in the septal and apical regions and increased perfusion indicating increased oxygen consumption in the anterior and inferior regions. A viability defect can be observed in the septum. In this region baseline perfusion is decreased, but perfusion reserve is normal. A decreased perfusion reserve area is found in the anterior region. The combination of a viability defect in the septum and a mismatch defect in the anterior region indicates myocardial ischemia and fibrosis in different myocardial regions despite normal coronary arteries. The color scales at the right side of the perfusion polar map is as indicated in figure 3. The color scale at the right side of the ^{18}FDG polar map indicates glucose uptake in μmol/min/100 g of myocardial tissue. Regions as indicated in figure 2.   (see for colourplate of this figure page 246).

systolic obstruction of the septal arteries. In younger patients also sudden death is a more frequent event, possibly due to lethal arrhythmias elicited by ischemia and/or reperfusion. During the natural course of the disease myocardial fibrosis may develop gradually in the ischemic areas resulting in a progressive deterioration of left ventricular systolic function. These fibrotic areas may function as arrhythmogenic foci able to trigger ventricular arrhythmias at any time, whereas the extent of myocardial fibrosis determines the potential but infrequent occurrence of left ventricular dilatation with symptoms of heart failure. Diastolic dysfunction, which is the most characteristic finding in hypertrophic cardiomyopathy patients, may be caused by myocardial ischemia at younger age, and by myocardial fibrosis at older age next to increased wall thickness.

Conclusion

The present study showed that with PET using $^{13}NH_3$ for myocardial perfusion imaging and ^{18}FDG for glucose uptake imaging, especially when analyzed with our automated parametric polar map display, the blood flow and metabolic condition of the myocardium in patients with hypertrophic cardiomyopathy can be studied accurately and extensively. *Myocardial fiber disarray* can be recognized as areas with increased resting perfusion, while *myocardial ischemia* can be detected by decreased reaction of perfusion during a dipyridamole stress test associated with sustained or increased ^{18}FDG uptake. *Myocardial fibrosis* can be demonstrated as areas with a metabolic ^{18}FDG uptake defect. The condition of the myocardium in patients with hypertrophic cardiomyopathy is the most important prognostic determinant, and the presence and extent of myocardial ischemia as a potentially treatable cause of symptoms and sudden death has distinct therapeutic implications. For instance, the PET finding of myocardial ischemia may institute anti-ischemic therapy. Therefore, in symptomatic hypertrophic cardiomyopathy patients, myocardial ischemia and metabolism should preferably be studied by positron emission tomography.

References

1. Maron BJ, Bonow RO, Cannon RO, Leon MB, Epstein SE. Hypertrophic cardiomyopathy. Interrelations of clinical manifestations, pathophysiology, and therapy. N Engl J Med 1987;316:780-89,844-52.
2. Camici P, Chiriatti G, Lorenzoni R et al. Coronary vasodilation is impaired in both hypertrophied and non-hypertrophied myocardium of patients with hypertrophic cardiomyopathy: a study with nitrogen-13 ammonia and positron emission tomography. J Am Coll Cardiol 1991;17:879-86.
3. Perrone-Filardi P, Bacharach SL, Dilsizian V, Panza JA, Maurea S, Bonow RO. Regional systolic function, myocardial blood flow and glucose uptake at rest in hypertrophic cardiomyopathy. Am J Cardiol 1993;72:199-204.
4. Kagaya Y, Ishide N, Takeyama D et al. Differences in myocardial fluoro-18 2-deoxyglucose uptake in young versus older patients with hypertrophic cardiomyopathy. Am J Cardiol 1992;69:242-6.
5. Nienaber CA, Gambhir SS, Vaghaiwalla Mody F, Ratib R, Huang SC. Regional myocardial blood flow and glucose utilization in symptomatic patients with hypertrophic cardiomyopathy. Circulation 1993;87:1580-90.
6. Blanksma PK, Willemsen ATM, Meeder JG et al. Quantitative myocardial mapping of perfusion and metabolism using parametric polar map displays in cardiac PET. J Nucl Med 1995;36:1-6.
7. Schelbert HR, Phelps ME, Huang SC et al. N-13 ammonia as an indicator of myocardial blood flow. Circulation 1981;63:1259-72.
8. Wisenberg G, Schelbert HR, Hoffman EJ et al. In vivo quantification of regional myocardial blood flow by positron emission tomography. Circulation 1981;63:1248-58.
9. Sha A, Schelbert HR, Schwaiger M et al. Measurement of regional myocardial blood flow with N-13 ammonia and positron emission tomography in intact dogs. J Am Coll Cardiol 1985;5:92-100.
10. Bellina CR, Parodi O, Camici P et al. Simultaneous in vitro and in vivo validation of nitrogen-13-ammonia for the assessment of regional myocardial blood flow. J Nucl Med 1990;31:1335-43.
11. Krivokapich J, Huang SC, Phelps ME et al. Estimation of myocardial metabolic rate for glucose using fluorodeoxyglucose. Am J Physiol 1980;238:E69.
12. Ratib O, Phelps ME, Huang SC, Henze E, Sellin C, Schelbert HR. The deoxyglucose method for the estimation of local myocardial glucose metabolism with positron emission tomography. J Nucl Med 1982;23:577.
13. Porenta G, Kuhle W, Czernin J et al. Semiquantitative assessment of myocardial blood flow and viability using polar map displays of cardiac PET images. J Nucl Med 1992;33:1628-36.
14. Patlak CS, Blasberg RG, Fenstermacher JD. Graphical evaluation of blood-to-brain transfer constants from multiple time uptake data. J Cerebral Blood Flow Metab 1985;5:584-90.
15. Gambhir SS, Schwaiger M, Huang SC et al. Simple non-invasive quantitative method for measuring myocardial glucose utilization in humans employing positron emission tomography and fluorine-18 desoxyglucose. J Nucl Med 1989;30:359-66.
16. Hicks RJ, Herman WH, Kalff V et al. Quantitative evaluation of regional substrate metabolism in the human heart by positron emission tomography. J Am Coll Cardiol 1991;18:101-11.

12   TREATMENT OF HYPERTROPHIC OBSTRUCTIVE CARDIOMYOPATHY WITH PACING

Lukas Kappenberger, Xavier Jeanrenaud,
and Nicole Aebischer

Introduction

Hemodynamic, metabolic or genetic disorders can lead to hypertrophy of the heart muscle. The hypertrophy is, whatever its cause, the source of symptoms such as dyspnea, syncope, angina or sudden death. Primary hypertrophic cardiomyopathy may present under 3 different forms: apical hypertrophy, diffuse hypertrophy, and asymmetric septal hypertrophy. This last form, when associated with obstruction, is referred as hypertrophic obstructive cardiomyopathy, a disease with a significant morbidity and mortality. The most common causes of mortality, with a reported annual of rate 3 to 8%,[1] are sudden cardiac death due to arrhythmias or congestive heart failure. Medical therapy is considered as initial treatment and includes betablockers, calcium antagonists and disopyramid.[2,3] For drug refractory patients, surgical therapy consisting of septal myotomy, myotomy-myectomy and eventually mitral valve replacement or repair has been performed with good results.[4] However, morbidity and mortality due to this intervention is not negligible.[5]

Over the last few years, hypertrophic obstructive cardiomyopathy has been proposed as a new indication for cardiac pacing, even in the absence of conduction system disease.[6,7] It has been shown to be effective in reducing the subaortic pressure gradient during hemodynamic investigations and also in relieving symptoms. Although the effect of single chamber right ventricular pacing on left ventricular outflow tract gradient has been reported many years ago,[8] this treatment was not considered valuable at long term due to reduced cardiac output. With the evolution of dual chamber pacemaker (DDD), this old idea could be reconsidered and proposed as a long-term treatment, as no hemodynamic deterioration was observed during acute testing with preservation of atrioventricular synchrony.[9] In this chapter we will analyze the mechanisms leading to acute hemodynamic improvement in patients with hypertrophic obstructive cardiomyopathy and discuss the mechanisms which might explain the long-term benefit of this promising new therapy.

149

E. E. van der Wall et al. (eds.), Cardiac Positron Emission Tomography, 149–155.
© 1995 Kluwer Academic Publishers.

Hemodynamic modification of acute pacing intervention

Hemodynamic studies have shown that approximately 75% of patients with classic hypertrophic obstructive cardiomyopathy develop a significant drop in the resting left ventricular outflow tract pressure gradient during DDD pacing.[6,7] This beneficial effect is seen only with an optimal atrioventricular (AV) delay. The optimal AV delay should be long enough to allow optimal left ventricular filling, and short enough to permit full ventricular capture. These two features are clue factors to the mechanisms of pacing in hypertrophic obstruction. Full cardiomyopathy ventricular capture by apical stimulation of the right ventricular apex results in early activation of the left ventricular apical region. It could be documented with angiographic analysis, that early apical activation, called apical pre-excitation, leads to emptying of the apical chamber before bulging of the ventricular septum occurs. Most of the left ventricular stroke volume is therefore ejected before septal activation occurs associated with obstruction of the outflow tract. Another mechanism might be a slower contraction of the myocardium due to a slower electrical activation by non His-Purkinje system (HPS). This "betablocker-like effect" of pacing might reduce contractility and thereby blood flow velocity and therefore the gradient within the obstructed area. The fourth effect is indirectly related to the outflow activation sequence and reduced contractility. A clue factor in hypertrophic obstructive cardiomyopathy is the anterior position of the mitral valve. If the channel between mitral valve and the hypertrophied septum is too narrow, a Venturi effect contributes to further aspiration of the mitral valve, referred to as systolic anterior motion (SAM). With pacing however, as flow velocities are reduced and septal bulging occurs late, mitral valve anterior motion will appear later, and the duration of the septum-mitral valve contact will be shortened.

The atrial contribution in the non-compliant left ventricle is of further importance. It is well known that a reduction in left ventricular volume increases the left ventricular outflow tract pressure gradient, as during the Valsalva manoeuvre or the inhalation of amylnitrit. Timed atrial systole increases left ventricular end-diastolic volume. It is conceivable that a larger left ventricular cavity results in a wider outflow tract, at least at the beginning of systolic contraction, resulting in less obstruction. Therefore careful attention has to be given when analyzing pacing effects in relation to a well timed atrial contraction. In our experience the reduction in left ventricular outflow pressure gradient varied greatly with the programmed AV delay.[6] Left ventricular outflow tract pressure gradient dropped progressively from 80 ± 41 mmHg during pacing at 90 beats/minute to 61 ± 37 mmHg during DDD pacing with AV interval of 50-90 milliseconds ($P < 0.002$) to 52 ± 35 mmHg during DDD pacing with an AV interval 90-100 milliseconds ($P < 0.002$) and than rose again to 62 ± 46 mmHg during DDD pacing with an AV interval of 100 to 150 milliseconds ($P < 0.009$). This U-curved correlation between AV interval and gradient reflects the situation between Scylla and Charybdis, where to much of AV shortening is as deleterious as incomplete left ventricular capture with to long AV intervals. Note that in these experiments, the cardiac output and mean arterial pressure remained unchanged. At the individual optimal AV interval, the left ventricular outflow tract gradient falls significantly by 43% from 82 ± 42 mmHg during AAI pacing to 47 ± 34 mmHg during DDD pacing ($P < 0.002$). Based on these observations, actually confirmed by other groups performing similar experiments,[7,10] the use of long-term pacing to treat outflow tract obstruction in drug refractory patients, before undergoing surgery, seemed appropriate and was therefore offered to a limited number of patients. The result of these are reported in the following section.

Permanent pacing in hypertrophic cardiomyopathy

In the 8 patients permanently implanted with DDD pacing, the pressure gradient obtained by echo-Doppler examination immediately after permanent implantation was similar to the one obtained a few days before, during the acute hemodynamic measurements.[6] All patients remained on verapamil and betablocker treatment after pacemaker implantation and had the AV interval programmed to the optimal value which was 63±80 milliseconds on average. In all patients, there was a striking improvement, particularly with respect to angina which improved from NYHA class 3.0 to 0.9 and dyspnea which improved from NYHA class 2.6 to 1.7.

Doppler evaluation was repeated at mid-term (11±10 months) and long-term (44±11 months) follow-up. At long-term follow-up, the mean resting left ventricular outflow tract pressure gradient was 17±10 mmHg, which was significantly lower than the mid-term follow-up, or immediately after implant. When the pacemaker was switched off after one year of pacing, the mean resting outflow tract pressure gradient rose only to 31±36 mmHg, which was significantly lower than at the start of the study. Similarly, Fananapazir et al.[7] observed a reduction of the resting outflow tract pressure gradient compared to pre-implantation value already at six weeks after pacemaker implantation, when the pacemaker was switched off. Several patients with syncopes prior to permanent pacemaker implantation were reported free of syncopal episode after this intervention. Similarly, episodes of atrial fibrillation seem to be less common. Two observations made in patients with the loss of full ventricular pre-excitation due to shortening of the intrinsic AV interval are very instructive. Both patients were limited during a pre-implantation exercise test due to dyspnea and lightheadedness. The symptoms occurred at an exercise level below 100 watts. After pacemaker implantation, exercise tolerance dramatically improved, and both patients could exceed 150 watts. However, if during exercise the intrinsic PR interval shortened and the QRS complex changed from pacemaker activated to narrowed HPS-activation, syncope occurred in both due to dramatic drop in blood pressure. Although there was no immediate echocardiographer available at that moment, the symptomatology was compatible with recurrence of severe outflow tract obstruction. This observation shows the importance of optimal pacemaker set-up in hypertrophic obstructive cardiomyopathy. Although the basic principle is that of a dual chamber pacemaker, the condition to warrant full ventricular capture throughout the full heart rate spectrum and even during exercise is essential. The atrial activity is detected with delay only and ·a short programmed AV interval during atrial sensing does not implicit a short mechanically AV delay. Therefore AV intervals programmed as short as 25 milliseconds might be necessary. Moreover a rate adaptive AV delay is a useful additional feature in view of the above mentioned experiences. As many patients remain on drug treatment, at least during the first few months after pacemaker implantation (mainly to maintain a prolonged PR interval), chronotropic incompetence is frequently encountered.[11] It could be argued whether this chronotropic incompetence is a consequence of the drug or is related to hypertrophic cardiomyopathy. In any case, a rate responsive mode might be an additional useful feature. As atrial arrhythmias are a common complication in hypertrophic obstructive cardiomyopathy, although less common after pacing, we have to be prepared for sudden acceleration of the atrial rhythm. Patients with hypertrophic obstructive cardiomyopathy will be very sensitive to sudden rate acceleration and a system with automatic mode-switching or fall-back, to control rate of ventricular pacing during supraventricular tachyarrhythmias, is recommended.

The optimal AV interval

The selection of a complex and multiprogrammable dual chamber rate responsive pacemaker gives the opportunity to adapt the AV delay as discussed above. As long as there is a normal PR interval, the optimal AV delay will always be a compromise. On one hand, it must be as late as possible to have the full benefit of atrial systole which is of paramount importance in the uncompliant ventricle, such as in hypertrophic obstructive cardiomyopathy, and on the other hand, it should be short enough to result in full ventricular capture which can be easily identified on the ECG, when the QRS complex is as large as possible. It might be possible that in order to fulfil the second criteria, the resulting PR interval will be too short with regard to the hemodynamic effect of atrial contribution. Under these circumstances, AV nodal ablation might be of additional benefit. In fact, it has been reported that radiofrequency AV nodal ablation might be useful in this situation to achieve optimalization of the AV interval and so to ensure pacemaker control of ventricular depolarization.[12] Such an approach can lead to significant improvement in patients who fail to benefit from pacing alone. These problems in choosing optimal interval will be even more pronounced during rapid heart rate such as during exercise. To warrant appropriate function over the whole range of frequencies, patients must therefore undergo an exercise test to determine the optimal AV delay and whether they can maintain a paced ventricular rhythm at all times.

Reflections on long-term evolution

Having adapted the pacemaker treatment to optimize the acute hemodynamic parameters, long-term treatment has shown to be even more beneficial than the acute testing would anticipate. It is our impression that the reduction of the subaortic obstruction diminishes the stimulus for septal hypertrophy, for example by reducing the sheer forces that stimulate growth. On the other hand, electrical stimulation of the heart changes completely the activation sequence, not only in regard of the electric wave front but also, however not investigated at all, with regard to left ventricular mechanism and motion. It is anticipated that such important influences will result in remodelling of the left ventricle. In fact, it has been shown in animal experiments that pacing results in a different geometry of left ventricular muscle mass.[13] Observations published so far in humans do not yet allow the same conclusions. In contrast, the clinical evolution is well proven[6,7,14] and shows unanimously an important reduction of the typical symptoms of hypertrophic obstructive cardiomyopathy. Apart from these subjective criteria, McDonald et al.[14] could document an impressive improvement in exercise tolerance. Note that these results have been mainly obtained while continuing the medical treatment with calcium antagonist and betablocking agents. Comparing our clinical results obtained by drug and pacemaker therapy to surgical therapy, as reported in the literature, reveals that both are equally beneficial.[4,15] It is evident however that pacemaker implantation is a small step resulting in minimal morbidity and no mortality. The surgical approach which includes myotomy, myectomy, and eventually mitral valve replacement is of course a major intervention. Pacemaker therapy could be considered, in the view of the observations described so far, as a first line treatment for drug refractory cases, and surgery only reserved for those patients who remain symptomatic. It is noteworthy to state however that none of the patients selected so far in our study,[6] had to undergo later a surgical intervention for this disease although they were primarily referred to the centers for this indication.

How to explain the effect of pacing in hypertrophic obstructive cardiomyopathy

Five different mechanisms have to be considered as having potential impact on acute modification of left ventricular functions.

First: the modification of the activation sequence of the left ventricle results in a delayed septal activation, and therefore obstruction of the outflow tract occurs only late in systole. This allows the major part of the stroke volume to be ejected before septal bulging or systolic anterior motion of the mitral valve occurs.

Second: the change in septal motion will modify mitral valve movement. Systolic anterior displacement of the anterior mitral valve leaflet will occur later during systole and the obstruction period will be shortened.

Third: as mitral valve incompetence in hypertrophic obstructive cardiomyopathy is considered to be a consequence of abnormal left ventricular geometry and aspiration of the mitral valve leaflet towards the septum, changing mitral valve and septal movement will result in reduced valve incompetence.

Fourth: with electrical stimulation, the time to full depolarization of the left ventricle is importantly delayed. This delayed spread-out will result in a delayed mechanical activation. The overall contraction period will be prolonged, reducing thereby maximal contractility and ejection velocity. This parameter, considered generally to be a negative effect of pacing might correct the hypercontractility in hypertrophic cardiomyopathy. It has been argued that this mechanism should also be helpful in non-obstructive hypertrophic cardiomyopathy but so far this hypothesis could not be proven.

Fifth: an altered activation sequence, delayed contraction, and reduced contractility will result in reduced flow velocity. As flow velocity is defining the gradient, the sheer forces on the septum and the Venturi effect on the mitral valve must have an important influence on the gradient. To simplify, pacing can be considered as having a betablocker-like effect on myocardial contractility parameters.

In conclusion we could show that pacing acutely reduces deleterious hemodynamic effects associated with hypertrophic obstructive cardiomyopathy. This effect, when applied on a long-term basis with the implantation of a pacemaker, results in further hemodynamic, but also clinical and symptomatic improvement. It appears that angina, dyspnea, episodes of atrial fibrillation, and syncope are all beneficially influenced with this treatment. Little is known about the potential mechanisms leading to this convincing clinical results. Therefore further studies are urgently needed, not only comparing the different therapeutic possibilities for this disease, but also evaluating the principles of pacemaker induced modifications of myocardial function.

References

1. Duport GM, Valeix B, Lefevre J et al. Intérêt de la stimulation ventriculaire droite permanente dans la cardiomyopathie obstructive. Nouv Presse Med 1978;32:2868-9.
2. Harrison DC, Braunwald E, Glick G, Mason DT, Chidsey CA, Ross Jr J. Effects of beta-adrenergic blockade on the circulation, with particular references to observations in patients with hypertrophic subaortic stenosis. Circulation 1964;29:84-98.
3. Kaltenbach M, Hopf R, Kober G, Bussmann W-D, Keller M, Petersen Y. Treatment of hypertrophic obstructive cardiomyopathy with verapamil. Br Heart J 1979;42:35-42.
4. Ten Berg JM, Suttorp MJ, Knaepen PJ, Ernst S, Vermeulen FEE, Jaarsma W. Hypertrophic obstructive cardiomyopathy: initial results and long-term follow-up after morrow septal myectomy. Circulation 1994;90:1781-5.
5. McIntosh CL, Maron BJ. Current operative treatment of obstructive hypertrophic cardiomyopathy. Circulation 1988;78:487-95.
6. Jeanrenaud X, Goy JJ, Kappenberger L. Effects of dual-chamber pacing in hypertrophic obstructive cardiomyopathy. Lancet 1992;339:1318-23.
7. Fananapazir L, Cannon RO, Tripodi D, Panza JA. Impact of dual-chamber permanent pacing in patients with obstructive hypertrophic cardiomyopathy with symptoms refractory to verapamil and b-adrenergic blocker therapy. Circulation 1992;85:2149-61.
8. Hassenstein P, Wolter HH. Therapeutische Beherrschung einer bedrohlichen Situation bei der idiopatischen hypertrophischen Subaortenstenose. Verh Dtsch Ges Kreislaufforsch 1967;33:242-6.
9. Duck JH, Hutschenreiter W, Pankau H, Trenchmann H. Vorhofsynchrone Ventrikelstimulation mit verjkurtzer AV verzogerungszeit als therapieprinzip der hypertrophischen obstruktiven kardiomyopathie. Z Gesamte Inn Med 1984;39:437-47.
10. Erwin J, McWilliams E, Gearty G, Maurer B. Haemodynamic and symptomatic improvement using dual chamber pacing in hypertrophic cardiomyopathy. Br Heart J 1985;54:641A (Abstract).
11. Slade AKB, Keeling PJ, Prased K, Page C, McKenna WJ. Hypertrophic cardiomyopathy: pacing and defibrillator therapy. J Am Coll Cardiol 1994;1A-484A,705-1 (Abstract).
12. Page A, Boudaut R, Bemurat M, Clementy J, Levy S, Besse P. Importance of sequential atrioventricular pacing in obstructive myocardiopathy with atrioventricular block. Arch Mal Coeur 1979;72:1253-58.
13. Prinzen FW, Augustijn CH, Arts T, Allessie MA, Reneman RS. Redistribution of myocardial fiber strain and blood flow by asynchronous activation. Am J Physiol 1990;259:H300-8.
14. McDonald K, McWilliams E, OKeefe B, Maurer B. Functional assessment of patients treated with permanent dual chamber pacing as a primary treatment for hypertrophic cardiomyopathy. Eur Heart J 1988;9:893-98.
15. Seiler C, Hess OM, Schoenbeck M et al. Long-term follow-up of medical versus surgical therapy for hypertrophic cardiomyopathy: a retrospective study. J Am Coll Cardiol 1991;17:634-42.

13 HEART FAILURE AND THE CARDIAC BETA-ADRENOCEPTOR

Otto-Erich Brodde

Introduction

In the human heart contractility and heart rate are regulated by receptor systems that act through accumulation of intracellular cAMP (G_s-protein coupled), by receptor systems that act through inhibition of cAMP formation (G_i-protein coupled) and by receptor systems that act independently of cAMP formation possibly through the phospholipase C/diacylglycerol/inositol-1,4,5-triphosphate (PLC/DAG/IP3)-pathway (Figure 1). Among all these receptors the ß-adrenoceptor-G_s-protein-adenylate cyclase-cAMP system is the most powerful physiological mechanism to alter acutely contractility and heart rate. This chapter, deals with the properties of ß-adrenoceptors in the human heart and their alterations in chronic heart failure.

ß₁- and ß₂-adrenoceptors in the nonfailing human heart

In the human heart both, ß₁- and ß₂-adrenoceptors coexist; this has been first demonstrated by radioligand binding studies, and was subsequently confirmed by functional experiments.[1-4] The number of ß-adrenoceptors is quite evenly distributed in right and left atrial and ventricular tissue; however, the proportion of ß₂-adrenoceptors is somewhat higher in the atria (approximately 1/3 of the total ß-adrenoceptor population) than in ventricular myocardium (about 20% of the total ß-adrenoceptor population,[5,6] and may be even higher (up to 50%) in the atrio-ventricular conducting system.[7]

Both ß₁- and ß₂-adrenoceptors couple to adenylate cyclase and cause increases in the intracellular amount of cAMP.[8-11] Interestingly, in the human heart adenylate cyclase is preferentially activated by ß₂-adrenoceptor stimulation although ß₁-adrenoceptors predominate: in human right atrial membranes ß₂-adrenoceptor selective agonists such as fenoterol, procaterol and terbutaline caused activation of adenylate cyclase activity

E. E. van der Wall et al. (eds.), Cardiac Positron Emission Tomography, 157–169.

Receptor Systems in the Human Myocardium

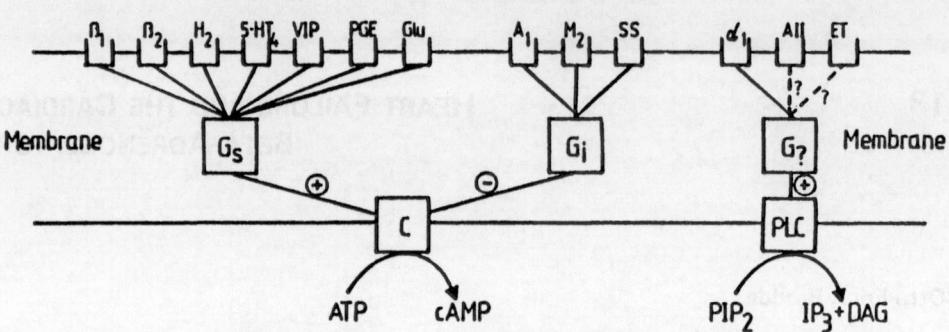

Positive Inotropic Effect (% of Isoprenaline·Maximum)

	Right Atrium	Ventricular Myocardium
H_2	80-85%	30-40%
$5\text{-}HT_4$	25-55%	??? (0)
VIP	???	40%
PGE_1	???	???
Glu	???	???
α_1	???	15-45%
A II	30-45%	??? (0)
ET-1	35-45%	???

Figure 1. Receptor systems and their signal-transduction mechanisms in the non-failing human heart. For details see text.
Abbreviations: β_1, β_2, α_1 = β_1-, β_2- and α_1-adrenoceptors; H_2 = histamine H2-receptors; $5\text{-}HT_4$ = $5\text{-}HT_4$-receptors; VIP = vasoactive intestinal peptide receptors; PGE_1 = prostaglandin E_1-receptors; Glu = glucagon receptors; A_1 = adenosine A_1-receptors; M_2 = muscarinic M_2-receptors; SS = somatostatin-receptors; A II = angiotensin II-receptors; ET = endothelin-receptors; G_S = stimulatory guanine nucleotide binding protein; G_i = inhibitory guanine nucleotide binding protein; C = catalytic unit of adenylate cyclase; PLC = phospholipase C; PIP_2 = phosphatidylinositol 4,5-bis-phosphate; DAG = 1,2-diacylglycerol; IP3 = inositol-1,4,5-trisphosphate;
ISO = isoprenaline; $\oplus$ = activation; $\ominus$ = inhibition.
Right atrium = positive inotropic effects were determined on isolated electrically driven right atria from patients without apparent heart failure undergoing coronary artery bypass grafting. Ventricular myocardium = positive inotropic effects were determined on isolated electrically driven right and left ventricular preparations obtained from would-be cardiac transplant donors.
From Brodde et al.[1]

that amounted to about 50-70% of that of isoprenaline[8,12,13] although only 30% of the total ß-adrenoceptor population is of the ß$_2$-subtype. Similarly, in ventricular membranes of the human heart the ß$_2$-adrenoceptor agonists terbutaline and zinterol caused 50% of maximal isoprenaline activation,[3,13] and isoprenaline, adrenaline, and noradrenaline evoked their stimulatory effects on adenylate cyclase activity predominantly via ß$_2$-adrenoceptor stimulation[3,10] although only 20% of the whole ß-adrenoceptor population is of the $ß_2$-subtype. The mechanism underlying the different coupling efficiencies of human cardiac $ß_1$- and $ß_2$-adrenoceptors to adenylate cyclase is not known at present. However, Green et al.[14] recently showed that in the mammalian fibroblast cell line CHW-1102 transfected with $ß_1$- or $ß_2$-adrenoceptor cDNA's the $ß_2$-adrenoceptor exhibited a much greater functional coupling to the adenylate cyclase than the $ß_1$-adrenoceptor. Similarly, Levy et al.[15] recently expressed human $ß_1$- and $ß_2$-adrenoceptors in permanent cell lines and found that activation of $ß_2$-adrenoceptors causes much larger activation of adenylate cyclase than did $ß_1$-adrenoceptors. Thus, it might be a general phenomenon that $ß_2$-adrenoceptors couple more efficiently to adenylate cyclase than $ß_1$-adrenoceptors.

In vitro experiments have convincingly shown that both $ß_1$- and $ß_2$-adrenoceptors mediate the positive inotropic effects of ß-adrenoceptor agonists in isolated electrically driven atrial and ventricular preparations[2,4,5,10,16] this has recently also been demonstrated in single myocytes from human ventricle.[17] Among the classical catecholamines isoprenaline and adrenaline cause their positive inotropic effects via stimulation of $ß_1$- and $ß_2$-adrenoceptors, while noradrenaline, the endogenous transmitter of the sympathetic nervous system, evokes its positive inotropic effect nearly exclusively via $ß_1$-adrenoceptor stimulation.[10,18] In right and left atria $ß_1$- and $ß_2$-adrenoceptor stimulation can evoke maximum positive inotropic effects, while on the right and left ventricle only $ß_1$-adrenoceptor stimulation can evoke maximum positive inotropic effects and $ß_2$-adrenoceptor stimulation has only submaximal positive inotropic effects.[3,10,18]

In vivo experiments in humans have confirmed that $ß_2$-adrenoceptors can mediate positive chronotropic and inotropic effects of ß-adrenoceptor agonists. Several studies have shown that isoprenaline-induced tachycardia in humans is mediated by both $ß_1$-and $ß_2$-adrenoceptors to about the same degree, while exercise-induced tachycardia (which is mainly due to neuronally released noradrenaline), is mediated solely by $ß_1$-adrenoceptor stimulation[5,19] - in close agreement with the in vitro data on isolated human right atria.

Moreover, in healthy volunteers the positive chronotropic effect caused by intravenous infusions of terbutaline was only marginally affected by the $ß_1$-adrenoceptor selective antagonists atenolol and bisoprolol given in doses that markedly inhibited $ß_1$-adrenoceptor mediated effects (Figure 2).[13,20,21] Finally, Hall et al.[22] have demonstrated that the positive chronotropic effect of salbutamol induced by injections into the right coronary artery of patients with chronic stable angina (thereby avoiding any systemic effects) was not affected by the $ß_1$-adrenoceptor selective antagonist practolol, but was significantly antagonized by propranolol indicating that it is mediated exclusively by cardiac $ß_2$-adrenoceptor stimulation. It is interesting to note, however, that - in contrast to the in vitro data - adrenaline appears to cause its positive chronotropic effect in vivo solely via cardiac $ß_2$-adrenoceptor stimulation. Thus, several authors have shown, that adrenaline-induced tachycardia is not affected by $ß_1$-selective antagonists such as metoprolol,[23] atenolol,[24] or bisoprolol[25] (Figure 2), but is completely abolished by the $ß_2$-selective antagonist ICI 118,551,[26] or by the non-selective ß-adrenoceptor antagonist propranolol[25] (Figure 2).

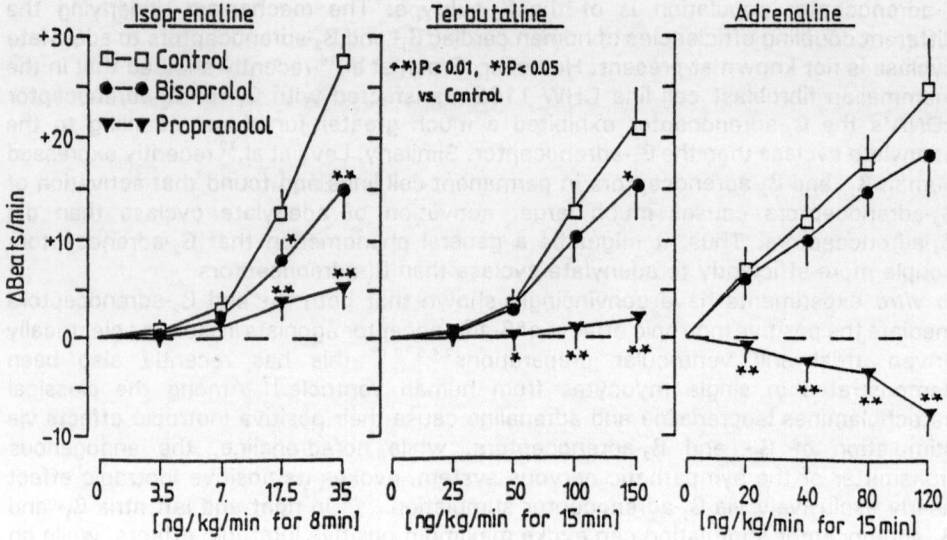

Figure 2. Effect of bisoprolol (15 mg orally 2 hours before infusion) or propranolol (5 mg i.v. 45 min before infusion) on isoprenaline-(left panel), terbutaline- (middle panel) or adrenaline- (right panel) infusion-induced increase in heart rate in 8 healthy male volunteers. Ordinate: Increase in heart rate in Δ beats/min; Abscissae: dose of the agonists in ng/kg/min. Means ± S.E.M. Modified from Daul et al.[25]

Using the β_2-adrenoceptor agonist terbutaline, at least two groups have convincingly shown that cardiac β_2-adrenoceptors can in vivo mediate also positive inotropic effects.[13,21] Moreover, Schäfers et al.[13] recently compared in healthy volunteers the positive chronotropic and inotropic effects induced by infusions of isoprenaline and terbutaline; they found that at doses that caused the same increase in heart rate isoprenaline caused larger positive inotropic effects than did terbutaline (Figure 3) - in close agreement with the in vitro observation that in human right atrium both β_1- and β_2-adrenoceptors cause maximal positive inotropic effects while in the ventricular myocardium only β_1-adrenoceptor stimulation caused maximal positive inotropic effects, and β_2-adrenoceptor stimulation evoked only submaximal positive inotropic effects.

Thus, the human heart shows quite a unique feature when compared with the heart of commonly used laboratory animals: it contains, in addition to β_1-adrenoceptors, a considerable amount of functional β_2-adrenoceptors that cause positive inotropic and chronotropic effects in vitro and in vivo. Moreover, in the human heart catecholamines activate adenylate cyclase mainly via β_2-adrenoceptor stimulation, although β_1-adrenoceptors predominate. And finally, the human heart does contain only a few spare receptors for β-adrenoceptor-mediated positive inotropic effects.[27-29] Because of this lack of a considerable receptor reserve any decrease in β-adrenoceptor number or reduction in coupling of the receptor to the adenylate cyclase will automatically lead to a reduction in functional responses to β-adrenoceptor stimulation.

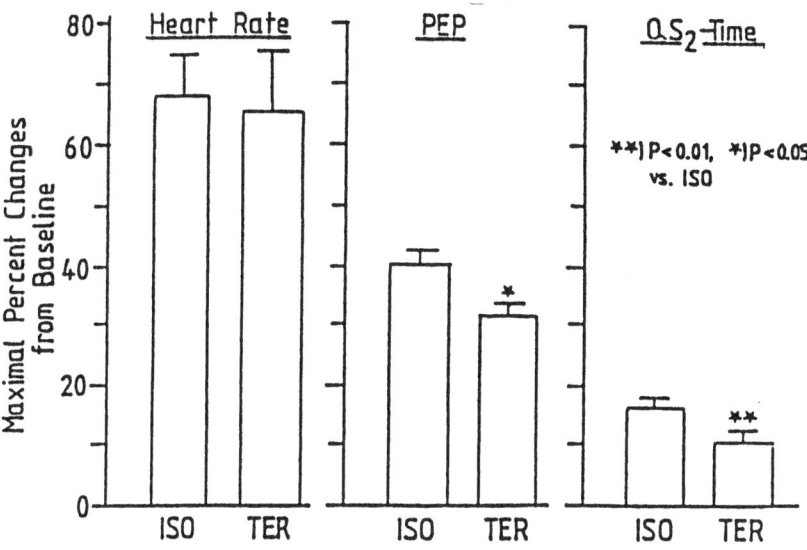

Figure 3. *Isoprenaline (ISO)- and terbutaline (TER)-infusion-induced maximal increases in heart rate and maximal shortening of pre-ejection-period (PEP) and heart-rate corrected QS$_2$-time in 7 male healthy volunteers. Ordinate: maximal increase in heart rate (left panel), and shortening of PEP (middle panel) and QS$_2$-time (right panel) expressed as maximal percent changes from baseline. Means ± S.E.M. Recalculated from Schäfers et al.[13]*

ß$_1$- and ß$_2$-adrenoceptors in the failing human heart

In chronic heart failure an increase in the activity of the sympathetic nervous system compensatorily to the reduced cardiac output seems to be initially a mechanism of the organism to aid the failing heart, but will subsequently lead to a down-regulation of cardiac ß-adrenoceptors.[16] Increased sympathetic activity in patients with chronic heart failure has been directly demonstrated in studies with peroneal nerve recordings of sympathetic efferent nerve traffic.[30] Furthermore, various authors have shown that in patients with chronic heart failure plasma noradrenaline levels are elevated,[31] and it has been suggested that plasma noradrenaline may serve as a predictor of the prognosis of the patients.[32] The mechanism underlying the increase in plasma catecholamines in chronic heart failure is not completely understood at present. It may be due to an increase in noradrenaline spillover from organs showing increased sympathetic drive such as heart and kidney[33,34] and a decrease in noradrenaline clearance.[34] Moreover, several studies have shown that in patients with chronic heart failure neuronal uptake of noradrenaline (uptake1) is markedly impaired.[5] This may lead to the well known finding that in chronic heart failure cardiac noradrenaline stores are (at least partly) depleted whereas plasma noradrenaline levels are elevated.[35,36] Thus, an enhanced release of endogenous noradrenaline and simultaneously a decreased cardiac neuronal uptake of noradrenaline may well lead to a prolonged increase in synaptic cleft noradrenaline concentrations. Since chronic exposure of a cell to agonists causes desensitization and finally down-regulation of cell-surface receptors,[37-39] it is well conceivable that under these pathological conditions cardiac ß-adrenoceptors are down-regulated.

This has in fact been first shown by Bristow et al.[40] who demonstrated by the use of radioligand binding studies that in severe heart failure the number of cardiac ß-adrenoceptors was markedly depressed when compared with non-failing hearts. Subsequently, many authors have confirmed these observations using different techniques: radioligand binding studies,[2,5,16] quantitative autoradiographic studies,[41] and very recently, in vivo positron emission tomography (PET) studies.[42]

However, β_1- and β_2-adrenoceptors are differentially changed in different forms of heart failure (Figure 4). While in all kinds of heart failure β_1-adrenoceptor number is decreased possibly because steady-state levels of β_1-adrenoceptor mRNA are reduced,[43,44] β_2-adrenoceptor number is unchanged in end-stage dilated cardiomyopathy[2,4,5,16] and possibly in aortic valve disease,[45,46] but it is decreased in mitral valve disease,[6,47] and in tetralogy of Fallot.[48] Divergent results have been reported on β_1- and β_2-adrenoceptor changes in end-stage ischemic cardiomyopathy: while Brodde et al.[48] and Steinfath et al.[46,49] found a concomitant decrease in β_1- and β_2-adrenoceptors in this disease, Bristow et al.[50,51] and Ungerer et al.[43] found only β_1-adrenoceptors to be decreased.

The decrease in ß-adrenoceptor number is accompanied by a reduction in isoprenaline-activated adenylate cyclase.[2,4,5] Since isoprenaline activates human cardiac adenylate cyclase mainly via β_2-adrenoceptor stimulation this indicates that even with an unchanged β_2-adrenoceptor number its function is reduced presumably because 1) recent data suggest that in end-stage dilated and ischemic cardiomyopathy steady state mRNA levels of ß-adrenergic receptor kinase (ARK) and the activity of ßARK are increased[43] leading to enhanced phosphorylation of both β_1- and β_2-adrenoceptors and by this to an uncoupling from the adenylate cyclase, and 2) several authors have convincingly demonstrated that in end-stage heart failure mRNA-levels[52,53] and tissue-amount of the cardiac inhibitory guanine nucleotide binding protein G_i is increased[5,54] thereby inhibiting cyclic AMP formation. In contrast to G_i-protein, human cardiac G_s-protein seems not be altered in chronic heart failure, as is the activity of the catalytic unit of the adenylate cyclase in end-stage heart failure obviously unchanged.[5,53]

Since the human heart contains only a few spare receptors for ß-adrenoceptor mediated positive inotropic effects it is not surprising that the reduced ß-adrenoceptor number and the impaired ability of ß-adrenoceptor stimulation to activate adenylate cyclase is accompanied by decreased contractile responses to ß-adrenoceptor agonists. Numerous authors have shown that in isolated electrically driven human myocardial preparations,[2,5,16] in single human cardiac myocytes,[55,56] and in vivo in patients with chronic heart failure[5,16,57] the positive inotropic and chronotropic effect to ß-adrenoceptor stimulation is decreased, while that to calcium^{2+} is only marginally affected. In all these studies it was consistently found that the extent of decrease in maximal positive inotropic effect (and in ß-adrenoceptor number) was directly related to the severity of the disease (judged clinically by NYHA classification, Figure 5). This is compatible with the view that the reason for the reduction in positive inotropic response to ß-adrenoceptor agonists is in fact the decrease in ß-adrenoceptor number.

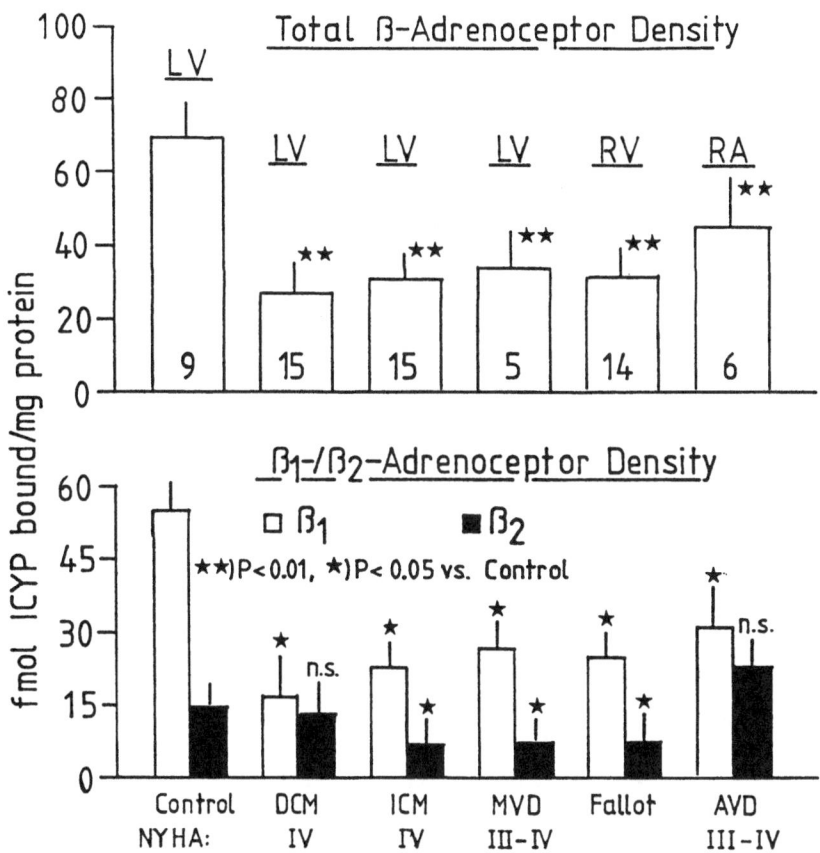

Figure 4. Total ß-, ß₁- and ß₂-adrenoceptor changes in different forms of heart failure. Upper panel: total ß-adrenoceptor density, determined from Scatchard-analysis of (-)-[¹²⁵I]iodocyanopindolol (ICYP) binding, in fmol ICYP specifically bound/mg protein. Lower Panel: ß₁- and ß₂-adrenoceptor densities in fmol ICYP specifically bound/mg protein. DCM = idiopathic dilated cardiomyopathy; ICM = ischemic cardiomyopathy; MVD = mitral valve disease; Fallot = tetralogy of Fallot; AVD = aortic valve disease. RA = right atrium; RV and LV = right and left ventricle. Means ± S.E.M., number of experiments at the bottom of the columns. From Brodde et al.[1]

Moreover, the in vitro studies on isolated human myocardial preparations clearly demonstrated that in all kinds of heart failure not only positive inotropic responses to ß₁-adrenoceptor stimulation were reduced (as to be expected, since ß₁-adrenoceptor number was consistently been found to be reduced, Figure 4) but also responses to

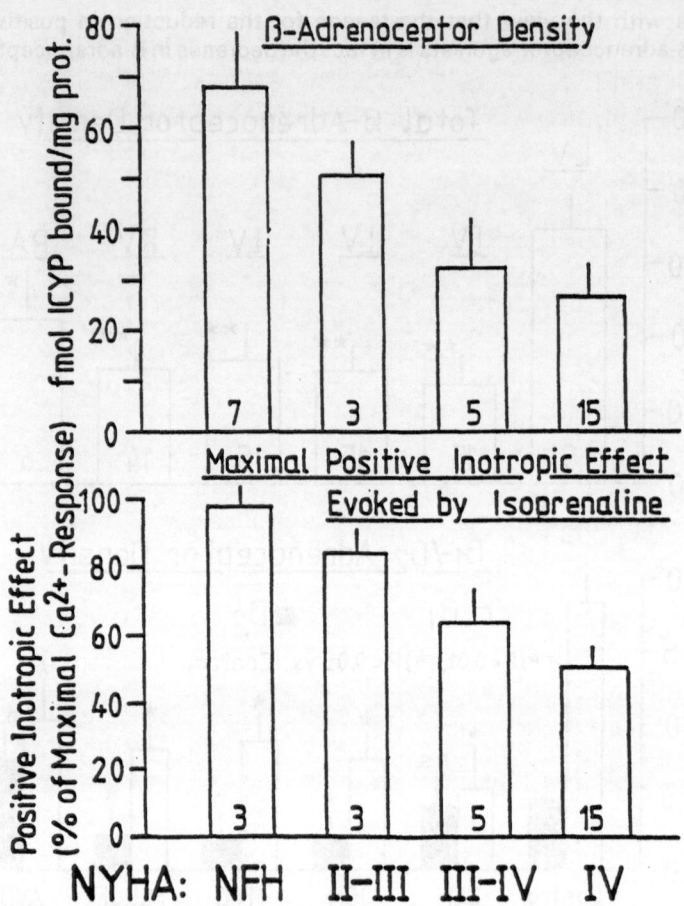

Figure 5. Left ventricular ß-adrenoceptor density (upper panel) and maximal positive inotropic effects evoked by isoprenaline on isolated electrically driven left ventricular preparations (lower panel) derived from patients with different degrees of heart failure (NFH = non-failing hearts; NYHA II-III and III-IV patients with mitral valve disease, NYHA IV: patients with end-stage dilated and/or ischemic cardiomyopathy). Ordinate, upper panel: Left ventricular ß-adrenoceptor density in fmol (-)-[125I]iodocyanopindolol (ICYP) specifically bound/mg protein; lower panel: Positive inotropic effect of isoprenaline in percent of maximal Ca^{2+}-response (that is not changed in end-stage heart failure).[5,16] Given are means ± SEM; number of experiments at the bottom of the columns. From Brodde et al.[47]

ß$_2$-adrenoceptor stimulation were diminished, presumably due to the uncoupling of the ß$_2$-adrenoceptors from the G$_s$-adenylate cyclase complex,[49-51] independently of whether ß$_2$-adrenoceptor number was reduced or not. From these findings it may be concluded that, if patients need acutely ß-adrenoceptor mediated positive inotropic support, non-selective full ß-adrenoceptor agonists should be more effective than partial ß-adrenoceptor agonists or ß$_1$- (or ß$_2$)- adrenoceptor selective agonists because stimulation of (even reduced or uncoupled) cardiac ß$_2$-adrenoceptors should cause positive inotropic effects additive to those via ß$_1$-adrenoceptor stimulation.

Conclusion

In the human heart there exist many receptor systems that regulate heart rate and contractility. Among these the ß-adrenoceptor-G-protein(s)-adenylate cyclase-cyclic AMP pathway is the most powerful mechanism to acutely increase contractility and heart rate. Compared to the heart of commonly used laboratory animals the human heart shows quite an unique feature: 1) it contains ß$_1$- and ß$_2$-adrenoceptors that both can mediate positive chronotropic and inotropic effects in vitro and in vivo; 2) ß$_2$-adrenoceptors are much more efficiently coupled to adenylate cyclase than ß$_1$-adrenoceptors; and 3) the human heart contains only a few spare receptors for ß-adrenoceptor-mediated positive inotropic effects and nearly all receptors must be occupied to reach maximal increases in force of contraction. Thus, any decrease in ß-adrenoceptor number and/or any situation which uncouples ß-adrenoceptors from the adenylate cyclase (for example in chronic heart failure) should automatically lead to a reduced positive inotropic response.

In chronic heart failure human cardiac ß$_1$-adrenoceptor number (because of the lack of spare receptors concomitantly inotropic responsiveness) is decreased presumably due to down-regulation by the - locally in the heart - enhanced released endogenous noradrenaline which is a rather selective ß$_1$-adrenoceptor agonist.[58] Cardiac ß$_2$-adrenoceptor number may or may not be reduced; however, its functional responsiveness is impaired possibly due to the increased amount and mRNA levels of the inhibitory G-protein G$_i$ and/or to enhanced phosphorylation by ßARK and, by this, uncoupling from the adenylate cyclase.

References

1. Brodde O-E, Hillemann S, Kunde K, Vogelsang M, Zerkowski H-R. Receptor systems affecting force of contraction in the human heart and their alterations in chronic heart failure. J Heart Lung Transplant 1992;11:S164-S74.
2. Jones CR, Molenaar P, Summers RJ. New views of human cardiac ß-adrenoceptors. J Mol Cell Cardiol 1989;21:519-35.
3. Bristow MR. Myocardial cell surface membrane receptors in heart failure. Heart Failure 1989;5:47-50.
4. Bristow MR, Hershberger RE, Port JD et al. ß-adrenergic pathways in nonfailing and failing human ventricular myocardium. Circulation 1990;82(Suppl I):I-12-I-25.
5. Brodde O-E. ß$_1$- and ß$_2$-Adrenoceptors in the human heart: properties, function, and alterations in chronic heart failure. Pharmacol Rev 1991;43:203-42.
6. Steinfath M, Lavicky J, Schmitz W, Scholz H, Döring V, Kalmar P. Regional distribution of ß$_1$- and ß$_2$-adrenoceptors in the failing and nonfailing human hearts. Eur J Clin Pharmacol 1992;42:607-12.
7. Elnatan J, Molenaar P, Summers RJ. Density and distribution of ß-adrenoceptor subtypes in human atrioventricular conducting system. Clin Exp Pharmacol Physiol 1991;(Suppl 18):16 (Abstract).
8. Brodde O-E, O'Hara N, Zerkowski H-R, Rohm N. Human cardiac ß-adrenoceptors: both ß$_1$- and ß$_2$-adrenoceptors are functionally coupled to the adenylate cyclase in right atrium. J Cardiovasc Pharmacol 1984;6:1184-91.
9. Bristow MR, Hershberger RE, Port JD, Minobe W, Rasmussen R. ß$_1$- and ß$_2$-adrenergic receptor-mediated adenylate cyclase stimulation in nonfailing and failing human ventricular myocardium. Mol Pharmacol 1989;35:295-303.
10. Kaumann AJ, Hall JA, Murray KJ, Wells FC, Brown MJ. A comparison of the effects of adrenaline and noradrenaline on human heart: the role of ß$_1$- and ß$_2$-adrenoceptors in the stimulation of adenylate cyclase and contractile force. Eur Heart J 1989;10(Suppl B):29-37.
11. Ikezono K, Michel MC, Zerkowski H-R, Beckeringh JJ, Brodde O-E. The role of cyclic AMP in the positive inotropic effect mediated by ß$_1$- and ß$_2$-adrenoceptors in isolated human right atrium. Naunyn-Schmiedeberg's Arch Pharmacol 1987;335:561-6.
12. Waelbroeck M, Taton G, Delhaye M et al. The human heart beta-adrenergic receptors. II. Coupling of beta2-adrenergic receptors with the adenylate cyclase system. Mol Pharmacol 1983;24:174-82.
13. Schäfers RF, Adler S, Daul A et al. Positive inotropic effect of the beta2-adrenoceptor agonist terbutaline in the human heart: effects of long-term beta1-adrenoceptor antagonist treatment. J Am Coll Cardiol 1994;23:1224-33.
14. Green SA, Holt BD, Liggett SB. ß$_1$- and ß$_2$-adrenergic receptors display subtype-selective coupling to G$_S$. Mol Pharmacol 1992;41:889-93.
15. Levy FO, Zhu X, Kaumann AJ, Birnbaumer L. Efficacy of ß$_1$-adrenergic receptors is lower than that of ß$_2$-adrenergic receptors. Proc Natl Acad Sci 1993;90:10798-802.
16. Feldman AM, Bristow MR. The ß-adrenergic pathway in the failing human heart: implications for inotropic therapy. Cardiology 1990;77(Suppl 1):1-32.
17. Del Monte F, Kaumann AJ, Poole-Wilson PA, Wynne DG, Pepper J, Harding SE. Coexistence of functioning ß$_1$- and ß$_2$-adrenoceptors in single myocytes from human ventricle. Circulation 1993;88:854-63.
18. Motomura S, Zerkowski H-R, Daul A, Brodde O-E. On the physiologic role of beta-2

adrenoceptors in the human heart: in vitro and in vivo studies. Am Heart J 1990;119:608-19.

19. McDevitt DG. In vivo studies on the function of cardiac ß-adrenoceptors in man. Eur Heart J 1989;10(Suppl B):22-8.

20. Strauss MH, Reeves RA, Smith DL, Leenen FHH. The role of cardiac beta-1 receptors in the hemodynamic response to a beta-2 agonist. Clin Pharmacol Ther 1986;40:108-15.

21. Levine MAH, Leenen FHH. Role of ß1-receptors and vagal tone in cardiac inotropic and chronotropic responses to a ß2-agonist in humans. Circulation 1989;79:107-15.

22. Hall JA, Petch MC, Brown MJ. Intracoronary injections of salbutamol demonstrate the presence of functional ß2-adrenoceptors in the human heart. Circ Res 1989;65:546-53.

23. Johnsson G. Influence of metoprolol and propranolol on hemodynamic effects induced by adrenaline and physical work. Acta Toxicol 1975;36(Suppl):59-68.

24. Leenen FHH, Chan YK, Smith DL, Reeves RA. Epinephrine and left ventricular function in humans: effects of beta-1 vs nonselective beta-blockade. Clin Pharmacol Ther 1988;43:519-28.

25. Daul A, Hermes U, Schäfers RF, Wenzel R, Von Birgelen C, Brodde O-E. The ß-adrenoceptor subtype(s) mediating adrenaline- and dobutamine-induced blood pressure and heart rate changes in healthy volunteers. Int J Clin Pharmacol Ther 1995;in press.

26. Brown MJ, Brown DC, Murphy MB. Hypokalemia from beta2-receptor stimulation by circulating epinephrine. N Engl J Med 1983;309:1414-9.

27. Kaumann AJ, Lemoine H, Schwederski-Menke U, Ehle B. Relations between ß-adrenoceptor occupancy and increases of contractile force and adenylate cyclase activity induced by catecholamines in human ventricular myocardium. Acute desensitization and comparison with feline ventricle. Naunyn-Schmiedeberg's Arch Pharmacol 1989;339:99-112.

28. Schwinger RHG, Böhm M, Erdmann E. Evidence against spare or uncoupled ß-adrenoceptors in the human heart. Am Heart J 1990;119:899-904.

29. Brown L, Deighton NM, Bals S et al. Spare receptors for ß-adrenoceptor-mediated positive inotropic effects of catecholamines in the human heart. J Cardiovasc Pharmacol 1992;19:222-32.

30. Leimbach WN, Wallin G, Victor RG, Aylward PE, Sundlof G, Mark AL. Direct evidence from intraneuronal recordings for increased central sympathetic outflow in patients with heart failure. Circulation 1986;73:913-9.

31. Cohn JN. Abnormalities of peripheral sympathetic nervous system control in congestive heart failure. Circulation 1990;82(Suppl I):I-59-I-67.

32. Cohn JN, Levine TB, Olivari MT et al. Plasma norepinephrine as a guide to prognosis in patients with chronic congestive heart failure. N Engl J Med 1984;311:819-23.

33. Hasking GJ, Esler MD, Jennings GL, Burton D, Johns JA, Korner PI. Norepinephrine spillover to plasma in patients with congestive heart failure: evidence of increased overall and cardiorenal sympathetic nervous activity. Circulation 1986;73:615-21.

34. Davis D, Baily R, Zelis R. Abnormalities in systemic norepinephrine kinetics in human congestive heart failure. Am J Physiol 1988;254:E760-E6.

35. Chidsey CA, Braunwald E. Sympathetic activity and neurotransmitter depletion in congestive heart failure. Pharmacol Rev 1966;18:685-700.

36. Anderson FL, Port JD, Reid BB, Larrabee P, Hanson G, Bristow MR. Myocardial catecholamine and neuropeptide Y depletion in failing ventricles of patients with idiopathic dilated cardiomyopathy. Correlation with ß-adrenergic receptor down-regulation. Circulation 1992;85:46-53.

37. Stiles GL, Caron MG, Lefkowitz RJ. ß-Adrenergic receptors: biochemical mechanisms of physiological regulation. Physiol Rev 1984;64:661-743.
38. Lefkowitz RJ, Caron MG. Adrenergic-receptors: molecular mechanisms of clinically relevant regulation. Clin Res 1985;33:395-406.
39. Hausdorff WP, Caron MG, Lefkowitz RJ. Turning off the signal: desensitization of ß-adrenergic receptor function. FASEB J 1990;4:2881-9.
40. Bristow MR, Ginsburg R, Minobe W et al. Decreased catecholamine sensitivity and ß-adrenergic-receptor density in failing human hearts. N Engl J Med 1982;307:205-11.
41. Summers RJ, Molenaar P, Russell F et al. Coexistence and localization of ß₁- and ß₂-adrenoceptors in the human heart. Eur Heart J 1989;10(Suppl B):11-21.
42. Merlet P, Delforge J, Syrota A et al. Positron emission tomography with CGP 12177 to assess beta-adrenergic receptor concentration in idiopathic dilated cardiomyopathy. Circulation 1993;87:1169-78.
43. Ungerer M, Böhm M, Elce JS, Erdmann E, Lohse MJ. Altered expression of ß-adrenergic receptor kinase and ß₁-adrenergic receptors in the failing human heart. Circulation 1993;87:454-63.
44. Bristow MR, Minobe WA, Raynolds MV et al. Reduced ß₁ receptor messenger RNA abundance in the failing human heart. J Clin Invest 1993;92:2737-45.
45. Michel MC, Maisel AS, Brodde O-E. Mitigation of ß₁- and/or ß₂-adrenoceptor function in human heart failure. Br J Clin Pharmacol 1990;30(Suppl 1):37S-42S.
46. Steinfath M, Geertz B, Schmitz W et al. Distinct down-regulation of cardiac ß₁- and ß₂-adrenoceptors in different human heart diseases. Naunyn-Schmiedeberg's Arch Pharmacol 1991;343:217-20.
47. Brodde O-E, Zerkowski H-R, Doetsch N, Motomura S, Khamssi M, Michel MC. Myocardial beta-adrenoceptor changes in heart failure: concomitant reduction in beta1- and beta2-adrenoceptor function related to the degree of heart failure in patients with mitral valve disease. J Am Coll Cardiol 1989;14:323-31.
48. Brodde O-E, Zerkowski H-R, Borst HG, Maier W, Michel MC. Drug- and disease-induced changes of human cardiac ß₁- and ß₂-adrenoceptors. Eur Heart J 1989;10(Suppl B):38-44.
49. Steinfath M, Danielsen W, Von der Leyen H et al. Reduced α₁- and ß₂-adrenoceptor-mediated positive inotropic effects in human end-stage heart failure. Br J Pharmacol 1992;105:463-9.
50. Bristow MR, Anderson FL, Port JD et al. Differences in ß-adrenergic neuroeffector mechanisms in ischemic versus idiopathic dilated cardiomyopathy. Circulation 1991;84:1024-39.
51. Bristow MR, Minobe W, Rasmussen R et al. ß-adrenergic neuroeffector abnormalities in the failing human heart are produced by local rather than systemic mechanisms. J Clin Invest 1992;89:803-15.
52. Feldman AM, Cates AE, Bristow MR, Van Dop C. Altered expression of alpha-subunits of G-proteins in failing human hearts. J Mol Cell Cardiol 1989;21:359-65.
53. Eschenhagen T, Mende,U, Nose M et al. Increased messenger RNA level of the inhibitory G protein α subunit Gᵢα-2 in human end-stage heart failure. Circ Res 1992;70:688-96.
54. Feldman AM. Experimental issues in assessment of of G protein function in cardiac disease. Circulation 1991;84:1852-61.
55. Harding SE, Jones SM, O'Gara P, Vescovo G, Poole-Wilson PA. Reduced ß-agonist sensitivity in single atrial cells from failing human hearts. Am J Physiol 1990;259(Heart Circ Physiol 28):H1009-H14.
56. Vescovo G, Jones SM, Harding SE, Poole-Wilson PA. Isoproterenol sensitivity of isolated

cardiac myocytes from rats with monocrotaline-induced right-sided hypertrophy and heart failure. J Mol Cell Cardiol 1992;21:1047-61.

57. Gilbert EM, Port JS, Hershberger RE, Bristow MR. Clinical significance of alterations in the ß-adrenergic receptor-adenylate cyclase complex in heart failure. Heart Failure 1989;5:91-8.

58. Lands AM, Arnold A, McAuliff JP, Luduena FP, Brown TG. Differentiation of receptor systems activated by symathomimetic amines. Nature 1967;214:597-8.

14   STUDY OF CARDIAC RECEPTOR LIGANDS BY POSITRON EMISSION TOMOGRAPHY

Aren van Waarde, Philip H. Elsinga, Rutger L. Anthonio,
Ton J. Visser, Paul K. Blanksma, Gerben M. Visser,
Anne M.J. Paans, and Willem Vaalburg

Introduction

Changes in receptor populations may be early markers of disease, or indicators of the therapeutic success. A large research effort is therefore directed towards tomographic imaging of receptors and quantitative interpretation of these images in terms of receptor densities. Before human studies are possible, putative receptor-binding radiotracers should be thoroughly tested.

The testing of a radioligand for imaging purposes includes two distinct areas of research: 1) it should be demonstrated that the compound binds preferentially to the chosen receptor in intact animals or humans; 2) an experimental protocol should be designed that allows changes in receptor density (e.g. due to disease) to be determined with sufficient accuracy and sensitivity.[1,2] This chapter will discuss the use of labeled ß-adrenoceptor ligands for cardiac imaging, as an example of receptor imaging in general.

Is the ligand accumulated in tissue because of its interaction with receptors?

Demonstration of in vivo binding to a chosen receptor is rather complicated. The ligand may bind to functional receptors but also to plasma proteins and tissue components (proteins, phospholipids) which are not involved in signal transmission. Drugs may be transported by carrier protein(s) and they can accumulate in cells because of their physical properties (e.g. membrane transport of the uncharged molecule by passive diffusion followed by intralysosomal protonation.[3] Labeled metabolites may be formed in the liver and in extrahepatic tissues; these radioactive species will be released into blood and they can be taken up by the tissue under study. The contribution of nonspecific binding and metabolite uptake to radioactivity in the target tissue should be as small as possible if one wants to visualize ligand-receptor interaction.

E. E. van der Wall et al. (eds.), Cardiac Positron Emission Tomography, 171–182.
© 1995 Kluwer Academic Publishers.

Some generally-accepted criteria are commonly used to define receptor binding. Association of the ligand should occur with 1) high affinity, 2) high specificity, 3) saturability, 4) stereoselectivity, and 5) a distribution that is related to the physiological response.[1,4]

The affinity criterion

Radioligands should bind with high affinity to the observed sites (dissociation constant $K_d < 10^{-8}$ M). Ligand/receptor interaction must be the major mechanism underlying accumulation of radioactivity in the target tissue. The ratio of the concentrations of bound and free ligand is therefore a very important parameter. If equilibrium has been reached and a single, homogeneous class of binding sites is present, this ratio is described by the following expression:

$$\frac{[Bound]}{[Free]} = \frac{B_{max}}{K_d} - \frac{[Bound]}{K_d} \qquad (Ref.5)$$

The ratio of bound/free ligand (target-to-nontarget ratio or *'binding potential'*) is maximally equal to B_{max}/K_d (receptor density in the tissue under study divided by the affinity of the radioligand for these receptors). If $B_{max}/K_d < 1$, the radioligand will not be accumulated over plasma levels and external detection of receptor binding will not be feasible. B_{max} in most tissues is low (10^{-7}-10^{-10} mol/kg tissue mass). The dissociation constant of the ligand/receptor complex should therefore be also low (i.e. $< 10^{-8}$ M) to acquire a binding potential > 10, resulting in adequate contrast in positron emission tomography (PET) images.

Several low-affinity ($K_d > 10^{-9}$ M) ß-blockers were labeled with gamma-emitting or positron-emitting radionuclides. These include iodotyramine analogs of practolol and alprenolol, iododenopamine, iodometoprolol, carbon-11(^{11}C)-labeled atenolol, metoprolol and practolol besides fluorine-18(^{18}F)-fluorometoprolol (Table 1). Such derivatives were either not taken up by the heart, or radioactivity accumulated by mechanisms unrelated to ß-adrenoceptor binding. Metabolites may contribute to total radioactivity in blood while they do not bind to ß-adrenoceptors. Protein-bound radioligand in plasma may not be free to interact with ß-adrenoceptors in the heart. Thus, tissue/blood ratios can be much lower than B_{max}/K_d if the ligand is rapidly metabolized and if it is strongly bound to plasma proteins.[6]

The affinity of antagonists to a certain receptor is usually higher than that of agonists. Antagonists may bind to a single class of sites, but agonists induce transitions between affinity states (e.g. due to interaction of the ligand/receptor complex with G-proteins). Mathematical description of the binding of an agonist is therefore more complex than that of an antagonist. Most in vivo studies of receptors have been performed with antagonist radioligands.

Table 1. Physicochemical characteristics of β-adrenoceptor ligands

Ligand	Affinity in myocardial membranes (M)	B_{max}/K_d (in rat heart)	Log P (octanol:P_i buffer at pH 7.4)	References (use for imaging)	Subtype selectivity
Radioiodinated compounds (pilot studies for SPECT)					
125I-hydroxybenzylpindolol	6.3×10^{-11} [50]	95	+ 2.50 [51]	[8-11]	β₂ 2 x [11]
123I/125I-iodocyanopindolol	1.2×10^{-11} (±, [52])	500	+ 1.26 [53]	[23]	nonsel. [54]
123I-iododenopamine	5.1×10^{-8} [55]	0.12	+ 1.56 [55]	[55]	β₁ [55]
123I-iodometoprolol	1.4×10^{-7} (±, estim.)	0.04		[56]	β₁ [56]
125I/131I-iodopindolol	3×10^{-11} (-,[57])	200	+ 1.05 [51]	[13,58]	nonsel. [57]
125I-tyramine-alprenolol	2×10^{-7} [11]	0.03		[11]	β₂ 1.4 x [11]
125I-tyramine-practolol	2×10^{-5} [11]	0.0003		[11]	β₁ 5 x [11]
Positron-emitting and tritiated compounds (pilot studies for PET)					
11C-atenolol	3×10^{-7} (±, [51])	0.02	- 2.00..2.14 [51,59]	[15,60]	β₁ 29 x [51]
3H-bisoprolol	1.6×10^{-9} [61]	3.8	- 0.23 [62]	unpubl.	β₁ 63 x [61]
11C-carazolol	5.9×10^{-11} [42]	100	+ 1.36 [53]	[31,32]	β₂ 2 x [11]
11C-CGP 12177	3×10^{-10} [52,53]	20	- 0.49..0.55 [51,53]	[35,46,48,63]	β₁ 2.7 x [22]
11C-CGP 20712A	3×10^{-10} [64]	20	- 1.56 [65]	[19]	β₁ 10000 x [66]
3H-dihydroalprenolol	6×10^{-10} [53]	10	+ 1.32 [51,53]	[12]	β₁ 2.6 x [11]
18F-fluorocarazolol	1.1×10^{-10} (-, [42,67])	55	+ 2.2 [33]	[20,32,33]	nonselec. [42]
18F-fluorometoprolol	3.5×10^{-7} (±, [68])	0.02		[68]	β₁ 49 x [68]
11C-metoprolol	1.9×10^{-8} (-, [69])	0.3	- 0.28..0.31 [51,59]	[15]	β₁ 31 x [68]
11C-pindolol	4.5×10^{-10} (-, [52])	13	- 0.33 [59]	[70]	β₂ 2 x [71]
11C-practolol	8.6×10^{-7} (±, [72])	0.007	- 1.60 [73]	[74]	β₁ 51 x [54]
11C-propranolol	3×10^{-10} (-, [72])	20	+ 1.21 [59]	[14]	nonselec. [75]

The selectivity criterion

In vivo blocking (or displacement) using selective drugs is a widely employed method of proving that a specific receptor interaction causes tissue uptake of a radioligand. Accumulation of radioactivity that cannot be blocked or displaced with the appropriate drugs is called *nonspecific* (i.e. not receptor-mediated) *binding.* In successful imaging studies, such binding contributes little to radioactivity in the region-of-interest (i.e. < 20%). Nonspecific binding is related to ligand lipophilicity (octanol:buffer partition coefficients)[7] and to the injected dose (in nmol/kg body mass).

Many ß-adrenoceptor ligands show relatively high nonspecific binding. Initial biodistribution studies used the potent radioligand ^{125}I-hydroxybenzylpindolol (IHYP).[8] If a filter assay was performed on tissue homogenates prepared 5-20 minutes after ligand injection, specific binding of IHYP to ß-adrenoceptors was detected in brain, heart and lung but not in liver. This binding could be blocked by co-injection of ß-adrenergic drugs (propranolol, sotalol and isoprenaline) but not by the *a*-antagonist phentolamine. Experiments with isolated perfused hearts indicated that the apparent off-rate of bound IHYP was increased by drugs which interact with ß-adrenoceptors but not by nonspecific displacing agents.[9] Upregulation of cardiac ß-adrenoceptors in thyroxin-treated animals was detectable, using isolated hearts, IHYP and an external gamma probe.[9] Occupancy of pulmonary ß-adrenoceptors by unlabeled propranolol or adrenaline could be assessed by measuring displacement of bound IHYP.[10] However, *total* radioactivity in organs of *intact animals* was not reduced by propranolol treatment with exception of a slight (< 50%) decrease in the lung. Imaging of cardiac ß-adrenoceptors with IHYP was therefore impossible.[8,11]

Although IHYP is potent enough to accumulate in tissues by its interaction with receptors, strong nonspecific binding results in poor signal-to-noise ratios. Receptor imaging with labeled bisoprolol (Table 1), dihydroalprenolol (DHA),[12] iodine-131 (^{131}I)-iodopindolol (IPIN),[13] ^{11}C-propranolol[4,14-16] or ^{11}C-CGP 20712A[17-19] has failed for the same reason. Propranolol shows a high pulmonary uptake which precludes imaging of the heart and which is largely unaffected after treatment with other ß-blockers.[4,16] About 50% of myocardial CGP-20712A uptake can be blocked by treatment of animals with unlabeled propranolol or ß$_1$-adrenoceptor binding drugs,[17,19] but similar blocking occurs after predosing with ß$_2$- or *a*-adrenoceptor antagonists.[18] Myocardial binding of CGP 20712A is therefore largely nonspecific.

Using specific agonists and antagonists, we have shown that myocardial and pulmonary uptake of $S(-)-^3$H-CGP 12177 and S-1'-^{18}F-fluorocarazolol in intact rats reflects radioligand binding to ß-adrenoceptors.[18,20] Tissue uptake at intervals more than 15 minutes post injection is mainly determined by the apparent receptor density and not by blood flow.

The saturability criterion

In vivo saturation curves can provide information on the density of binding sites in various tissues and the apparent affinity of the radioligand to these sites. Data thus obtained can be compared to results of in vitro binding assays. As uptake is generally measured in excised tissue, the construction of saturation curves is quite laborious and requires the use of many experimental animals. Such curves have therefore been published for relatively few radioligands.

Law[21] assessed the effect of coinjection of unlabeled (-)-CGP 12177 on tissue uptake of ^{3}H-CGP 12177 in conscious rats. The data were best fit to a single, homogeneous class of binding sites. B_{max} values of 45 and 6 pmol/g wet weight were obtained in lung and heart, respectively. The apparent affinity of the radioligand to cardiac ß-adrenoceptors (predominantly $ß_1$, K_d 1.3 nmol/kg body weight) was higher than that to pulmonary ß-adrenoceptors (predominantly $ß_2$, K_d 2.5 nmol/kg body weight). These in vivo results compare favourably with in vitro estimations of receptor density and ligand affinity. CGP 12177 is known to be 2-3 times more potent at $ß_1$- than at $ß_2$-adrenoceptors.[22]

Sisson et al.[23] administered increasing doses of (-)-^{125}I-iodocyanopindolol (ICYP) to rats and examined myocardial ^{125}I-uptake by postmortem *ex vivo* counting. The data were best fit to two sites: one with high affinity and low capacity (apparent K_d 22 nmol/kg body weight, B_{max} 6.2 pmol/g), the other with low affinity and high capacity (apparent K_d 0.9 μmol/kg body weight and B_{max} 110 pmol/g). The former site is a ß-adrenoceptor, as various agonists and antagonists had the expected pharmacological effects. The latter may be a non-ß-adrenergic binding site which is present in the heart.[24] Ligand binding to this site will be negligible at the dose used in a ^{123}I-ICYP single photon emission computed tomography (SPECT) image.

Relatively low apparent in vivo K_d's of labeled ß-adrenoceptor ligands may be a consequence of the fact that a large fraction of radioactivity in blood is not free but bound to erythrocytes (CGP 12177, ICYP) and plasma proteins (ICYP).[25]

The stereoselectivity criterion

If tissue uptake of a radioligand is due to its interaction with receptors, the binding should display stereoselectivity. Nonspecific binding or binding to non-ß-adrenergic sites is usually not stereospecific.[26-30] A test for stereoselectivity can be performed in two different ways: 1) active and inactive enantiomers of the radioligand can be synthesized and their biodistributions compared, or 2) active and inactive enantiomers of an unlabeled antagonist can be used to block ligand uptake and their blocking potencies assessed.

Both techniques have been employed to validate SPECT and PET radioligands. Berridge et al.[31,32] synthesized the *R*- and *S*-enantiomers of ^{11}C-carazolol. The *S*-enantiomer was avidly taken up by heart and lung, but the *R*-enantiomer was not accumulated above blood levels in the target organs. Hughes et al.[13] detected specific binding of ^{131}I-*l*-pindolol in rabbit lung and heart (ca. 50% of total uptake), whereas ^{131}I-*d*-pindolol uptake was wholly nonspecific. Zheng et al.[33] produced the *R*- and *S*-enantiomers of ^{18}F-fluorocarazolol. Myocardial and pulmonary binding of the *S*-enantiomer were strongly reduced by propranolol treatment, but biodistribu-tion of the *R*-enantiomer was not affected. Law[21] compared cardiac and pulmonary uptake of (-)- and (±)-^{3}H-CGP 12177 in rats. Tissue/plasma ratios of the active isomer were > 2-fold higher than those of the racemate. Similar results have been published for myocardial binding of (-)- and (±)-^{125}I-iodocyanopindolol.[23]

Barnes and Karliner[12] examined the effect of *L*- and *D*-propranolol on the biodistribution of ^{3}H-dihydroalprenolol (DHA). L-propranolol was approximately 100-fold more potent than D-propranolol to block cardiac and pulmonary ^{3}H-DHA uptake. We obtained similar results for blocking of the in vivo binding of S-^{18}F-fluorocarazolol.[20]

These data suggest that ^{11}C-carazolol, ^{18}F-fluorocarazolol and ^{11}C-CGP 12177 are useful ligands for PET imaging of ß-adrenoceptors. Dihydroalprenolol and iodopindolol are less suitable because they show high nonspecific binding.[12,13] Biodistribution studies with ^{125}I-iodocyanopindolol indicate that the ^{123}I- or ^{131}I-labeled compound has some potential for cardiac SPECT.[23]

Binding related to the physiological response

If a radioligand is bound to functional receptors, a relationship should exist between its binding and the physiological response. In the case of cardiac ß-adrenoceptor ligands, this can be demonstrated by simultaneously measuring 1) displacement of bound radioligand by an unlabeled antagonist and 2) heart rate. Seto et al.[34] have shown that displacement of bound ^{11}C-CGP 12177 by unlabeled ß-blockers in dog heart is synchronous with the development of bradycardia. This observation suggests that ^{11}C-CGP 12177 binds to signal-transducing sites in the intact animal.

Metabolism

Rapid metabolism of a radioligand is generally undesirable. It complicates assessment of the arterial input function of tracer-kinetic models and it may lead to uptake of labeled metabolites by the target tissues which will increase 'nonspecific binding'.

Metabolite analysis of ß-adrenoceptor ligands has resulted in conflicting findings. Some workers[35-37] reported very rapid metabolism of ^{11}C-CGP 12177 in rats, dogs and human volunteers whereas others could not reproduce these results and observed slow metabolism in all species.[38-40] Berridge et al.[32] found that ^{11}C- and ^{18}F-analogues of c-arazolol were relatively stable upon injection in mice and pigs but in our studies,[41-43] we noted rapid degradation of ^{18}F-fluorocarazolol in rats and sheep.

As none of the research groups detected significant cardiac or pulmonary uptake of labeled metabolites upon injection of ^{11}C-CGP 12177 or S-1'-^{18}F-fluorocarazolol, radioactivity in these tissues seems to represent bound ligand which facilitates modeling.[17,32,34,38,41-43] However, the arterial input of such models is hard to determine and is still controversial.

Sensitivity of ligand binding to changes in receptor density

Myocardial uptake of S-^{11}C-CGP 12177 has been shown to be sensitive to changes in receptor density. Chemical sympathectomy in dogs results in rapid (< 10 days) upregulation of myocardial ß-adrenoceptors which can be assessed by PET.[44] Idiopathic dilated cardiomyopathy is associated with a loss of cardiac ß-adrenoceptors which is measurable in humans using PET, CGP 12177 and a graphical method.[45,46] The diffuse reduction of myocardial ß-adrenoceptors in patients with hypertrophic cardiomyopathy[47,48] and corticosteroid- or ß-agonist-induced alterations of pulmonary ß-adrenoceptors in asthmatics[49] are also reflected by changed in vivo binding of CGP-12177.

The effect of subtype-selective ß-adrenoceptor-blocking drugs on the biodistribution of S-^{18}F-fluorocarazolol suggests that myocardial and pulmonary binding of this ligand will reflect changes in tissue B_{max}.[20] It is not yet known whether receptor density can be estimated from fluorocarazolol-PET images with sufficient precision to detect ß-adrenoceptor alterations in heart failure.

Conclusion

Many ß-adrenoceptor ligands have been labeled with gamma- or positron-emitting radionuclides and evaluated for imaging purposes. Most of them proved unsuitable because of low affinity, high nonspecific binding, lack of selectivity, or a combination of these factors. Only CGP 12177, ^{11}C-carazolol, and ^{18}F-carazolol seem to meet all the criteria for successful imaging. Metabolism and tracer-kinetic modelling of these compounds should be further investigated.

Acknowledgements

T.J. Visser was financially supported by the Netherlands Asthma Foundation.

References

1. Eckelman WC. The testing of putative receptor binding radiotracers in vivo. In: Diksic M, Reba RC, editors. Radiopharmaceuticals and brain pathology studied with PET and SPECT. Boca Raton, FL: CRC Press, 1991: 41-68.
2. Eckelman WC. The application of receptor theory to receptor-binding and enzyme-binding oncologic radiopharmaceuticals. Nucl Med Biol 1994;21:759-69.
3. Cramb G. Selective lysosomal uptake and accumulation of the ß-adrenergic antagonist propranolol in cultured and isolated cell systems. Biochem Pharmacol 1986;35:1365-72.
4. Syrota A. Investigation of myocardial receptors by PET in heart diseases. In: Heiss WD, editors. Clinical Efficacy of Positron Emission Tomography. Dordrecht: Martinus Nijhoff, 1987:253-63.
5. Scatchard G. The attractions of proteins for small molecules and ions. Ann N Y Acad Sci 1949;51:660-72.
6. Gibson RE, Eckelman WC, Rzeszotarski WJ et al. Radiotracer localization by ligand-receptor interactions. In: Colombetti LG, editor. Principles of Radiopharmacology, Volume 2. West Palm Beach, FL: CRC Press, 1979:7-40.
7. Hellenbrecht D, Lemmer B, Wiethold G, Grobecker H. Measurement of hydrophobicity, surface activity, local anaesthesia and myocardial conduction velocity as quantitative parameters of the nonspecific membrane affinity of nine ß-adrenergic blocking agents. Naunyn Schmiedebergs Arch Pharmacol 1973;277:211-26.
8. Bylund DB, Charness ME, Snyder SH. Beta adrenergic receptor labeling in intact animals with ^{125}I-hydroxybenzylpindolol. J Pharmacol Exp Ther 1977;201:644-53.
9. Hughes B, Bergmann SR, Corr PB, Sobel BE. External detection of ß-adrenoreceptors with ^{125}I-hydroxybenzylpindolol in isolated perfused hearts. Nucl Med Biol 1986;13:565-71.
10. Homcy CJ, Strauss HW, Kopiwoda S. Beta receptor occupancy: assessment in the intact animal. J Clin Invest 1980;65:1111-8.
11. Eckelman WC, Gibson RE, Vieras F, Rzeszotarski WJ, Francis BE, Reba RC. In vivo receptor binding of iodinated ß-adrenoceptor blockers. J Nucl Med 1980;21:436-42.
12. Barnes PJ, Karliner JS. In vivo identification and distribution of α- and ß-adrenoceptors in rat heart and lung. Pharmacology 1982;24:321-7.
13. Hughes B, Marshall DR, Sobel BE, Bergmann SR. Characterization of ß-adrenoreceptors in vivo with iodine-131 pindolol and gamma scintigraphy. J Nucl Med 1986;27:660-7.
14. Berger G, Mazière M, Prenant C, Sastre J, Syrota A, Comar D. Synthesis of ^{11}C-propranolol. J Radioanal Chem 1982;74:301-4.
15. Antoni G, Uhlin J, Långström B. Synthesis of the ^{11}C-labelled ß-adrenergic receptor ligands atenolol, metoprolol and propranolol. Appl Radiat Isot 1989;40:561-4.
16. Syrota A. Positron Emission Tomography: Evaluation of cardiac receptors. In: Marcus ML, eds. Cardiac Imaging. Philadelphia, PA: W.B.Saunders, 1991:1256-70.
17. Van Waarde A, Meeder JG, Blanksma PK et al. Suitability of CGP12177 and CGP26505 for quantitative imaging of ß-adrenoceptors. Nucl Med Biol 1992;19:711-8.
18. Van Waarde A, Meeder JG, Blanksma PK et al. Uptake of radioligands by rat heart and lung in vivo: CGP12177 does and CGP26505 does not reflect binding to ß-adrenoceptors. Eur J Pharmacol 1992;222:107-12.

19. Elsinga PH, Van Waarde A, Visser GM, Vaalburg W. Synthesis and preliminary evaluation of (R,S)-1-[2-((carbamoyl-4-hydroxy)phenoxy)-ethylamino]-3-[4-(1-^{11}C-methyl-4-trifluoromethyl-2-imidazolyl) phenoxy]-2-propanol (^{11}C-CGP 20712A) as a selective ß$_1$-adrenoceptor ligand for PET. Nucl Med Biol 1994;21:211-7.
20. Van Waarde A, Elsinga PH, Brodde OE, Visser GM, Vaalburg W. Myocardial and pulmonary uptake of S-1'-^{18}F-fluorocarazolol in intact rats reflects radioligand binding to ß-adrenoceptors. Eur J Pharmacol 1995;(in press).
21. Law MP. Demonstration of the suitability of CGP 12177 for in vivo studies of ß-adrenoceptors. Br J Pharmacol 1993;109:1101-9.
22. Nanoff C, Freissmuth M, Schutz W. The role of a low ß$_1$-adrenoceptor selectivity of ^{3}H-CGP-12177 for resolving subtype-selectivity of competitive ligands. Naunyn Schmiedebergs Arch Pharmacol 1987;336:519-25.
23. Sisson JC, Wieland DM, Koeppe RA et al. Scintigraphic portrayal of ß-receptors in the heart. J Nucl Med 1991;32:1399-407.
24. Björnerheim R, Golf S, Hansson V. Specific non-ß-adrenergic binding sites for ^{125}I-iodocyanopindolol in myocardial membrane preparations: a comparative study between human, rat, and porcine hearts. Cardiovasc Res 1991;25:764-73.
25. Raffel DM, Holden JE, De Jesus OT, Endres CJ, Pooley RA. Plasma free fraction as determinant of in vivo vs in vitro equilibrium dissociation constants of receptor binding ligands: Direct experimental validation. J Nucl Med 1991;32:1004-5 (Abstract).
26. Kerry R, Scrutton MC. Binding of ^{3}H-dihydroalprenolol and ^{3}H-acetobutolol to human blood platelets is not related to occupancy of ß-adrenoceptors. Thromb Res 1983;29:583.
27. Krawietz W, Erdmann E. Specific and nonspecific binding of ^{3}H-dihydroalprenolol to cardiac tissue. Biochem Pharmacol 1979;28:1283-8.
28. Dax EM, Partilla JS, Gregerman RI. The (-) ^{3}H-dihydroalprenolol binding to rat adipocyte membranes: an explanation of curvilinear Scatchard plots and implications for quantitation of ß-adrenoceptors. J Lipid Res 1982;23:1001-7.
29. Dax EM, Partilla JS, Gregerman RI. Quantitation of ß-adrenergic receptors in liver membranes with ß-adrenergic antagonists: only stereospecific displacement defines the ß-receptor. J Recept Res 1981;2:267-83.
30. O'Hara N, Brodde OE. Identical properties of (±) and (-) ^{125}I-iodocyanopindolol to ß$_2$-adrenoceptors in intact human lymphocytes. Arch Int Pharmacodyn Ther 1984;272:24-39.
31. Berridge MS, Cassidy EH, Terris AH, Vesselle JM. Preparation and in vivo binding of ^{11}C-carazolol, a radiotracer for the ß-adrenergic receptor. Nucl Med Biol 1992;19:563-9.
32. Berridge MS, Nelson AD, Zheng LB, Leisure GP, Miraldi F. Specific ß-adrenergic receptor binding of carazolol measured with PET. J Nucl Med 1994;35:1665-76.
33. Zheng LB, Berridge MS, Ernsberger P. Synthesis, binding properties, and ^{18}F labeling of fluorocarazolol, a high-affinity ß-adrenergic receptor antagonist. J Med Chem 1994;37:3219-30.
34. Seto M, Syrota A, Crouzel C et al. Beta-adrenergic receptors in the dog heart characterized by ^{11}C-CGP12177 and PET. J Nucl Med 1986;27:949 (Abstract).
35. Delforge J, Syrota A, Lançon JP et al. Cardiac ß-adrenergic receptor density measured in vivo using PET, CGP 12177, and a new graphical method. J Nucl Med 1991;32:739-48.
36. Delforge J, Nakajima K, Syrota A et al. PET investigation of ß-adrenergic receptors using CGP12177. J Nucl Med 1989;30:825 (Abstract).

37. Mazière B, Cantineau R, Coenen HH et al. PET radiopharmaceutical metabolism - plasma metabolite analysis. In: Stöcklin G, Pike VW, editors. Radiopharmaceuticals for Positron Emission Tomography, Methodological Aspects. Dordrecht: Kluwer Academic Publishers, 1993:151-78.
38. Jones HA, Rhodes CG, Law MP et al. Rapid analysis for metabolites of ^{11}C-labelled drugs: fate of ^{11}C-S-4-(tert.-butylamino-2-hydroxypropoxy)- benzimidazol-2-one in the dog. J Chromatogr 1991;570:361-70.
39. Luthra SK, Osman S, Steel CJ et al. Comparison of S-^{11}C-CGP12177 metabolism in rat, dog and man using solid phase extraction and HPLC. J Label Comp Radiopharm 1992;31:518-20 (Abstract).
40. Van Waarde A, Anthonio RL, Visser TJ et al. Quantification of a carbon-11-labelled ß-adrenoceptor ligand, S-(-)-CGP 12177, in plasma of humans and rats. J Chromatogr 1995;(in press).
41. Elsinga PH, Van Waarde A, Vos MG et al. PET imaging of pulmonary ß-adrenoceptors with S-^{18}F-fluorocarazolol. J Nucl Med 1994;35:257P (Abstract).
42. Elsinga PH, Vos MG, Braker AH et al. Improved synthesis and evaluation of (S,S)- and (S,R)-^{18}F-fluorocarazolol, ligands for the visualization of ß-adrenergic receptors. J Label Comp Radiopharm 1994;35:148-9 (Abstract).
43. Van Waarde A, Elsinga PH, Anthonio RL et al. Quantification of a fluorine-18-labelled ß-adrenoceptor ligand, S-1'-^{18}F-fluorocarazolol, in plasma of humans, rats and sheep. J Chromatogr 1995;(ms in preparation).
44. Valette H, Delforge J, Merlet P, Crouzel C, Fuseau C, Syrota A. Up-regulation of myocardial ß-adrenergic receptors early after sympathetic chemical denervation in dogs assessed with PET and C-11 CGP 12177. J Nucl Med 1993;34:45P-6P (Abstract).
45. Merlet P, Dubois-Randé JL, Adnot S et al. Myocardial ß-adrenergic desensitization and neuronal norepinephrine uptake function in idiopathic dilated cardiomyopathy. J Cardiovasc Pharmacol 1992;19:10-6.
46. Merlet P, Delforge J, Syrota A et al. Positron emission tomography with ^{11}C-CGP-12177 to assess ß-adrenergic receptor concentration in idiopathic dilated cardiomyopathy. Circulation 1993;87:1169-78.
47. Lefroy DC, De Silva R, Choudhury L et al. Myocardial ß-adrenoceptor density is reduced in hypertrophic cardiomyopathy. Circulation 1992;86:I-246 (Abstract).
48. Lefroy DC, De Silva R, Choudhury L et al. Diffuse reduction of myocardial ß-adrenoceptors in hypertrophic cardiomyopathy: a study with positron emission tomography. J Am Coll Cardiol 1993;22:1653-60.
49. Qing F, Sriskandan S, Rhodes CG et al. Alveolar ß-adrenergic receptor density in asthmatic subjects before and during corticosteroid and ß-agonist therapy: preliminary studies using positron emission tomography (PET) and ^{11}C-S-CGP12177. Thorax 1992;47:871 (Abstract).
50. Robberecht P, Delhaye M, Taton G et al. The human heart ß-adrenergic receptors. I. Heterogeneity of the binding sites: presence of 50% ß$_1$- and 50% ß$_2$-adrenergic receptors. Mol Pharmacol 1983;24:169-73.
51. Abrahamsson T, Ek B, Nerme V. The ß$_1$- and ß$_2$-adrenoceptor affinity of atenolol and metoprolol. A receptor-binding study performed with different radioligands in tissues from the rat, the guinea pig and man. Biochem Pharmacol 1988;37:203-8.
52. Raffel DM. In vivo receptor pharmacology studies with ß-adrenergic receptors in isolated perfused rat heart. University of Wisconsin, Madison WI: PhD thesis, 1991:1-219.
53. Staehelin M, Simons P, Jaeggi K, Wigger N. CGP-12177. A hydrophilic

ß-adrenergic receptor radioligand reveals high affinity binding of agonists to intact cells. J Biol Chem 1983;258:3496-502.

54. Engel G, Hoyer D, Berthold R, Wagner H. ($\pm$)[125]Iodocyanopindolol, a new ligand for ß-adrenoceptors: Identification and quantitation of subclasses of ß-adrenoceptors in guinea pig. Naunyn Schmiedebergs Arch Pharmacol 1981;317:277-85.

55. Bertaux M, Brutesco C, Loc'h C, Valette H, Mazière B. Preparation of ^{123}I-iododenopamine: A potential radiotracer for myocardial ß-adrenergic receptor studies. J Label Comp Radiopharm 1992;31:533-4 (Abstract).

56. Du J, Jin X, Yuan S. Preparation of ^{123}I-labeled metoprolol with iodine monochloride process. 10th Int Symp Radiopharm Chem, Kyoto 1993;226 (Abstract).

57. Juberg EN, Minneman KP, Abel PW. $ß_1$- and $ß_2$-adrenoceptor binding and functional response in right and left atria of rat heart. Naunyn Schmiedebergs Arch Pharmacol 1985;330:193-202.

58. Tondo L, Conway PG, Brunswick DJ. Labeling in vivo of ß-adrenergic receptors in the central nervous system of the rat after administration of ^{125}I-iodopindolol. J Pharmacol Exp Ther 1985;235:1-9.

59. Harada S, Ban T, Fujita T, Koshiro A. Negative inotropic effects and the hydrophobicity of ß-adrenergic blocking agents. Arch Int Pharmacodyn Ther 1981;252:262-71.

60. Agon P, Goethals P, Van Haver D, Kaufman JM. Permeability of the blood-brain barrier for atenolol studied by positron emission tomography. J Pharm Pharmacol 1991;43:597-600.

61. Kaumann AJ, Lemoine H. Direct labelling of myocardial $ß_1$- adrenoceptors. Comparison of binding affinity of [3]H-(-)-bisoprolol with its blocking potency. Naunyn Schmiedebergs Arch Pharmacol 1985;331:27-39.

62. Recanatini M. Partition and distribution coefficients of aryloxypropanolamine ß-adrenoceptor antagonists. J Pharm Pharmacol 1992;44:68-70.

63. Ueki J, Rhodes CG, Hughes JMB et al. In vivo quantification of pulmonary ß-adrenoceptor density in humans with (S)-^{11}C-CGP-12177 and PET. J Appl Physiol 1993;75:559-65.

64. Borea PA, Amerini S, Masini I et al. $ß_1$- and $ß_2$-adrenoceptors in sheep cardiac ventricular muscle. J Mol Cell Cardiol 1992;24:753-63.

65. Pauwels PJ, Leysen JE, Janssen PA. ß-Adrenoceptor-mediated cAMP accumulation in cardiac cells: effects of nebivolol. Eur J Pharmacol 1989;172:471-9.

66. Dooley DJ, Bittiger H, Reymann NC. CGP 20712 A: a useful tool for quantitating $ß_1$- and $ß_2$-adrenoceptors. Eur J Pharmacol 1986;130:137-9.

67. Kinsey BM, Barber R, Tewson TJ. Synthesis of fluorine-18 fluorocarazolol: A ligand for the ß-adrenergic receptor. J Label Comp Radiopharm 1992;31:298-300 (Abstract).

68. De Groot TJ, Van Waarde A, Elsinga PH, Visser GM, Brodde OE, Vaalburg W. Synthesis and evaluation of 1'-^{18}F-fluorometoprolol as a potential tracer for the visualization of ß-adrenoceptors with PET. Nucl Med Biol 1993;20:637-42.

69. Wahlund G, Nerme V, Abrahamsson T, Sjöquist PO. The $ß_1$- and $ß_2$-adrenoceptor affinity and $ß_1$-blocking potency of S- and R-metoprolol. Br J Pharmacol 1990;99:592-6.

70. Prenant C, Sastre J, Crouzel C, Syrota A. Synthesis of ^{11}C-pindolol. J Label Comp Radiopharm 1987;24:227-32.

71. Wuppermann D, Zimmermann F, Friedrich L. Vergleich der Wirksamkeit von Alprenolol, Bunitrolol, Ethaverin, Oxprenolol, Papaverin, Practolol, Pindolol,

Pronethalol, Propranolol, Toliprolol und Verapamil auf die ß-Rezeptoren des Herzens und Bronchialsystems. Arzneimittelforschung 1978;28:794-8.

72. Barnett DB, Rugg EL, Nahorski SL. Direct evidence of two types of ß-adrenoceptor binding site in lung tissues. Nature 1978;273:166-8.
73. Hellenbrecht D, Enenkel J. Estimation of the nonspecific cardiovascular toxicity of ß-adrenoceptor blocking drugs with different hydrophobic properties in the cat. Arzneimittelforschung 1984;34:980-3.
74. Berger G, Prenant C, Sastre J, Syrota A, Comar D. Synthesis of a ß-blocker for heart visualization: ^{11}C-practolol. Appl Radiat Isot 1983;34:1556-7.
75. Tsuchihashi H, Nakashima Y, Kinami J, Nagatomo T. Characteristics of ^{125}I-iodocyanopindolol binding to ß-adrenergic and serotonin-1B receptors of rat brain: selectivity of ß-adrenergic agents. Jpn J Pharmacol 1990;52:195-200.

15   ASSESSMENT OF SYMPATHETIC CARDIAC INNERVATION BY SCINTIGRAPHIC TECHNIQUES

Götz Münch, Ngoc Nguyen, Don Wieland,
and Markus Schwaiger

Introduction

Modulation of the cardiac sympathetic nervous system, by various pharmacologic means, has been shown to influence the outcome of patients in numerous clinical trials. Nevertheless, knowledge of sympathetic activation in heart disease, insights about changes in the presynaptic and postsynaptic sympathetic nervous system in cardiomyopathy and autonomic dysfunction in diabetes mellitus or patients after heart transplantation have only been derived from animal studies. Data from investigations in patients are sparse and mostly obtained with invasive techniques. With the introduction of scintigraphic techniques, noninvasive evaluation of the sympathetic nervous system became possible. Development of tracers selective for the investigation of the presynaptic nervous system and postsynaptic receptors have allowed for differential assessment of changes in the sympathetic nervous system under different pathophysiological conditions in-vivo. This chapter focuses on the evaluation of the sympathetic innervation of the heart with scintigraphic techniques.

Physiology of cardiac sympathetic innervation

Presynaptic site
The heart is innervated by both sympathetic and parasympathetic nerve fibers. Parasympathetic innervation originates from the medulla and passes through the right and left vagal nerves, which further divide into the superior and inferior cardiac nerves. Parasympathetic fibers primarily modulate the activity of the sino-atrial (SA) node and the atrio-ventricular (AV) node function and innervate the atria; whereas vagal fibers to the ventricles are sparse. Sympathetic innervation includes four or five thoracic ganglia as well as the superior, middle, and inferior cervical ganglia. The superior, middle, and inferior cardiac nerves originate from their respective ganglia and form the cardiac plexus of the heart. Sympathetic nerves also control the SA node and AV node

183

E. E. van der Wall et al. (eds.), Cardiac Positron Emission Tomography, 183–199.
© 1995 Kluwer Academic Publishers.

together with parasympathetic nerves. The fibers branch and end as sympathetic nerve terminals in the myocardium of the atria and ventricles.

The most important neurotransmitter in the heart is norepinephrine since epinephrine release during nerve activation is negligible.[1] Biosynthesis of norepinephrine (Figure 1) starts with the aminoacid tyrosine, which is enzymatically converted to DOPA and then to dopamine. Dopamine is actively transported into storage vesicles and transformed to norepinephrine by the vesicular enzyme dopamine-ß-hydroxylase (DBH). In the sympathetic nerve terminals, norepinephrine is stored in granules until it is released during nerve activation. The release of norepinephrine is proportional to the neuronal firing rate. Depending on the neuronal activation, a certain amount of transmitter granules fuse with the cell membrane of the presynaptic sympathetic nerve varicosity, and release norepinephrine into the neuronal cleft by an exocytotic, energy and calcium-dependent process, which is modulated by multiple presynaptic receptors.[2] Furthermore, it has been shown that norepinephrine modulates its own release either by autoinhibitory a_2 adrenoceptor stimulation[3] or by facilatory $ß_2$ adrenoceptors.[4] Acetylcholine from adjacent parasympathetic neurons via m-cholinoreceptors, adenosine from the transsynaptic myocytes via A1 receptors, and angiotensin II via Angiotensin II receptors by paracrine regulation are also known to participate in the regulation of norepinephrine release via presynaptic receptors.[3] In addition, other presynaptic receptor systems are being currently investigated.

The biological action of norepinephrine in the synaptic cleft is terminated mainly by reuptake into the presynaptic sympathetic nerve ending by the uptake-1 carrier, which is dependent on energy rich phosphates and a sodium gradient across the plasma membrane.[5] Structurally related amines including epinephrine, dopamine, guanethidine and metaraminol are also transported by uptake-1, which can be inhibited by cocaine and desipramine. In addition to neuronal uptake via uptake-1, a quantitatively less significant transport protein, uptake-2, removes norepinephrine from extracellular space in non-neuronal tissue.[6]

Norepinephrine in the cytosol of the sympathetic nerve endings is transported into the granule by an active process, which can be inhibited by reserpine. Free cytosolic norepinephrine is rapidly degraded to dihydroxyphenylglycol (DPG) by monoamino-oxidase (MAO). Removal of the lipophilic DPG through the presynaptic cell membrane into the extracellular space performed is by passive diffusion.

Postsynaptic site
Norepinephrine as well as circulating epinephrine interact with adrenoceptors in the heart at various structural levels, which include the myocardium, conduction system and blood vessels. Adrenergic receptors are located perivascularly to control blood flow of the coronary artery. These perivascular receptors consist mainly of the a_1 and $ß_2$ adrenoceptor type. The conduction system also depends on nerval input via adrenergic receptors to regulate heart rate and refractoriness. In the SA and AV nodes, $ß_2$ adrenoceptors prevail. However, the highest proportion of all adrenoceptors in the heart are located on the myocytes and regulate contractility. In addition to $ß_1$ and $ß_2$ adrenoceptors,[7] a_1 receptors also play an important role in controlling myocardial contraction.[8] Apart from the sympathetic system, multiple receptor systems in the human myocardium including histamine, serotonine (5 HT), Angiotensin I and II, vasoactive intestinal polypeptide (VIP), substance P and calcitonin gene-related peptide

have been discovered.[9] Changes in these receptors in patients with heart failure and other cardiovascular diseases is a broad and intensive field of scientific investigation.

SYMPATHETIC NERVE TERMINAL

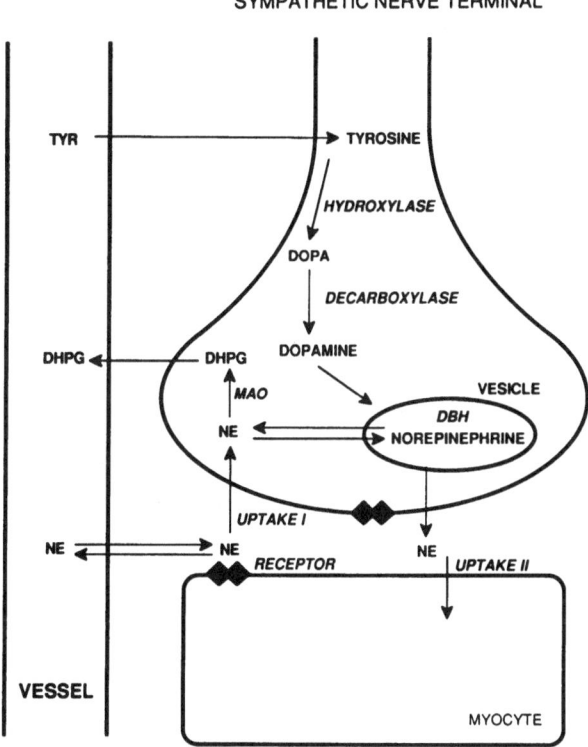

Figure 1. Diagram of the fate of norepinephrine in the sympathetic nerve terminal.

Pathophysiological changes in cardiac disease

In patients with heart failure, plasma norepinephrine concentrations are significantly elevated as a consequence of sympathetic activation.[10] Enhanced sympathetic activity is believed to be a major factor contributing to deterioration of the myocardial performance in these patients. As a result of increased synaptic norepinephrine levels, postsynaptic receptors are desensitized. The number of β_1 receptors available for norepinephrine interaction is decreased by internalization into cytoplasmatic compartments. Enhanced degradation or reduced synthesis of ß-receptors, as shown by decreased receptor mRNA, additionally reduces the number of ß-receptors.[11] Furthermore, functional coupling of β_2 receptors to intracellular postreceptor mechanisms is changed. As inhibitory G proteins coupled to adenylyl cyclase gain increasing influence over stimulatory G proteins, a decrease in intracellular cAMP results.[12] Receptors (mainly β_2) are functionally uncoupled by phosphorylation with a specific ß-adrenergic receptor kinase (bARK) or proteinekinase A and C.[13] Clinical relevance of these biochemical changes has been demonstrated in various studies which prove beneficial effects of chronic beta-adrenergic blockade in patients with cardiomyopathies.[14]

Changes in presynaptic sympathetic nerve endings in patients with cardiomyopathy have also been described. In patients with cardiomyopathy, the number of sympathetic nerve endings in the myocardium tends to become sparse.[15] This discrepancy between increased catecholamine concentrations and decreasing density of sympathetic neurons was explained by a downregulation of uptake carriers with decreasing clearance of norepinephrine from the site of action.[16] In a recent investigation, Böhm et al.[17] demonstrated a decrease in uptake-1 carrier density by radioligand binding in left ventricular preparations from patients with congestive cardiomyopathy.

In acute ischemic heart disease, the systemic and cardiac sympathetic nervous system is activated as shown by increased plasma catecholamine levels and increased norepinephrine release from the ischemic myocardium by a non-exocytotic, metabolically induced process.[5] The increase in catecholamine concentrations may generate malignant arrhythmias or cause myocardial necrosis.[18,19]

In chronic ischemic syndromes, heart failure develops and results in an ischemic cardiomyopathy. Differences in receptor desensitization between idiopathic and ischemic cardiomyopathy have also been reported. ß$_1$ adrenoceptors are downregulated in both pathological states; whereas, ß$_2$ receptors are reduced in ischemic cardiomyopathy but are unchanged in idiopathic/congestive heart failure. Due to inhomogeneous sympathetic denervation following myocardial infarction, a supersensitivity to circulating catecholamine with the capacity for generating arrhythmias may result as previously shown in the experimental setting.[20]

Radiotracers

Positron emission tomography (PET) and single photon emission computed tomography (SPECT) have been shown to be useful tools for in-vivo investigations of changes in the sympathetic nervous system in patients. Arising from the complexity of the sympathetic system, there are different demands on scintigraphic radiotracers for pre- or postjunctional sympathetic specificity. For validation of results, it must be taken into account that synthesis and degradation of sympathetic transmitters occur in vivo at different turn-over rates and at different sites.

Presynaptic site
The first radiotracer to selectively mark sympathetic presynaptic nerve endings was developed in the early 1980s at the University of Michigan. Iodine-123 meta-iodobenzylguanedine (^{123}I-MIBG), an analog of the antihypertensive drug guanethidine, was used for selective mapping of the cardiac sympathetic nerve endings using SPECT.[21] ^{123}I-MIBG is transported and stored into the presynaptic sympathetic nerve ending as a "false neurotransmitter", and it is most likely released in a similar manner as endogenous norepinephrine.[22,23] However, ^{123}I-MIBG has not only affinity to presynaptic sympathetic nerves, but also a low affinity for postsynaptic adrenergic receptors, which presents a disadvantage for the selectivity of the radioligand.

With the development of PET, improved imaging technology has become available that permits in-vivo regional quantification of tissue tracer concentrations.[24] The first success in the development of PET tracers for sympathetic nerve mapping was achieved by labeling norepinephrine with carbon-11 (^{11}C).[25] Rapid degradation of this ligand by endogenous enzymes MAO and COMT, however, made the interpretation of scintigraphic results difficult. Studies with fluorine-18 (^{18}F)-labeled dopamine, a norepinephrine precursor, showed uptake, storage and transformation to norepinephrine by DBH.[26] However, comparison of the tissue content of tritiated dopamine and ^{18}F-dopamine concentration revealed inconsistent and low affinity for uptake and metabolism by DBH. These drawbacks in the development of an in-vivo marker for presynaptic sympathetic nerve endings were overcome by using an structural analog of norepinephrine. ^{18}F-labeled metaraminol, a false neurotransmitter, was developed as a potential tracer for PET. Studies with this tracer in rats with pharmacological inhibition of uptake-1 and vesicular storage showed similar characteristics of ^{18}F metaraminol to that of norepinephrine.[27,28] Due to the presence of the alpha methyl group, metaraminol is resistant to metabolic breakdown by MAO, and with the absence of the catechol group, it is also resistant to COMT metabolism (Figure 2).

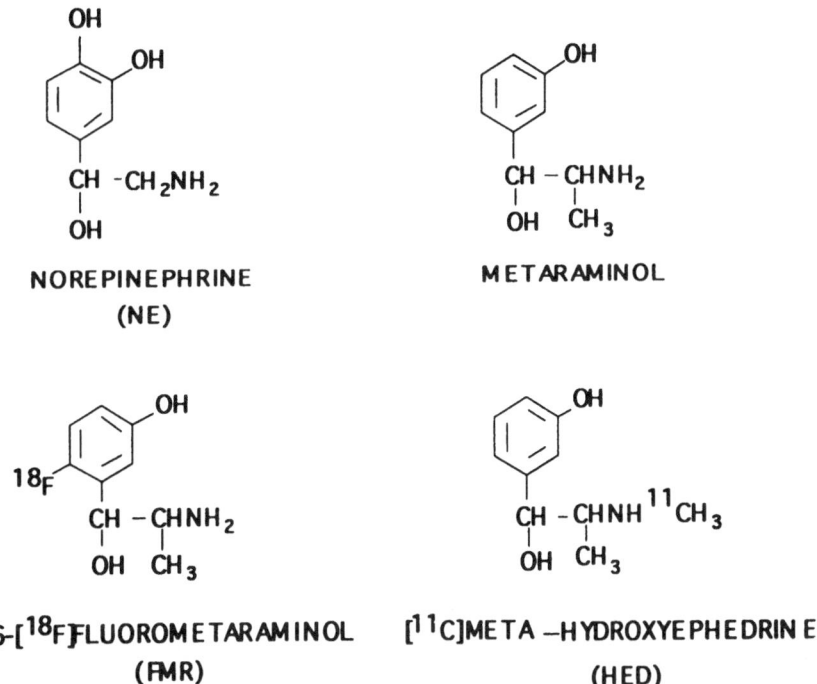

Figure 2. Chemical structures of norepinephrine and radiolabeled norepinephrine analogs.

Unfortunately, the inherent problem of low specific activity of only approximately 1-15 Ci/mmol could not be solved. Therefore, clinical application of ^{18}F-metaraminol failed due to pharmacological effects in patients following injection of ^{18}F-metaraminol with sufficient radioactivity for good image quality.

Another norepinephrine analog, ^{11}C-hydroxyephedrine (HED), was developed at the University of Michigan by direct reaction of the free base of metaraminol with ^{11}C-CH$_3$-I in dimethylformamide for PET imaging of sympathetic nerve terminals.[29] Unlike ^{18}F metaraminol, HED was synthesized with a specific activity ranging from 500 to 2000 Ci/mmol, which was suitable for clinical applications. HED has been shown to have similar uptake and storage mechanisms as endogenous catecholamines.[30] In animal studies, significant reduction in ^{11}C-HED retention by uptake-1 blockade with desipramine as well as inhibition of vesicular storage by reserpine were demonstrated.[31] It has also been shown, in the isolated working rat heart, that circulating norepinephrine competes with HED for uptake sites, which may complicate interpretation of PET results under conditions of increased plasma catecholamine levels.[32] In contrast to directly labeled catecholamines, the noradrenaline analogs are not metabolized by cytosolic MAO.[33] However, analysis of metabolites in blood revealed degradation of HED. Early after injection 85% of the blood activity was HED, which decreased to 52% after 20 minutes, indicating metabolism by a different enzyme, i.e. COMT[34]. Studies in a chronic dog model confirms specific uptake of HED into sympathetic nerve terminals with little non-neuronal accumulation.[28] A close correlation between HED tissue retention and histologically determined tissue norepinephrine content has also been shown. In normal healthy volunteers the tracer showed avid uptake into the heart with rapid clearance from the blood (Figure 3a). Relative tracer retention in the myocardium, expressed as percentage of peak myocardial activity, was about 80 % at 60 minutes after tracer injection, indicating a long tissue half-life. Patients with recent cardiac transplant, however, showed HED retention of only 18% of the maximum myocardial activity (Figure 3b), indicating little non-neuronal tracer accumulation.[35] Thus far, HED is the only clinically proven PET tracer for presynaptic sympathetic imaging in patients and seems to be an ideal in-vivo marker for evaluating the integrity of the sympathetic neurons.

Postsynaptic site
Knowledge about changes in postsynaptic receptor characteristics has been primarily obtained from in-vitro studies in animal models or from biopsy material and postmortem investigations in humans. However, with the development of radio-labeled receptor ligands for scintigraphy, the investigation of density and location of receptors in organs in patients in vivo became possible. Radiolabeled ligands for muscarinic-cholinergic, ß-adrenergic and dopamine receptors have been synthesized.[30] For quantification of receptors, mathematical model for quantification of ß-adrenoceptors has been established. For ß-adrenoceptors the SPECT tracer ^{123}I-iodocyanopindolol, a nonselective beta-adrenoceptor antagonist, was synthetized. In-vivo quantification of ß-receptors by SPECT was achieved in dogs using a three compartment model and 7 increasing doses of ^{123}I-iodocynopindolol.[37]

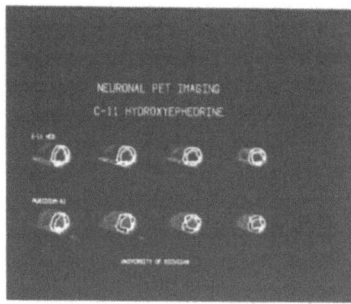

Figure 3a. Short axis cardiac PET images of a healthy volunteer. Top row images show homogenous HED uptake as an illustration of sympathetic innervation. Bottom images of Rubidium-82 uptake illustrates corresponding normal myocardial blood flow.

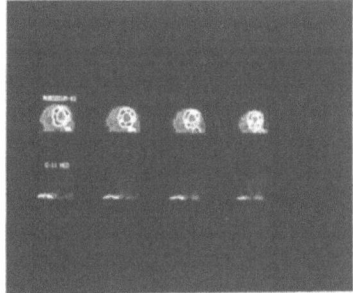

Figure 3b. Short axis cardiac PET images of a patient with recent cardiac transplant. Top images show normal blood flow as illustrated by-Rubidum-82; while bottom images show significant decrease in HED uptake.

For PET investigations Delforge et al.[38] used a compartmental model for reliable in-vivo quantification of receptor density in the dog heart. They investigated m-cholinoceptors with ^{11}C-labeled methylquinuclidinyl benzilate (MQNB), an antagonist of the muscarinic receptor that is not susceptible to metabolism. A comparable or even higher quantity of m-cholinoceptors in comparison to previous in- vitro findings with the tritiated ligand was found. For in-vivo assessment of ß-adrenoceptors, antagonists including propranolol, practolol, pindolol and CGP-12177 have been labeled with ^{11}C. Of these PET tracers, the hydrophilic ß antagonist CGP-12177 presents the greatest advantages concerning affinity, specifity and hydrophility. The synthesis of ^{11}C-CGP-12177 and the development of a new graphical method made quantitative in-vivo assessment of ß-adrenoceptors with PET clinically applicable.[39] Moreover, the hydrophilic ligand ^{11}C-CGP-12177 does not bind to receptors that are translocated into the cytoplasma due to downregulation. With this technique absolute quantity (Bmax) of the active receptors located on the surface of the plasma membrane could be determined in-vivo. Myocardial ß-adrenergic receptor density have been shown to differ among species. The highest values with 311 fmol/mg protein was reported in the dog heart; whereas receptor density in the rat and rabbit was 150 and 152 fmol/mg protein,respectively.

Clinical application of tracer approaches

The prognosis of patients with ischemic and congestive heart failure is mainly influenced by sudden cardiac death due to malignant arrhythmias and by the progression of pump failure of the left ventricle.[40] Heterogeneity of sympathetic innervation resulting in a supersensitivity to electrical stimulation have been demonstrated in animal studies. Inoue et al showed that dogs with autonomic heterogeneity were increasingly prone to ventricular fibrillation after programmed ventricular stimulation compared to sham operated animals.[20] In patients, detection of heterogeneity of sympathetic innervation by PET investigations may help to identify high risk patients for sudden cardiac death.

Deterioration of pump function in patients with heart failure is correlated to increased circulating norepinephrine.[41] The impairment of norepinephrine uptake and the resulting decrease in clearance from the synaptic cleft could be a major factor contributing to receptor desensitizing. Thus far, clinical PET data in diabetes mellitus, transplant patients, arrhythmia, infarction, long QT-syndrome, cocaine abusers and hypertrophic and congestive cardiomyopathy are available.

Presynaptic site

For the understanding of sympathetic dysfunction in ischemic cardiomyopathy, pathophysiology in acute ischemic syndromes must be investigated in order to elucidate this dynamic process leading to arrhythmias and deterioration of left and right ventricular function. Dysfunction of the presynaptic sympathetic nerve endings after acute myocardial ischemia have been shown with both SPECT and PET using various radiotracers in animal studies and in patients.

In experimentally induced myocardial infarctions in dogs, SPECT with ^{123}I-MIBG showed reduction in ^{123}I-MIBG uptake in areas with normal perfusion. Supersensitivity to electrical stimulation in areas of sympathetic denervation with normal perfusion was also demonstrated.[42] Similarly, in patients after myocardial infarction, sympathetic denervation was confirmed by the absence of ^{123}I-MIBG uptake in noninfarcted areas with normal thallium-201 uptake. However, a relationship between denervation and inducible ventricular tachycardias in these patients was not verified.[43]

These qualitative changes were confirmed with ^{18}F metaraminol and PET in open chest dogs models. Following 30 minutes of left anterior descendens coronary artery occlusion, a significant reduction in tracer accumulation in the ischemic area was shown. Comparisons with histologically measured norepinephrine content revealed a significant but weak correlation between histology and PET findings. As ^{18}F-metaraminol is transported and stored by the endogenous systems, it was concluded that the decrease in ^{18}F-metaraminol distribution in the dog heart after myocardial infarction was due to impaired uptake mechanism, storage mechanism and partially sympathetic denervation.[44] These findings of sympathetic changes in uptake and storage are in accordance with increased plasma norepinephrine concentration after acute ischemic syndromes. The increase in plasma norepinephrine concentration may induce malignant arrhythmias and may be of major importance for the initialization of the vicious circle leading to receptor desensitizing and deterioration of pump function in ischemic cardiomyopathy.

The first studies with HED in combination with PET for assessment of sympathetic prejunctional dysfunction in patients after myocardial infarction undergoing thrombolytic therapy showed a larger area of abnormal HED retention compared to the area of abnormal blood flow representing myocardial scar (Figure 4). Especially in patients with-non-Q-wave infarctions, the difference between neuronal injury and myocardial scar was shown (Figure 5). In a follow-up study, no change in the neuronal scar was detected, suggesting no relevant reinnervation in the first eight months after myocardial infarction.[45] The area of sympathetic denervation in intact myocardium with normal perfusion may induce malignant arrhythmias due to postsynaptic supersensitivity.

In order to evaluate the hypothesis of denervation supersensitivity as a mechanism for malignant arrhythmias, patients with sustained ventricular tachycardias after myocardial infarction were investigated. Patients referred for placement of an implantable defibrillator were examined with HED and PET, which showed significant reduction in HED retention in the infarcted area. Electrophysiological investigations also showed a prolonged refractory period in areas with decreased HED retention. However, the refractory period did not change significantly with norepinephrine infusion. These data did not demonstrate supersensitivity to norepinephrine in denervated segments. Nevertheless, the correlation between scintigraphically identified sympathetic dysfunction and electrophysiologic signs for arrhythmogenity may be helpful in evaluating the relationship between the sympathetic nervous system and ventricular arrhythmias.[46] Furthermore, PET with HED may be a useful tool to identify high risk patients for implantation of an internal cardioverter defibrillator.

In patients with idiopathic cardiomyopathy, sympathetic neuronal dysfunction was demonstrated with ^{123}I-MIBG and SPECT, showing decreased radiotracer distribution in the heart.[47] Elevated concentration of plasma norepinephrine, in these patients, competes with ^{123}I-MIBG for uptake into the presynaptic neuron. Although this group found only a partial correlation between increased plasma norepinephrine levels and decreased ^{123}I-MIBG uptake, they could not exclude the possibility of competitive displacement of ^{123}I-MIBG by endogenous norepinephrine at the uptake sites. Therefore, discrimination between impaired uptake function and decreased ^{123}I-MIBG uptake due to increased competition between endogenous norepinephrine and ^{123}I-MIBG in patients with cardiomyopathy is difficult. An additional factor that complicates interpretation of the scintigraphic results is the thinning of sympathetic nerve in the myocardium.[15] Further investigations are required to elucidate this problem with tracers for vesicular storage, ie. tetrabenazine, which is currently being developed.[48]

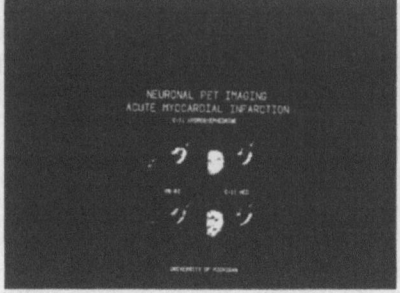

Figure 4. Long axis PET images of a patient with acute myocardial infarction. Left images show myocardial blood flow with Rb-82, and right images illustrate HED uptake. The arrows indicate the area with perfusion defect, shown by Rb-82 image, with relatively larger neuronal abnormality shown by reduced HED uptake.

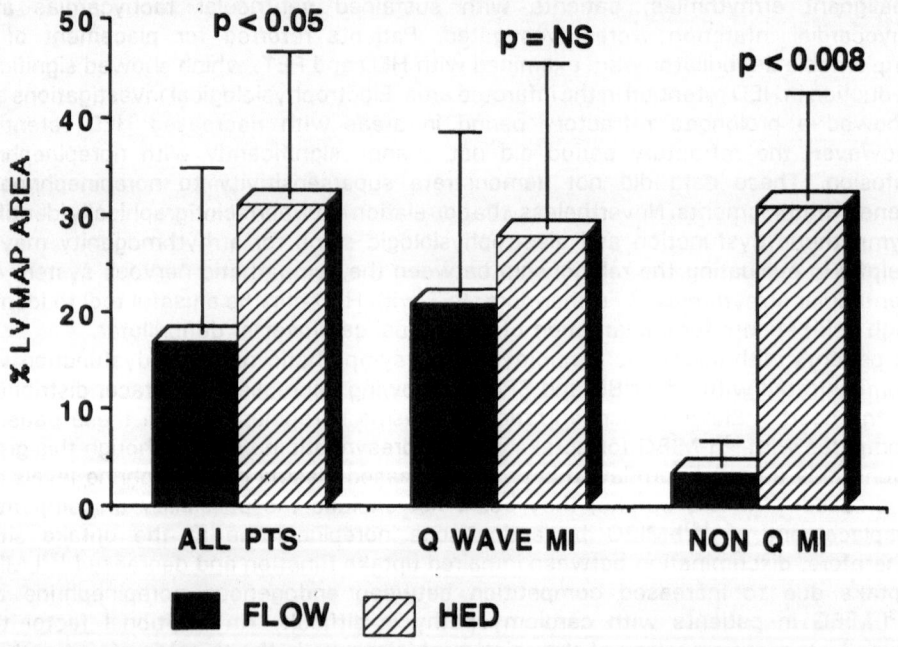

Figure 5. Extent of abnormal scintigraphic distribution of HED and $^{13}NH_3$ (blood flow) expressed as percentage of the left ventricle map area in patients with non-Q wave and Q wave infarctions. Filled bar represent myocardial blood flow, and hatched bar represent HED uptake. Patients with non-Q wave myocardial infarction have significantly larger defect in HED uptake compared to defect in blood flow.

In order to evaluate these findings for clinical relevance, a comparison between ^{123}I-MIBG uptake and various noninvasive techniques including echocardiography, radionuclide left ventriculography or chest X-ray for the prognosis of patients with cardiomyopathy was performed. The results from SPECT investigation showed a higher correlation to survival of patients with cardiomyopathy, compared to the other techniques.[49] An additional investigation demonstrated a good correlation between decreased ^{123}I-MIBG uptake with decreased inotropic response to ß-adrenoceptor stimulation and the increase of the plasma norephephrine concentration. They concluded that desensitization of ß-receptors is related to an impaired uptake mechanism and increased norepinephrine availability. According to these data, the impairment of the uptake mechanism seems to be the first and most important step for the process of increased sympathetic activity in patients with dilative cardiomyopathy.[50] Schwaiger et al.[51] also reported similar findings with HED using PET in patients with dilated cardiomyopathy (Figure 6). Due to the importance of the sympathetic nervous system in the development of cardiac failure, MIBG scintigraphy and PET with HED may be valuable tools in prognostic evaluation of patients for the assessment of the urgency of cardiac transplant.

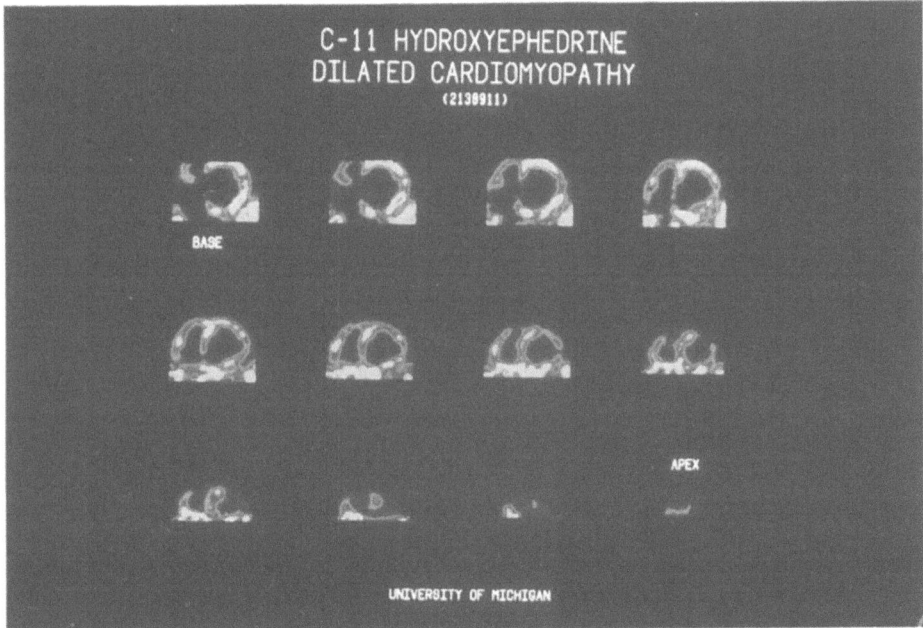

Figure 6. Shortaxis cardiac images with HED using PET in a patient with dilated cardiomyopathy, showing nonhomogenous distribution of the tracer. (see for colourplate of this figure page 246).

Impairment of the sympathetic nerve endings has also been described in other wide spread diseases. Autonomic neuropathy in patients with diabetes mellitus is well known and has been thought to be responsible for the poor prognosis of patients suffering, for example, from postural hypotension. Until recently, only indirect assessment of autonomic neuropathy by functional tests was possible. However, Allman et al.[52] demonstrated regional reduction in HED retention using PET in 8 diabetic patients with evident autonomic neuropathy compared to normal control subjects, but not in 5 diabetic patients without clinical signs of autonomic abnormalities (Figure 7). The differentiation between impaired uptake and storage or loss of neurons was not possible with HED, and mechanisms of diabetic neuropathy are not fully understood. Metabolic alterations due to increase in glucose metabolism via aldose reductase/sorbitol pathway are currently discussed as a major factor contributing to neuronal damage in diabetes.[53] Inhibitors of the aldose reductase have shown promising results in the treatment of diabetic neuropathy. As PET seems to be more sensitive for investigation of autonomic neuropathy than functional tests, assessment of autonomic neuropathy using PET could identify patients for the indication of aldose reductase medication. Furthermore, follow-up studies with HED and PET during treatment could help to assess autonomic nerve function in patients with diabetes.

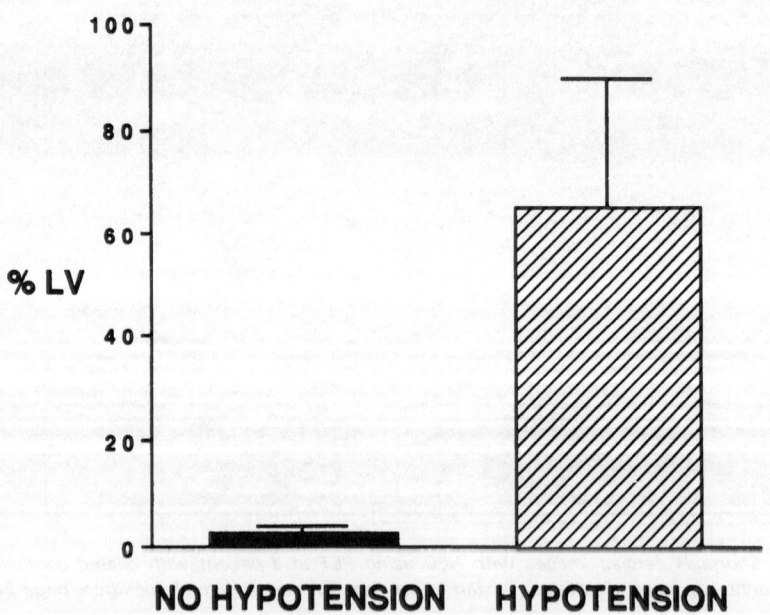

Figure 7. Extent of abnormal HED distribution shown as percent of left ventricle map area in patients with diabetic neuropathy. The filled bar represents patients without autonomic abnormality (no hypotension), while hatched bar represents patients with autonomic dysfunction indicated by hypotension.

In patients with heart transplants, increase in cardiac output is mainly achieved by increase in stroke volume; whereas increase in heart rate and contraction force is limited by autonomic denervation. Heart rate variability in these patients appears to improve over time as a sign for sympathetic reinnervation. In experimental models, reinnervation has been shown 9-12 months after surgery; however, reinnervation in patients remains controversial. With HED and PET, it was demonstrated that patients with recent cardiac transplantation showed significant reduction in HED uptake compared to control subjects (Figure 3); whereas patients with transplantation longer than 2 years showed signs of sympathetic reinnervation. Although HED retention in these patients was still significantly less than controls,[35] it was the first in-vivo assessment of sympathetic reinnervation with functioning uptake and vesicular storage of norepinephrine in patients with heart transplants for longer than 2 years.

As cardiac adverse effects including myocardial ischemia, pulmonary edema and aortic rupture have been ascribed to the inhibition of norepinephrine uptake in drug abusers, the influence of cocaine on catecholamine uptake and storage was investigated using HED and PET. Due to uptake-1 blockade by cocaine, HED retention was significantly reduced in dogs after administration of cocaine. This demonstrated the reliability of HED as a tool for the assessment of cocaine drug effects on myocardial catecholamine uptake and storage (Figure 8).[54]

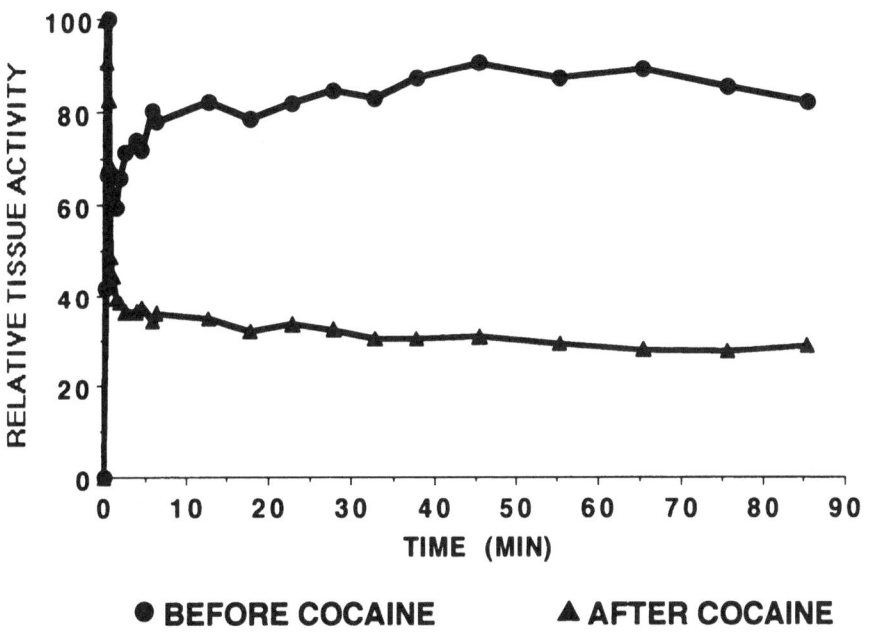

Figure 8. Representative time activity curves of HED before and after intravenous cocaine injection in dogs illustrated as percent of maximum tissue activity. Tissue retention of HED is significantly reduced after cocaine injection compared to a study before cocaine injection.

Postsynaptic site

Investigation of postsynaptic receptors with radiolabeled tracers suitable for PET has been a domain of neurologic investigations. Although ^{11}C labeled tracers including ^{11}C-MQNB for m-cholinoceptors, ^{11}C-CGP-12177 for ß-adrenoceptors, and ^{11}C-prazosin for a-adrenoceptors are available, only few investigations of receptors in the heart using PET have been published. Quantitative assessment of m-cholinoceptors in the dog heart with ^{11}C-MQNB reported absolute receptor density and dissociation constant comparable to in-vitro labeling was shown.[38] More recently, in-vivo investigation of m-cholinoceptors in patients was also reported.[55]

Animal studies of ß-adrenoceptors using PET have been reported.[56] Recent investigations by Merlet and coworkers[57] with ^{11}C-CGP-12177 showed a 53 % decrease in the number of ß-adrenoceptors in patients with idiopathic cardiomyopathy. Furthermore, the in-vivo results matched precisely in most patients with intra-individual comparison of in-vitro labeling of myocardial biopsies with ^{3}H-CGP-12177. This non-invasive investigation of ß-adrenoceptors in patients with dilated cardiomyopathy is in accordance with previous in-vitro studies. Due to the hydrophilic nature of ^{11}C-CGP-12177, binding to the surface ß-adrenoceptors may be measured. Therefore, reliable numbers of the active receptors may be determined by PET in patients without invasive preparations. This technique offers a useful tool for the investigation of changes in receptor densities together with functional studies in patients under certain pathophysiological states. Direct assessment of the density of the different receptor types may help in clinical situations to determine specific pharmacological treatment and follow-up studies.

Conclusions

Evaluations of the sympathetic nervous system using SPECT and PET have been demonstrated to be useful in the understanding of pathophysiological diseases affecting the sympathetic nervous system. Changes in norepinephrine uptake and storage during myocardial ischemia and in idiopathic and ischemic cardiomyopathy can be scintigraphically characterized in patients. It has also been shown that increased synaptic norepinephrine due to impaired uptake mechanism may play a major role in the development of arrhythmias and the deterioration of pump function in these patients. However, clinical application of neuronal imaging of the heart has not yet been established. The most promising application is the prognostic evaluation of patients with cardiomyopathy. Scintigraphic results may help to improve selection of patients for heart transplantation by identifying high risk groups for early mortality. However, further studies are required to define the relationship between scintigraphic signs of regional denervation and incidence of arrhythmias or even sudden death.

References

1. Esler M, Jennings G, Lambert G, Meredith I, Horne M, Eisenhofer G. Overflow of catecholamine neurotransmitters to the circulation: source, fate, and functions. Physiol Rev 1990;70:963-85.
2. Langer SZ. Presynaptic regulation of the release of catecholamines. Pharmacol Rev 1980;32:337-62.
3. Starke K, Gothert M, Kilbinger H. Modulation of neurotransmitter release by presynaptic autoreceptors. Physiol Rev 1989;69:864-989.
4. Majewski H, Tung LH, Rand MJ. Adrenaline activation of prejunctional beta-adrenoceptors and hypertension. J Cardiovasc Pharmacol 1982;4:99-106.
5. Schomig A. Catecholamines in myocardial ischemia. Systemic and cardiac release. Circulation 1990;82(Suppl 3):II13-II22.
6. Russ H, Gliese M, Sonna J, Schomig E. The extraneuronal transport mechanism for noradrenaline (uptake2) avidly transports 1-methyl-4-phenylpyridinium (MPP+). Naunyn Schmiedebergs Arch Pharmacol 1992;346:158-65.
7. Brodde OE, Zerkowski HR, Borst HG, Maier W, Michel MC. Drug- and disease-induced changes of human cardiac beta 1- and beta 2-adrenoceptors. Eur Heart J 1989;10(Suppl B):38-44.
8. Böhm M, Diet F, Feiler G, Kemkes B, Erdmann E. Alpha-adrenoceptors and alpha-adrenoceptor-mediated positive inotropic effects in failing human myocardium. J Cardiovasc Pharmacol 1988;12:357-64.
9. Gulbenkian S, Saetrum Opgaard O, Ekman R et al. Peptidergic innervation of human epicardial coronary arteries. Circ Res 1993;73:579-88.
10. Cohn JN, Levine TB, Olivari MT et al. Plasma norepinephrine as a guide to prognosis in patients with chronic congestive heart failure. N Engl J Med 1984;311:819-23.
11. Muntz KH, Zhao M, Miller JC. Downregulation of myocardial beta-adrenergic receptors. Receptor subtype selectivity. Circ Res 1994;74:369-75.
12. Ungerer M, Bohm M, Elce JS, Erdmann E, Lohse MJ. Altered expression of beta-adrenergic receptor kinase and beta 1-adrenergic receptors in the failing human heart. Circulation 1993;87:454-63.
13. Lohse MJ. Molecular mechanisms of membrane receptor desensitization. Biochim Biophys Acta 1993;1179:171-88.
14. Anonymous. A randomized trial of beta-blockade in heart failure. The Cardiac Insufficiency Bisoprolol Study (CIBIS). CIBIS Investigators and Committees. Circulation 1994;90:1765-73.
15. Amorim DS, Olsen EG. Assessment of heart neurons in dilated (congestive) cardiomyopathy. Br Heart J 1982;47:11-8.
16. Petch MC, Nayler WG. Uptake of catecholamines by human cardiac muscle in vitro. Br Heart J 1979;41:336-9.
17. Böhm M, La Rosee K, Schwinger RH. Evidence for a reduced norepinephrine uptake-1 in failing human myocardium. Circulation 1994;90:I-547 (Abstract).
18. Corr PB, Gillis RA. Autonomic neural influences on the dysrhythmias resulting from myocardial infarction. Circ Res 1978;43:1-9.
19. Van Vliet PD, Burchell HB, Titus JL. Focal myocarditis associated with pheochromocytoma. N Engl J Med 1966;274:1102-8.
20. Inoue H, Zipes DP. Results of sympathetic denervation in the canine heart: supersensitivity that may be arrhythmogenic. Circulation 1987;75:877-87.
21. Wieland DM, Brown LE, Rogers WL et al. Myocardial imaging with a radioiodinated norepinephrine storage analog. J Nucl Med 1981;22:22-31.

22. Tobes MC, Jaques S Jr, Wieland DM, Sisson JC. Effect of uptake-one inhibitors on the uptake of norepinephrine and metaiodobenzylguanidine. J Nucl Med 1985;26:897-907.

23. Nakajo M, Shimabukuro K, Yoshimura H et al. Iodine-131 metaiodobenzylguanidine intra- and extravesicular accumulation in the rat heart. J Nucl Med 1986;27:84-9.

24. Hoffmann EJ, Phelps ME. Positron emission tomography: principles and quantitation. In: Phelps ME, Mazziotta JC, Schelbert HR, editors. Positron emission tomography and autoradiography: principles and applications for the brain and heart. New York: Raven Press, 1986:237-87.

25. Fowler JS, Wolf AP, Christman DR, MacGregor RR, Ansari A, Atkins H. Carrier-free 11C-labeled catecholamines. In: Subramanian G, Rhodes BA, Cooper JF, Sodd VJ, editors. Radiopharmaceuticals. New York: Society of Nuclear Medicine, 1975:196-204.

26. Eisenhofer G, Hovevey-Sion D, Kopin IJ et al. Neuronal uptake and metabolism of 2- and 6-fluorodopamine: false neurotransmitters for positron emission tomographic imaging of sympathetically innervated tissues. J Pharmacol Exp Ther 1989;248:419-27.

27. Wieland DM, Rosenspire KC, Hutchins GD et al. Neuronal mapping of the heart with 6-[18F]fluorometaraminol. J Med Chem 1990;33:956-64.

28. Hutchins GD, Schwaiger M, Haka MS, Rosenspire KC, Wieland DM. Compartmental analysis of the behavior of catecholamine analogs in myocardial tissue. J Nucl Med 1989;30:735 (Abstract).

29. Rosenspire KC, Schwaiger M, Mangner TJ, Hutchins GD, Sutorik A, Kuhl DE. Metabolic fate of [13N]ammonia in human and canine blood. J Nucl Med 1990;31:163-7.

30. Wieland DM, Hutchins GD, Rosenspire KC et al. [C-11]Hydroxyephedrine (HED): a high specific activity alternative to 6-[F-18]fluorometaraminol (FMR) for heart neuronal imaging. J Nucl Med 1989;30:767-8.

31. DeGrado TR, Toorongian SA, Hutchins GD, Wieland DM, Schwaiger M. Characterization of C-11 m-hydroxyephedrine (HED) kinetics in isolated rat hearts. J Nucl Med 1992;33:870-1 (Abstract).

32. DeGrado TR, Hutchins GD, Toorongian SA, Wieland DM, Schwaiger M. Myocardial kinetics of carbon-11-meta-hydroxyephedrine: retention mechanisms and effects of norepinephrine. J Nucl Med 1993;34:1287-93.

33. Chakraborty PK, Gildersleeve DL, Toorongian SA, Kilbourn MR, Schwaiger M, Wieland DM. Synthesis of [11C]epinephrine and other biogenic amines by direct methylation of normethyl precursors. J Label Compounds Radiopharm 1992;32:172-3.

34. Rosenspire KC, Pisani TL, Haka MS, Schwaiger M. Metabolic studies of the PET neuronal heart agent [C-11]-meta-hydroxyephedrine (MHED). J Nucl Med. In press

35. Schwaiger M, Hutchins GD, Kalff V et al. Evidence for regional catecholamine uptake and storage sites in the transplanted human heart by positron emission tomography. J Clin Invest 1991;87:1681-90.

36. Syrota A. Receptor binding studies in the living heart. New Concepts Card Imaging 1988;4:141-66.

37. Sisson JC, Wieland DM, Koeppe RA, Frey KA, Normolle DP. Defining beta adrenoceptors in the living heart with iodocynopindolol. In: Kuhl DE, editor. In vivo imaging of neurotransmitter functions in brain, heart, and tumors. Washington DC: American College of Nuclear Physicians, 1991

38. Delforge J, Janier M, Syrota A et al. Noninvasive quantification of muscarinic receptors in vivo with positron emission tomography in the dog heart. Circulation 1990;82:1494-504.

39. Delforge J, Syrota A, Lancon JP et al. Cardiac beta-adrenergic receptor density measured in vivo using PET, CGP 12177, and a new graphical method. J Nucl Med 1991;32:739-48.

40. Kannel WB, Thomas HE Jr. Sudden coronary death: the Framingham Study. Ann N Y Acad Sci 1982;382:3-21.
41. Schwaiger M, Kalff V, Rosenspire K et al. Noninvasive evaluation of sympathetic nervous system in human heart by positron emission tomography. Cirvulation 1990;82:1681-90.
42. Minardo JD, Tuli MM, Mock BH et al. Scintigraphic and electrophysiological evidence of canine myocardial sympathetic denervation and reinnervation produced by myocardial infarction or phenol application. Circulation 1988;78:1008-19.
43. Stanton MS, Tuli MM, Radtke NL, Heger JJ et al. Regional sympathetic denervation after myocardial infarction in humans detected noninvasively using I-123-metaiodobenzylguanidine. J Am Coll Cardiol 1989;14:1519-26.
44. Schwaiger M, Guibourg H, Rosenspire K et al. Effect of regional myocardial ischemia on sympathetic nervous system as assessed by fluorine-18-metaraminol. J Nucl Med 1990;31:1352-7.
45. Allman KC, Stevens MJ, Wieland DM et al. Noninvasive assessment of cardiac diabetic neuropathy by carbon-11 hydroxyephedrine and positron emission tomography. J Am Coll Cardiol 1993;22:1425-32.
46. Calkins H, Allman K, Bolling S et al. Correlation between scintigraphic evidence of regional sympathetic neuronal dysfunction and ventricular refractoriness in the human heart. Circulation 1993;88:172-9.
47. Henderson EB, Kahn JK, Corbett JR et al. Abnormal I-123 metaiodobenzylguanidine myocardial washout and distribution may reflect myocardial adrenergic derangement in patients with congestive cardiomyopathy. Circulation 1988;78:1192-9.
48. DaSilva JN, Kilbourn MR, Koeppe RA, Sherman P, Pisani T, Mangner TJ. In vivo mouse brain biodistribution and monkey PET imaging of [C-11]tetrabenazine: a new PET marker for monoaminergic neurons. J Nucl Med 1992;33:870 (Abstract).
49. Merlet P, Dubois-Rande JL, Adnot S et al. Myocardial beta-adrenergic desensitization and neuronal norepinephrine uptake function in idiopathic dilated cardiomyopathy. J Cardiovasc Pharmacol 1992;19:10-6.
50. Merlet P, Valette H, Dubois-Rande JL et al. Prognostic value of cardiac metaiodobenzylguanidine imaging in patients with heart failure. J Nucl Med 1992;33:471-7.
51. Schwaiger M, Hutchins G, Rosenspire K, Haka M, Wieland DM. Quantitative evaluation of the sympathetic nervous system by PET in patients with cardiomyopathy. J Nucl Med 1990;31:792 (Abstract).
52. Allman KC, Wieland DM, Muzik O, Degrado TR, Wolfe ER Jr, Schwaiger M. Carbon-11 hydroxyephedrine with positron emission tomography for serial assessment of cardiac adrenergic neuronal function after acute myocardial infarction in humans. J Am Coll Cardiol 1993;22:368-75.
53. Tomlinson DR, Stevens EJ, Diemel LT. Aldose reductase inhibitors and their potential for the treatment of diabetic complications. Trends Pharmacol Sci 1994;15:293-7.
54. Melon PG, Nguyen N, DeGrado TR, Mangner TJ, Wieland DM, Schwaiger M. Imaging of cardiac neuronal function after cocaine exposure using carbon-11 hydroxyephedrine and positron emission tomography. J Am Coll Cardiol 1994;23:1693-9.
55. Delforge J, Le Guludec D, Syrota A et al. Quantification of myocardial muscarinic receptors with PET in humans. J Nucl Med 1993;34:981-91.
56. Law MP. Demonstration of the suitability of CGP 12177 for in vivo studies of beta-adrenoceptors. Br J Pharmacol 1993;109:1101-9.
57. Merlet P, Delforge J, Syrota A et al. Positron emission tomography with 11C CGP-12177 to assess beta-adrenergic receptor concentration in idiopathic dilated cardiomyopathy. Circulation 1993;87:1169-78.

16

Rutger L. Anthonio, Aren van Waarde, Antoon T.M. Willemsen,
Jan Pruim, Wiek H. van Gilst, Paul K. Blanksma,
Willem Vaalburg, and Kong I. Lie

Introduction

In the last decades increasing information has become available on changes in cardiac receptors during pathophysiological circumstances. With the advent of positron emission tomography (PET) imaging it is now theoretically possible to measure receptor density noninvasively in vivo. In the field of sympathetic innervation and postsynaptic cardiac ß-adrenoceptors in the heart, the first data using the PET technique have been published. Beta-adrenoceptors have been quantified by in vitro binding assays and changes in ß-adrenoceptor density have been associated with congestive heart failure,[1,2] myocardial ischemia,[3,4] cardiomyopathy,[5,6] valvular diseases,[7] hypertension,[8] diabetes,[9,10] hyperthyroidism[11] and chronic drug administration.[12,13] Cardiac ß_1-adrenoceptors exert positive inotropic, lusitropic, and chronotropic effects, whereas cardiac ß_2-adrenoceptors mainly have positive chronotropic and vasodilatory effects. Alteration in number of these receptors will affect cardiac function, especially since the human heart has a small receptor reserve for ß-agonists.[2]
This chapter will give a brief overview of 1) several experimental models and clinical pathophysiologic circumstances, in which ß-adrenoceptor density is changed, and 2) the first clinical PET ß-adrenoceptor measurements in healthy volunteers and patients.

Experimental factors causing altered cardiac ß-receptor densities

Several causative factors may induce changes of membrane-bound ß-adrenoceptor density. These can be divided into different groups: 1) heart failure, 2) ischemia, 3) hypertension, and 4) toxic damage. Most studies have employed radioligand binding techniques, but autoradiographic methods were also used to measure ß-adrenoceptor density. Heart failure causes downregulation[1,2] or no change in

E. E. van der Wall et al. (eds.), Cardiac Positron Emission Tomography, 201–210.

ß-adrenoceptor density.[14] Ischemia will cause upregulation of membrane bound ß-adrenoceptors,[3,4] and a downregulation of vesicular ß-adrenoceptors.[3,14] However, some studies also find downregulation of ß-adrenoceptors in ischemic hearts.[15] Experimental hypertension and pressure overload cause upregulation of sarcolemmal ß-adrenoceptors.[16,17] Conflicting results may be explained by the fact that long-lasting ischemia or hypertension proceeding to heart failure may cause downregulation of ß-adrenoceptors whereas short-term ischemia may cause upregulation. Alterations in ß-adrenoceptor density are strongly influenced on the model used and are dependent on variability in severity of heart failure in the groups studied. Table 1 gives a brief overview of changes in in vitro studies, using different models.

Table 1 Experimental in vitro B_{max} studies

disease	B_{max} alteration	Reference
heart failure	→ ↓	14,36,37,38
ischemia	→ ↑ ↓	4,15,39,40,41
hypertension	→ ↑ ↓	16,17,42,43,44,45
toxic (i.e. adriamycin)	↓	46,47
diabetes	↓	9,10

→ = no change in Bmax, ↓ = decrease of B_{max}, ↑ = increase of B_{max}, B_{max} = ß-adrenoceptor density

Clinical diseases and factors causing altered cardiac ß-receptor densities

Most pathophysiologies with altered ß-adrenoceptor densities, are diseases in which the clinical syndrome 'heart failure' finally is present. Until now most clinical ß-adrenoceptor densities in patients are assessed using in vitro assays on blood cells. A few studies use cardiac biopsies or autopsy material for binding studies. Most biopsy material was obtained from patients suffering from idiopathic dilated cardiomyopathy. In the diagnostic procedure a biopsy is a common method in these patients, to identify a cause for cardiac dilation. Therefore cardiac tissue is easily obtained for further research. 'Normal values' for B_{max} are obtained in biopsies from donor hearts and in lymphocytes of healthy volunteers. Table 2 gives a brief overview of ß-receptor density changes in different clinical circumstances. Several general reviews describing the changes occurring in different heart diseases are available.[18-21]

Table 2 Human (clinical) in vitro B_{max} studies

disease	B_{max} alteration	Reference
ischemic cardiomyopathy	↓	6,19
dilated cardiomyopathy	↓	5,6,19
valvular disease	↓	7
exercise	↑	48

→ = no change in Bmax, ↓ = decrease of B_{max}, ↑ = increase of B_{max}, B_{max} = ß-adrenoceptor density

Methods for ß-adrenoceptor density measurement

Since the availability of radiolabeled ligands in the 1970s it has become possible to measure both ß-receptor density and affinity. Unfortunately the invasive character of the method, limits its applicability. For quantification of ß-adrenoceptor density, by this in vitro method, homogenates of cardiac tissue are required. These can only be obtained from cardiac biopsies, donor hearts or explanted hearts. Another more indirect method is the measurement of ß-adrenoceptors on blood cells (lymphocytes and platelets). Although easy to obtain, the interpretation of changes in blood cell receptor density can be difficult, because changes in these blood cells may not necessarily reflect changes in the heart.[22] Another problem with this method is, that only $ß_2$- and no $ß_1$-adrenoceptors are present on these cells.[22,23] Despite these limitations, binding studies on blood cells are often performed to elucidate receptor alterations in many cardiac and non-cardiac diseases. Beta-adrenoceptor density can also be measured by quantitative autoradiography. As tissue structure remains intact, it is possible to measure local changes (i.e., differences between subendocardial and endocardial layers) of ß-adrenoceptor density in different layers of cardiac tissue.[24] Unfortunately, this method has otherwise the same disadvantages as binding studies on tissue homogenates.
A totally different approach, without the disadvantages of in vitro assays, is the non-invasive analysis of receptors by PET. Using this method it is possible to quantify not only ß-adrenoceptor density but also the spatial distribution of ß-adrenoceptors in the heart. Because of technical difficulties, especially regarding radioligand synthesis, only limited data are available. The first PET center which successfully quantified ß-adrenoceptors was the group of Syrota et al.[25] in Orsay. Later the PET center in Hammersmith by Lefroy et al.[26] reported in vivo ß-adrenoceptor measurements using the same radiolabeled ligand and assay method. Since 1994 this method, developed by Orsay as modified in cooperation with the Hammersmith group,[27] is also available in Groningen.

PET to quantitate ß-adrenoceptor density

PET provides the opportunity to quantify ligand uptake in vivo. A useful ligand for quantification of receptor density has to meet several criteria. These criteria are extensively mentioned in the chapter 'Study of cardiac receptor ligands'.[28] In brief the main criteria are: 1) binding must occur with high affinity (K_d < 10^{-8}) to a signal-transducing site, 2) tissue uptake must represent (stereo)selective binding, 3) the binding must be saturable, 4) the ligand should clear rapidly from the circulation, to provide a sufficient contrast between the tissue and the blood, 5) radiolabeled metabolites must be formed slowly, or not at all, and they should not be extracted by the tissue of interest, and 6) there must be a correlation between binding and biological effect (i.e., displacement of the ligand is accompanied by the receptor-specific biological effect). A radioligand meeting these criteria is (S)-^{11}C-CGP12177 and first results have been published.[28-32] (S)-^{11}C-CGP12177 exhibits most criteria: It is a hydrophilic ß$_1$ and ß$_2$-adrenoceptor antagonist, which binds with a high specificity, selectivity and affinity to membrane bound receptors. Unfortunately Delforge et al.[25] found early metabolization of the ligand, and simple linear models, using plasma time-activity curves as input function of the myocardium could not explain the myocardial time-activity curve satisfactorily.

A method for quantification of ß-adrenoceptors is described by Delforge et al.[25] They developed a graphical method using a multiple injection protocol. Briefly, the method is based on a difference in kinetic behavior of the ligand when injected under different levels of high and low receptor occupation which is induced by injection of high and low amounts of (S)-^{11}C-CGP12177. Due to the different kinetic behavior under these conditions, two differently shaped time-activity curves are obtained. Using the differences between these two time-activity curves, an estimation of B'_{max} can be assessed.[27]

A schematic representation of the tissue response after both injections is shown in Figure 1. The time-activity curves of (S)-^{11}C-CGP12177 are measured in regions of interest encompassing myocardium of the left ventricle. The first injection and the second injection of respectively a high and low specific activity radioligand. The slope of the curves after the first and second injection is characterized by a rapid and a slow component corresponding to washout of free and bound ligand. Extrapolation of the slow component of both curves (respectively S_0 and S_1) to the moment of injection gives the concentration of bound ligand after the first (C_0) and second (C_1) injection. When these data are combined with the known dose at first (D_0) and second (D_1) injection and the specific activity at time of injection, B'_{max} can be calculated with Formula 1.

PET ß-adrenoceptor density measurements

Table III shows the current PET ß-adrenoceptor data in the literature and preliminary data from our institute. Delforge et al.[25] have demonstrated the suitability of the graphical method in dogs. In patients with idiopathic dilated cardiomyopathy,[33] they found a significantly decreased ß-adrenoceptor density. From these patients they

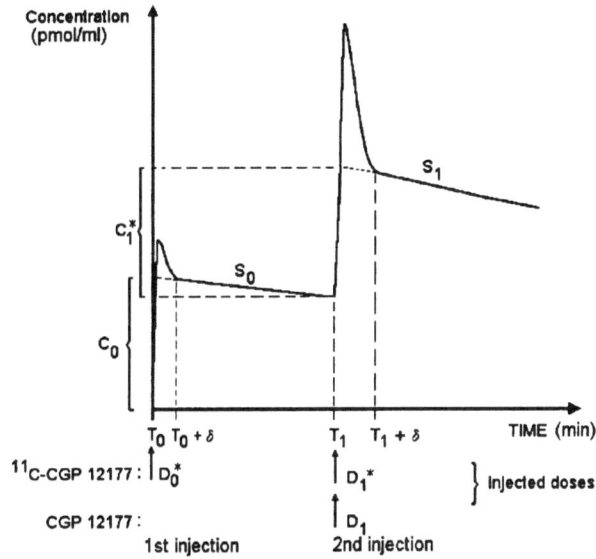

Figure 1. A schematic representation of the time-activity curves obtained after a two injection protocol with in the first injection a high specific activity (low mass) and in the second injection a low specific activity (high mass). B'_{max} = ß-adrenoceptor concentration, C_0^* = concentration of bound ligand after the first injection, C_1^* = concentration of bound ligand after the second injection, D_0^* = dose of (S)-^{11}C-CGP12177 in the first injection, D_1^* = dose of (S)-^{11}C-CGP12177 in the second injection, D_1 = dose (S)-CGP12177 in the second injection, S_0 = bound ligand concentration after the first injection, S_1 = bound ligand concentration after the second injection. (Reproduced with permission from[25])

$$(B'_{max}-C^*(T1-\varepsilon))(1-e^{\left(\dfrac{D_1^*+D_1}{D_0^*}\right)\log\left(\dfrac{B'_{max}-C_0^*}{B'_{max}}\right)})-C_1^*\left(\dfrac{D_1^*+D_1}{D_1^*}\right)=0$$

Formula 1. The correct B_{max} formula as developed by Delforge et al.[27] B'_{max} = ß-adrenoceptor concentration, C_0^* = concentration of bound ligand after the first injection, C_1^* = concentration of bound ligand after the second injection, $C^*(T1-\epsilon)$ = the concentration (S)-^{11}C-CGP12177 just before the second injection, D_0^* = dose of (S)-^{11}C-CGP12177 in the first injection, D_1^* = dose of (S)-^{11}C-CGP12177 in the second injection, D_1 = dose of (S)-CGP12177 in the second injection. (Reproduced with permission from[27])

Table 3 PET ß-adrenoceptor density studies

	B_{max}	Reference
Orsay	pmol/ml tissue	
dogs (n = 5)	31 ± 4	26
healthy volunteers (n = 7)	7.22 ± 0.75	34
HTX (n = 8)	7.25 ± 0.97	35
IDC (n = 10)	3.12 ± 0.51	34
Hammersmith	pmol/g tissue	
healthy volunteers (n = 8)	11.5 ± 2.18	26
HOCM (n = 11)	7.7 ± 1.86	26
Groningen	pmol/ml tissue	
healthy volunteers (n = 6)	3.5 ± 0.4	non published data

→ = no change in B_{max}, ↓ = decrease of B_{max}, ↑ = increase of B_{max}, B_{max} = ß-adrenoceptor concentration in pmol/ml tissue (Orsay, Groningen) or in pmol/g tissue (Hammersmith), IDC = idiopathic dilating cardiomyopathy patients, HOCM = hypertrophic obstructive cardiomyopathy patients, HTX = heart transplant patients

also obtained endomyocardial biopsies, and estimated B_{max} in vitro using ^{3}H-CGP12177. A good correlation between PET and in vitro data (r = 0.79, p = 0.019) was found. Moreover, ß-contractile responsiveness was measured in these patients, and a direct correlation between the receptor density acquired by PET and functional receptor status was noted (r = 0.83, p = 0.003). In post heart transplant patients they found no change in ß-adrenoceptor density, which is conceivable, since these hearts are denervated.[34] Lefroy et al.[26] measured PET ß-adrenoceptor density in patients with hypertrophic cardiomyopathy. They found a significantly decreased ß-adrenoceptor density in these patients (p < 0.001). ß-adrenoceptor density distribution was homogeneous despite differences in wall thickness. They found no elevated plasma catecholamines in these patients. We studied ß-adrenoceptor distribution in healthy volunteers, and constructed parametric polarmaps consisting of 480 segments of the left ventricle. With the same parametric polarmap construction as is used for ^{19}FDG and ^{13}NH3 studies in our institute B_{max} values were calculated for each segment by the graphical method as developed and corrected by Delforge et al.,[27] using the mean uptake in each segment.

The parametric polarmap construction

The construction of parametric polarmaps is described in the chapter 'Parametric imaging of myocardial perfusion and metabolism' by Willemsen et al.[35] In brief, the data of each study were reoriented to 10 short axis images, using a manually drawn long axis in the left ventricle. The myocardium in the different slices was divided in 48 segments (7.5° each). Time activity curves were obtained for all segments in all slices. For all frames polarmaps were calculated, using the same set of reorientation data. Thus for all segments of all slices dynamic tissue data were obtained yielding 480 separate segments. From these data dynamic parametric polarmaps were constructed. These polarmaps show the three dimensional ß-adrenoceptor density distribution of ß-adrenoceptors in 480 segments.

We thus found an average receptor density of 3.5 ± 4 pmol/ml tissue with an interindividual coefficient of variation of 30%. The differences in B_{max} values between the different groups may be explained by differences in correction methods for partial volume and spill-over effects. Merlet et al.[33] used echocardiographic estimated wall thickness and a recovery factor measured experimentally on a heart phantom. Lefroy et al.[26] corrected their data for blood volume using a $C^{15}O$ scan, and performed myocardial perfusion measurements. We corrected our data for blood volume with a theoretical blood volume of 5%, where as a partial volume correction was not applied.

Conclusions

Many new opportunities are in the scope of PET imaging. This modality may provide new insights in in vivo changes of cardiac ß-adrenoceptors. Using CGP-PET with standardized reorientation to 10 short axis slices, changes in ß-receptor distribution e.g. due to myocardial infarction and ischemia may be better identified and characterized. Because of its non-invasive character, PET also provides the possibility of serial measurements, and may elucidate the effects of different treatment strategies, in several heart diseases on cardiac ß-adrenergic receptors.

References

1. Bristow MR, Ginsburg R, Umans V et al. Beta$_1$- and beta$_2$- adrenergic-receptor subpopulations in nonfailing and failing human ventricular myocardium: coupling of both receptor subtypes to muscle contraction and selective beta 1-receptor down-regulation in heart failure. Circ Res 1986;59:297-309.
2. Brodde O-E, Zerkowski H-R, Borst HG, Maier W, Michel MC. Drug- and disease-induced changes of human cardiac ß$_1$- and ß$_2$-adrenoceptors. Eur Heart J 1989;10(Suppl B):38-44.
3. Maisel AS, Motulsky HJ, Insel PA. Externalization of β-adrenergic receptors promoted by myocardial ischemia. Science 1985;230:183-6.
4. Mukherjee A, Wong TM, Buja LM, Lefkowitz RJ, Willerson JT. Beta-adrenergic and muscarinic cholinergic receptors in canine myocardium. Effects of ischemia. J Clin Invest 1979;64:1423-8.
5. Heilbrunn SM, Shah P, Bristow MR, Valantine HA, Ginsburg R, Fowler MB. Increased ß-receptor density and improved hemodynamic response to catecholamine stimulation during longterm metoprolol therapy in heart failure from dilated cardiomyopathy. Circulation 1989;79:483-90.
6. Bristow MR, Anderson FL, Port JD et al. Differences in beta-adrenergic neuroeffector mechanisms in ischemic versus idiopathic dilated cardiomyopathy. Circulation 1991;84:1024-31.
7. Brodde OE, Zerkowski HR, Doetsch N, Motomura S, Khamssi M, Michel MC. Myocardial ß-adrenoceptor changes in heart failure: concomitant reduction in ß$_1$ and ß$_2$-adrenoceptor function related to the degree of heart failure in patients with mitral valve disease. J Am Coll Cardiol 1989;14:323-31.
8. Yamada S, Ishima T, Tomita T, Hayashi T, Okada T, Hayashi E. Alterations in cardiac α- and ß-adrenoceptors during the development of spontaneous hypertension. J Pharmacol Exp Ther 1984;228:454-9.
9. Heyliger CE, Pierce GN, Singal PK, Beamish RE, Dahalla NS. Cardiac α- and ß-adrenergic receptor alterations in diabetic cardiomyopathy. Basic Res Cardiol 1982;77:610-8.
10. Williams RS, Schaible TF, Scheuer J, Kenny R. Effects of experimental diabetes on adrenergic and cholinergic receptors of rat myocardium. Diabetes 1983;32:881-6.
11. Lefkowitz RJ, Caron MG, Stiles GL. Mechanism of membrane-receptor regulation. Biochemical, Physiological, and clinical insights derived from studies of the adrenergic receptors. N Engl J Med 1984;24:1570-9.
12. Maisel AS, Phillips C, Michel MC, Ziegler MG, Carter SM. Regulation of cardiac ß-adrenergic receptors by captopril. Implications for congestive heart failure. Circulation 1989;80:669-75.
13. Maisel AS, Motulsky HJ, Insel PA. Propranolol treatment externalizes ß-adrenergic receptors in guinea-pig myocardium and prevents further externalization by ischemia. Circ Res 1986;60:108-12.
14. Vleeming W, Van der Wouw PA, Te Biesebeek JD, Van Rooij HH, Wemer J, Porsius AJ. Density of ß-adrenoceptors in rat heart and lymphocytes 48 hours and 7 days after acute myocardial infarction. Cardiovasc Res 1989;23:859-66.
15. Rhee HM, Tyler L. Myocardial ischemia injury and ß-adrenergic receptors in perfused working rabbit hearts. Adv Exp Med Biol 1985;191:281-8.
16. Limas CJ. Increased number of ß-adrenergic receptors in the hypertrophied myocardium. Biochem Biophys Acta 1979;588:174-8.
17. Kumano K, Upsher ME, Khairallah PA. ß-Adrenergic receptor response coupling in

hypertrophied hearts. Hypertension 1993;5(Suppl I):I175-83.
18. Barnet DB. Myocardial ß-adrenoceptor function and regulation in heart failure: implications for therapy. Br J Clin Pharmacol 1989;27:527-37.
19. Brodde OE. Beta 1- and beta 2-adrenoceptors in the human heart: properties, function, and alterations in chronic heart failure. Pharmacol Rev 1991;43:203-42.
20. Bristow MR. The adrenergic nervous system in heart failure. N Engl J Med 1984;311:850-1.
21. Gopalakrishnan M, Triggle DJ. The regulation of receptors, ion channels, and G proteins in congestive heart failure. Cardiovasc Drug Rev 1990;8:255-302.
22. Brodde OE, Michel MC, Gordon EP, Sandoval A, Gilbert EM, Bristow MR. Beta-adrenoceptor regulation in the human heart: can it be monitored in circulating lymphocytes? Eur Heart J 1989;10(Suppl):B2-10.
23. Michel MC, Beckeringh JJ, Ikezono K, Kretsch R, Brodde OE. Lymphocyte beta 2-adrenoceptors mirror precisely beta 2-adrenoceptor, but poorly beta 1-adrenoceptor changes in the human heart. J Hypertens 1986;4(Suppl):S215-8.
24. Steinfath M, Lavicky J, Schmitz W, Scholtz H, Döring V, Kalmár P. Regional distribution of ß1 and ß2 adrenoceptors in the failing and nonfailing human heart. Eur J Clinical Pharmacol 1992;42:607-12
25. Delforge J, Syrota A, Lancon JP et al. Cardiac beta-adrenergic receptor density measured in vivo using PET, CGP 12177, and a new graphical method. J Nucl Med 1991;32:739-48.
26. Lefroy DC, De Silva R, Choudhury L et al. Diffuse reduction of myocardial beta-adrenoceptors in hypertrophic cardiomyopathy: a study with positron emission tomography. J Am Coll Cardiol 1993;22:1653-60.
27. Delforge J. Correction of a relationship that assesses beta-adrenergic receptor concentration with PET and carbon-11-CGP 12177. J Nucl Med 1994;35(5):921.
28. Van Waarde A. Study of cardiac receptor ligands. In: Van der Wall EE, Blanksma PK, Niemeyer MG, and Paans AMJ, editors. Cardiac positron emission tomography. Dordrecht: Kluwer Academic Publishers, 1995.
29. Jones HA, Rhodes CG, Law MP et al. Rapid analysis for metabolites of 11C-labelled drugs: fate of ¹¹C-S-4-(tert.-butylamino-2-hydroxypropoxy)-benzimidazol-2-one in the dog. J Chromatogr 1991;570:361-70.
30. Law MP. Demonstration of the suitability of CGP 12177 for in vivo studies of beta-adrenoceptors. Br J Pharmacol 1993;109:1101-9.
31. Van Waarde A, Meeder JG, Blanksma PK et al. Suitability of CGP-12177 and CGP-26505 for quantitative imaging of beta-adrenoceptors. Int J Rad Appl Instrum 1992;19:711-8.
32. Van Waarde A, Meeder JG, Blanksma PK et al. Uptake of radioligands by rat heart and lung in vivo: CGP 12177 does and CGP 26505 does not reflect binding to beta-adrenoceptors. Eur J Pharmacol 1992;222:107-12.
33. Merlet P, Delforge J, Syrota A et al. Positron emission tomography with 11C CGP-12177 to assess beta-adrenergic receptor concentration in idiopathic dilated cardiomyopathy. Circulation 1993;87:1169-78.
34. Merlet P, Benvenuti C, Valette H et al. ß-receptors in human transplanted heart assessed with positron emission tomography. First international congress of nuclear cardiology 1993;1:4302 (Abstract).
35. Willemsen A. Parametric imaging of myocardial perfusion and metabolism. In: Van der Wall EE, Blanksma PK, Niemeyer MG, and Paans AMJ, editors. Cardiac positron emission tomography. Dordrecht: Kluwer Academic Publishers, 1995.
36. Baumann G, Riess G, Erhardt WD et al. Impaired ß-adrenergic stimulation in the

uninvolved ventricle post-acute myocardial infarction: reversible defect due to excessive circulatory catecholamine-induced decline in number and affinity of ß-receptors. Am Heart J 1981;101:569-81

37. Baumann G, Felix SB, Reib G, Loher U, Ludwig L, Blomer H. Effective stimulation of cardiac contractility and metabolism by impromidine and dimaprit-two new H2 agonistic compounds in the surviving, catecholamine-insensitive myocardium after coronary occlusion. J Cardiovasc Pharmacol 1982;5:542-53.

38. Karliner JS, Stevens M, Grattan M, Woloszyn W, Honbo N, Hoffman JIE. Beta-adrenergic receptor properties of canine myocardium: effects of chronic myocardial infarction. J Am Coll Cardiol 1986;8:349-56.

39. Wolff AA, Hines DK, Karliner JS. Refined membrane preparations mask ischemic fall in myocardial ß-receptor density. Am J Physiol 1989;257:H1032-6.

40. Dominiak P, Turck D. Alterations of ß-adrenoceptors subsequent to myocardial infarction. Basic Res Cardiol 1986;81(Suppl 1):243-51.

41. Wolff AA, Karliner JS. H2-histaminergic and ß-adrenergic adenyl cyclase activation is maintained despite receptor changes and Gs dysfunction during acute myocardial ischemia. Clin Res 1988;36:328A (Abstract).

42. Foster KA, Hock CE, Reibel DK. Altered responsiveness of hypertrophied rat hearts to α- and ß-adrenergic stimulation. J Mol Cell Cardiol 1991;23:91-101.

43. Ganguly PK, Lee SL, Beamish RE, Dhalla NS. Altered sympathetic system and adrenoceptors during the development of cardiac hypertrophy. Am Heart J 1989;118:520-5.

44. Michel MC, Kanczik R, Khamssi M et al. α- and ß-adrenoceptors in hypertension. I. Cardiac and renal α1-, ß1, and ß2-adrenoceptors in rat models of acquired hypertension. J Cardiovasc Pharmacol 1989;13:421-31.

45. Chevalier B, Mansier P, Callens-El, Amrani F, Swynghedauw B. ß-adrenergic system is modified in compensatory pressure cardiac overload in rats: physiological and biochemical evidence. J Cardiovasc Pharmacol 1989;13:412-20.

46. Bocherens-Gadient SA, Quast U, Nussberger J, Brunner HR, Hof RP. Chronic adriamycin treatment and its effect on the cardiac beta-adrenergic system in the rabbit. J Cardiovasc Pharmacol 1992;19:770-8.

47. Yoshikawa T, Handa S, Suzuki M, Nagami K. Abnormalities in sympathoneuronal regulation are localized to failing myocardium in rabbit heart. J Am Coll Cardiol 1994;24:210-5.

48. Brodde OE, Daul A, Michel-Reher M et al. Agonist-induced desensitization of beta-adrenoceptor function in humans. Subtype-selective reduction in beta 1- or beta 2-adrenoceptor-mediated physiological effects by xamoterol or procaterol. Circulation 1990;81:914-21.

17

METHODOLOGICAL ISSUES IN REGIONAL MYOCARDIAL
PERFUSION IMAGING WITH POSITRON
EMISSION TOMOGRAPHY

Anne Bol, William Wijns, and Jacques A. Melin

Introduction

Positron emission tomography (PET) is currently the only technique available that permits the quantification of regional myocardial blood flow in vivo. Absolute PET measurements of nutrient tissue flow and flow reserve[1] have contributed significantly to the understanding of the mechanisms of various cardiac disorders such as ischemic heart disease, cardiac hypertrophy or microcirculatory disorders.[2] However these quantitative measurements are demanding and are currently performed adequately in a limited number of laboratories with particular expertise in instrumentation and tracer modelling. This chapter deals with several aspects of PET methodology in the evaluation of myocardial perfusion.

Instrumentation

Appropriate quantification of cardiac PET studies is based on the ability to accurately measure the arterial input function and the myocardial tissue concentration, generally as a function of time. In order to derive absolute values of myocardial blood flow, these quantities need to be incorporated into suitable physiologic models. However, before attempting to model the dynamic data obtained with PET, great care is required in every step that will ultimately yield quantitative images from the raw sinograms. This is especially true during cardiac studies where the tomograph often works at its performance limits. This paragraph deals with some important factors possibly responsible for distortion of the data during cardiac PET studies.

High count rates
The presence of the cardiac chambers in the imaged field of view allows the non-invasive determination of the arterial input curve. However, this causes the entire

E. E. van der Wall et al. (eds.), Cardiac Positron Emission Tomography, 211–220.

amount of injected activity to pass through the field of view producing very high count rates and particularly so when the tracer is injected as a short bolus.[3] Such high counting rates lead to two effects: a time varying loss of counts (dead-time losses) and a degradation of the image contrast due to increased random coincidences.

The dead-time losses are due to the time needed by the electronic system to process an event. Should another event occur during that time interval, the electronics would be unable to process it and that event would be lost. These losses increase with the count rate and alter the proportionality between the number of recorded true coincidences and the activity concentration. The dead-time losses depend on the capabilities of each tomograph. These losses can be estimated and corrected for quite accurately by measuring the single rates of the detectors. Nevertheless, it is important to operate the tomograph at count rates where one can be confident in the accuracy of the correction. Therefore, it is best to limit the amount of activity administered so that the magnitude of this correction is kept lower than a factor of two.

The random or accidental coincidences correspond to recorded coincidences due to 2 photons that do not come from the same annihilation. These coincidences contribute significantly to the degradation of the contrast in the reconstructed image. Their number depends linearly on the width of the coincidence window and quadratically on the amount of activity. The random coincidences can be estimated either by measuring the single rates of the detectors, knowing the width of the coincidence window, or by the delayed coincidence method. This correction may increase the noise in the images but if carefully performed, it should not introduce significant errors on the results of the quantification process.

Both dead-time and random coincidences effects are generally accounted for in commercially available tomographs. Nevertheless one should be aware of their respective magnitude in order to determine the optimal dose to be injected to obtain a maximum of useful data without induly increasing radiation exposure to the patient.

Attenuation

The attenuation represents the loss of detected events because of interactions of the emitted photons with the surrounding tissues. Because of the large size and the inhomogeneity of the chest, this effect is particularly important in cardiac studies where the attenuation factors are important (factors of 10 to 20 are common) and variable between adjacent structures. In principle, an accurate attenuation correction can be achieved with PET by means of an external transmission source (generally a rotating rod containing activity). The main cause of error in that measurement is patient motion during the course of the study, which produces a misalignment between attenuation and emission scans. This misalignment can lead to improper corrections resulting not only in erroneous absolute values but also in artefactual regional inhomogeneities. Different methods have been proposed to compensate for this misalignment[4,5] but they are not routinely applied. Therefore we must keep in mind this important source of error when interpreting myocardial images and instruct patients to maintain their position within the gantry during the entire course of the study.

Scatter

The two photons emitted after annihilation have a high probability to interact (mainly by Compton effect) with electrons from the tissue and change their direction. Some of these scattered photons can reach the detectors and produce a coincident event which would thus be registered on an erroneous line of response. This leads to a reduction in the contrast of the image by simulating activity in cold regions adjacent to hot areas. For cardiac studies, where regional defects are usually surrounded by normal regions, this effect can lead to misinterpretation of the images. In order to account for scatter, commercial scanners generally provide correction algorithms most of which were initially developed for brain imaging. Therefore, the application of these corrections to the chest where the activity is non uniformly distributed in a large and inhomogeneous area, is questionable and needs further validation.

Finite resolution effect

The spatial resolution is the ability of the imaging device to distinguish between small adjacent objects. The image resolution is limited 1) by the geometry of the gantry and the detectors, 2) by physical factors such as the positron range in tissue and the divergence of the two annihilation photons from exact colinearity, and 3) by the filtering of the data which is needed to obtain good quality images. The practical in-plane resolution of current PET scanners is on the order of 8 mm but, due to cardiac and respiratory motions, the resolution achieved in cardiac PET images is considerably poorer than the one obtained when imaging the brain. Moreover the finite resolution in the axial direction plays a role as well and, when reslicing a set of transaxial slices, its effect is added to the in-plane effect.

Finite resolution effects produce blurring of the images which affects the accuracy of quantitative cardiac data under the following circumstances:

1) when imaging an object whose dimensions are comparable or less than the resolution, the measured activity concentration will be underestimated (partial volume effect). The poorer the resolution or the smaller the object, the lower the fraction of recovered activity in a given region of interest. This effect is important for the heart due to the small thickness of the myocardial wall (typically around 10 mm in normal cases and often much thinner in ischemic heart diseases);

2) when imaging adjacent structures with very different levels of activity, a cross-contamination can occur, resulting in smearing of counts from the region of high activity into the region of low activity (spillover effect). Due to this effect, a defect region may appear falsely to have a non-zero concentration. Moreover, since the activity is moving from the ventricle to the myocardial wall during the course of cardiac studies, spillover produces a distortion of the recorded time-activity curves, overestimating the myocardial curve at the beginning and the cavity curve at later times.

A common clinical problem is to measure blood flow to dysfunctioning myocardial areas. In a dog model, artifactual reductions up to a 36 % decrease in apparent tracer concentration were caused by the reduced systolic thickening of areas made transiently akinetic.[6] In addition, the visual interpretation of uncorrected images has led to erroneous hypotheses regarding the severity of the flow deficits in "hibernating" myocardium. There is indeed increased evidence from appropriate quantitative measurements of residual flow that most "hibernating" areas have (near) normal perfusion.[7,8] Clearly, visual flow defects in asynergic areas need to be shifted upwards in order to account for the offset imposed by the partial volume effect.

The finite resolution effects are thus of major importance for quantification since they can lead to erroneous estimations of the activity concentrations both in the cardiac chambers (input curve) and in the myocardial tissue. If the actual geometric dimensions of the object and the resolution function of the scanner are known, one can attempt to correct for these effects. However, such corrections are complicated by cardiac and respiratory motion. Although gated data acquisition would solve these issues, this approach is not widely used because it is tedious and produces a loss in count information. An alternative method is to compensate for cardiac motion artifacts by artificially increasing the width of the resolution function.[9] Another method consists of including finite resolution effects as additional parameters in the operational equations of the models, as outlined below.

Tracer modelling

Assuming that the PET instrumentation is able to accurately measure the time course of both the arterial input function and the myocardial tissue concentration, absolute values of myocardial blood flow are obtainable by incorporating these quantities in a suitable physiologic model which takes into account the kinetics of the injected tracer. The ideal radiotracer for the quantification of myocardial perfusion should have the following characteristics: 1) be trapped in tissue in direct proportion to flow, 2) have minimal recirculation in the vascular system, 3) have a short physical half-life to allow for repeated studies. Labeled microspheres meet these criteria but the need for their intra-ventricular administration precludes routine utilization in man. The radiotracers commonly used to measure myocardial perfusion can be divided in two categories depending on their behavior in tissue after having diffused across the capillary membrane. The freely *diffusible tracers* are inert and simply washed out of the tissue, while the *extractable tracers* are trapped in the myocardium by energy-dependent mechanisms. Next, we will briefly discuss the main characteristics of the existing models together with their limitations. Their detailed description and mathematical formulations can be found in the corresponding referenced publications.[10-21]

Diffusible tracers

The methods developed for myocardial perfusion quantification using inert diffusible tracers, such as labeled water ($H_2^{15}O$) or equivalently labeled carbon dioxide ($C^{15}O_2$) are based on the principle of inert gas exchange developed by Kety.[10] The kinetic behavior of labeled water in tissue is described by a simple two-compartment model which allows the estimates of two physiologic parameters: myocardial blood flow and the partition coefficient of water between blood and tissue. Several investigators have developed and validated techniques for myocardial blood flow measurement either by intravenous injection of $H_2^{15}O$[11-13] or by continuous inhalation of $C^{15}O_2$.[14] These techniques are very similar from a mathematical point of view but their implementation varies considerably depending on the approach selected for correcting finite resolution effects. Both Iida et al.[11] and Araujo et al.[14] have added the myocardial recovery coefficient as a third parameter to be estimated when fitting the blood and tissue time-activity curves to the model. The spillover from blood pool into myocardial walls is measured by a separate scan following inhalation of $C^{15}O$. Bergmann et al.[12] estimated both correction factors (recovery and spillover) as additional fitted parameters. In these three studies, the partition coefficient cannot be separately identified and must therefore be kept constant at a theoretical value. In the fourth method, Bol et al.[13] used finite resolution correction factors obtained by an independent Monte Carlo method.[9] Time-activity curves are corrected before any fitting of the data to the model. This technique avoids the need to keep the partition coefficient constant. These four approaches have been validated in animal studies, showing good agreement with reference blood flow values obtained with labeled microspheres. Moreover, they all give myocardial blood flow estimates in humans, both at rest or under pharmacological stress, that are within the expected physiological range. Nevertheless, each method has limitations that are now discussed.

Continuous inhalation of $C^{15}O_2$ avoids high counting rates and thus errors due to random coincidences or dead-time of the system. However, for the same dose administered to the patient, the estimates of myocardial perfusion are less accurate than with a bolus injection, particularly at high flow. On the other hand, the bolus method allows shorter acquisition times, making easier repeat studies after acute interventions or the combination of perfusion measurements with metabolic studies using other tracers. Yet, it necessitates a PET system with high count rate capabilities and good temporal sampling. Depending on the different ways finite resolution effects are taken into account, the estimates of myocardial perfusion become sensitive either to the tracer uptake[13] or to the washout of the tracer.[11,12,14] In the latter, the variance of the estimates is increased whereas the first method is very much dependent on the exact knowledge of the heart dimensions. To this end, complementary data from other imaging modalities with better spatial resolution than PET are needed. Whatever method is used, the rapid tracer washout produces images with low contrast between tissue and blood. In order to draw the myocardial regions of interest, additional myocardial images obtained with other tracers are required, which increases the complexity of the acquisition protocol. An interesting alternative was recently proposed which facilitates left ventricular recognition by principal component analysis of the $C^{15}O_2$ data.[15]

Another issue is the possible effect of time discrepancies between input and myocardial time-activity curves on flow quantification using sharp bolus injections of $H_2^{15}O$.[16] Time shifts of 1 second can be measured under basal conditions when the left atrium is used for the arterial input. This can result in a systematic error in the flow estimates of 30% at most. When the arterial input is taken from a region of interest drawn over the left ventricular cavity, these errors become of much lesser importance.

Extractable tracers

At the present time, nitrogen-13 (^{13}N) ammonia is the most frequently used tracer of this type. It demonstrates a rather high first pass extraction (70 to 80%) and a rapid elimination from the blood. Therefore, it produces excellent quality images of the myocardium. However, like all tracers of this category, its extraction decreases non-linearly when flow increases. Moreover, its kinetic behavior depends on the conversion of ammonia into glutamine and is thus affected by the prevailing metabolic state of the myocardium. Absolute quantification of myocardial perfusion with such tracers requires therefore more complex models than when diffusible tracers are used.

Two methods have been developed for the measurement of myocardial blood flow with ^{13}N-ammonia.[17,18] Both of them have been successfully applied in animals and in human studies. The mathematical equations are basically similar but the model of Hutchins et al.[18] is more comprehensive. It contains three compartments: vascular ^{13}N-ammonia, extra-vascular ^{13}N-ammonia and metabolically trapped ^{13}N-glutamine. One parameter is added to the three rate constants in order to take into account the finite resolution effects. The need to correct for the presence of circulating metabolites constitutes a limitation to this model. Nevertheless, the magnitude of this correction is far less important in humans than in dogs or other smaller animals.

The method developed by Krivokapich et al.[17] is based on important assumptions that simplify the equations and reduce the model to a two-compartment model. It contains a single parameter (blood flow) and uses fixed values for the other quantities based on an empirical relationship between ammonia retention and microsphere blood flow derived from experiments in dogs. In order to avoid the need for metabolite correction, the method uses a short (90 seconds) study duration. The trade-off here is that images with lower counting statistics are obtained, which leads to greater variability in the results.

Rubidium-82(^{82}Rb)-chloride, another extractable tracer, seems very attractive for the evaluation of myocardial perfusion because it is generator-produced and has a very short half-life (75 seconds). This tracer also produces good contrast images in humans and has been, therefore, extensively used for qualitative flow imaging. To quantify myocardial blood flow, the kinetics of both extraction and retention of ^{82}Rb must be incorporated in the mathematical equations, leading to a two-compartment model.[19] This model has been successfully validated in dogs over a wide range of flow values, using different methods to correct for finite resolution effects.[19,20] Until now, quantitative estimates of flow with ^{82}Rb have not yet been obtained in human subjects.

Finally, the same kind of two-compartment model has been applied to studies with potassium-38 (^{38}K) since this tracer has a kinetic behavior which is very similar to ^{82}Rb, the potassium analogue. ^{38}K has a half-life of 8 minutes and its production requires a 30 MeV protons cyclotron. The absolute values of myocardial blood flow obtained with ^{38}K have been compared to microspheres and $H_2^{15}O$ estimates of flow over a range from 5 to 330 ml/100g/min.[21] The results show a good estimation of perfusion with ^{38}K in the regions with low (including infarcted areas) or normal flow. However, at higher flow rates, the estimates are far less accurate than those obtained with $H_2^{15}O$.

Clinical limitations

It is clear from the above that performing adequate quantification of regional myocardial blood flow with PET remains a complex and tedious procedure due to the numerous constraints imposed on data acquisition and analysis. The choice of the tracer and its way of administration will depend ultimately on a compromise based on experience, tracer availability, dosimetry and convenience. On top of the technical issues as delineated earlier, there are additional limitations when applying these measurements to physiological or pathophysiological conditions.

Variability and reproducibility

Given the tight coupling that exists in normal myocardium between supply and demand, flow values are strongly dependent on myocardial work. Differences in loading conditions and inotropic state between subjects likely contribute to the wide range of normal values observed in most studies.[2] Therefore, it is important to attempt to normalize baseline myocardial blood flow for the oxygen demand at the time of the measurement. A significant linear relationship between flow and rate-pressure product, which is known to be related to cardiac work and oxygen demand, has been reported.[22,23] One approach is to multiply baseline flow by the mean rate-pressure product in the subjects as a group and divide this value by the rate-pressure product in the individual patient.[24]

Flow values are also affected by physical training[25] and ageing. Baseline myocardial blood flow tends to increase linearly with age as a consequence of an age related increase in cardiac work.[23] In addition, a reduction in hyperemic flow in subjects older than 60 years has been recently reported.[22,26] Gender was not shown to significantly affect myocardial blood flow values, although the number of younger women studied remains limited.[23]

Comparable flow values were measured in dogs[13] and in normal human volunteers[27] when the results obtained with both ^{13}N-ammonia and $H_2^{15}O$ were directly compared. In the experimental myocardial infarction, ^{13}N-ammonia estimates were more comparable to microspheres than the data obtained with $H_2^{15}O$. Similar comparative studies have not yet been performed in abnormal myocardium in patients.

Surprisingly, to the best of our knowledge, no data are available on the short and long term variability of PET flow measurements in normal or diseased myocardium.

Tissue heterogeneity

In normal tissue, flow to the subendocardial layers is greater than to the subepicardium. The subendocardium is also known to be more sensitive to reductions in flow due to ischaemia or hypertrophy. Therefore, it would be of great interest to be able to measure the transmural perfusion gradient with PET. Unfortunately, this appears to be impossible with the currently available instrumentation with the exception of studying individuals with thickened myocardial walls, such as the septum in patients with hypertrophic cardiomyopathy. Subendocardial hypoperfusion (with a reduced subendocardial to subepicardial flow ratio) following intravenous dipyridamole has indeed been documented in a few of such cases.[28]

Using the microsphere technique and very small samples of tissue, Austin et al.[29] reported a large spatial heterogeneity of resting and maximal flow in normal dogs. This heterogeneity resulted in extreme values of "normal" coronary flow reserve ranging from 1.75 to 21.9. A similar profound spatial heterogeneity is likely to exist in humans but again, cannot be measured with PET because rather large regions of interest are needed in order to derive meaningful measurements.

For the same reasons, tissue heterogeneity becomes of even greater concern when normally perfused myocardium is intermixed with scarred or severely hypoperfused tissue. Such condition is frequently encountered in patients with reperfused myocardial infarction or chronic ischemic left ventricular dysfunction. Iida et al.[30] has proposed an elegant possible solution to this problem using $H_2^{15}O$, which is based on the principle that viable tissue is required for rapid transsarcolemmal exchange of water. In his model, the perfusable tissue fraction (g/ml) is measured from the blood pool ($C^{15}O_2$) and blood flow ($H_2^{15}O$) data and represents the fraction of tissue capable of exchanging water within a given region of interest. In fact, this index may provide a potential means for quantitatively discriminating the relative proportions of viable and non-viable tissue components within a given asynergic region.[31,32]

Conclusion

The good agreement obtained between microsphere measurements and the different PET methods for the assessment of myocardial perfusion demonstrates the ability of PET to quantitate blood flow noninvasively. However, each of these methods has limitations which are imposed either by the properties of the tracer and thus the characteristics of the model, or by the limitations of the imaging instrumentation. Up to now, no method of choice emerges. Rather, one has to compromise and select the most appropriate technique in each case, considering the performance characteristics of the tomograph, the availability of a given tracer, the clinical question to be addressed as well as the expertise and experience of the team.

References

1. Hoffman JIE. Maximal coronary flow and the concept of coronary vascular reserve. Circulation 1984;70:153-9.
2. Camici PG, Gropler RJ, Jones T et al. The impact of myocardial blood flow quantitation with PET on the understanding of cardiac diseases. Circulation;(Submitted).
3. Iida H, Takahashi A, Tamura Y, Ono Y, Lammertsma A. Myocardial blood flow: comparison of oxygen-15-water bolus injection, slow infusion and oxygen-15-carbon dioxide slow inhalation. J Nucl Med 1995;36:78-85.
4. Bettinardi V, Gilardi MC, Lucignani G et al. A procedure for patient repositioning and compensation for misalignement between transmission and emission data in PET heart studies. J Nucl Med 1993;34:137-42.
5. Bacharach S, Douglas M, Carson R et al. Three-dimensional registration of cardiac positron emission tomography attenuation scans. J Nucl Med 1993;34:311-21.
6. Parodi O, Schelbert HR, Schwaiger M, Hansen H, Selin C, Hoffman EJ. Cardiac emission computed tomography: underestimation of regional tracer concentrations due to wall motion abnormalities. J Comput Assist Tomography 1984;8:1083-92.
7. Vanoverschelde J-L, Wijns W, Depré C et al. Mechanisms of chronic regional postischemic dysfunction in humans. New insights from the study of noninfarcted collateral-dependent myocardium. Circulation 1993;87:1513-23.
8. Marinho NVS, Keogh BE, Costa DC, Ell PJ, Lammertsma AA, Camici PG. Hibernating myocardium: is it really due to chronic underperfusion? Circulation 1994;90:I-314.
9. Vanoverschelde J-L, Melin J, Bol A et al. Regional oxidative metabolism in patients with reperfused anterior myocardial infarction: relation to regional blood flow and glucose uptake. Circulation 1992;85:9-21.
10. Kety SS. Measurement of local blood flow by the exchange of an inert, diffusible substance. Methods Med Res 1960;8:228-36.
11. Iida H, Kanno I, Takahashi A et al. Measurement of absolute myocardial blood flow with $H_2^{15}O$ and dynamic positron emission tomography. Circulation 1988;78:104-15.
12. Bergmann SR, Herrero P, Markham J, Weinheimer CJ, Walsh MN. Noninvasive quantitation of myocardial blood flow in human subjects with oxygen-15-labeled water and positron emission tomography. J Am Coll Cardiol 1989;14:639-52.
13. Bol A, Melin J, Vanoverschelde J-L et al. Direct comparison of N-13 ammonia and O-15 water estimates of perfusion with quantification of regional myocardial blood flow by microspheres. Circulation 1993;87:512-25.
14. Araujo L, Lammertsma A, Rhodes C et al. Non invasive quantification of regional myocardial blood flow in coronary artery disease with oxygen-15-labeled carbon dioxide inhalation and positron emission tomography. Circulation 1991;83:875-85.
15. Boyd HL, Gunn RN, Marinho NVS et al. Left ventricular volumes and wall motion with gated Positron Emission Tomography: comparison with radionuclide angiography. Circulation 1994;90:I-364.
16. Herrero P, Hartman JJ, Senneff MJ, Bergmann SR. Effects of time discrepancies between input and myocardial time-activity curves on estimates of regional myocardial perfusion with PET. J Nucl Med 1994;35:558-66.
17. Krivokapich J, Smith GT, Huang SC et al. N-13 ammonia myocardial imaging at rest and with exercise in normal volunteers. Quantification of absolute myocardial perfusion with dynamic positron emission tomography. Circulation 1989;80:1328-37.
18. Hutchins GD, Schwaiger M, Rosenspire KC, Krivokapich J, Schelbert H, Kuhl DE. Noninvasive quantification of regional blood flow in the human heart using N-13 ammonia and dynamic positron emission tomographic imaging. J Am Coll Cardiol 1990;15:1032-

42.

19. Herrero P, Markham J, Shelton ME, Bergmann SR. Implementation and evaluation of a two-compartment model for quantification of myocardial perfusion with rubidium-82 and positron emission tomography. Circ Res 1992;70:496-507.
20. Frankar G, Bol A, Vanoverschelde J-L et al. Direct comparison of O-15 water and rubidium-82 for quantification of myocardial perfusion with PET. J Nucl Med 1992;33:884.
21. Bol A, Baudhuin T, De Pauw M et al. Quantification of absolute myocardial perfusion with potassium-38 and positron emission tomography. J Nucl Med 1993;34:86.
22. Uren NG, Camici PG, Wijns W et al. The effect of ageing on coronary flow reserve in man. Circulation 1993;88:I-171 (Abstract).
23. Czernin J, Muller P, Chan S et al. Influence of age and haemodynamics on myocardial blood flow and flow reserve. Circulation 1993;88:62-9.
24. Uren NG, Melin JA, De Bruyne B, Wijns W, Baudhuin T, Camici PG. Myocardial blood flow as a function of coronary stenosis severity in man. N Engl J Med 1994;330:1782-8.
25. Radvan J, Camici PG, Marwick T, Boyd H, Sheridan DJ. Physiological hypertrophy does not affect coronary flow reserve in man. Circulation 1993;88:I-214 (Abstract).
26. Senneff MJ, Geltman EM, Bergmann SR, Hartmann J. Noninvasive delineation of the effects of moderate aging on myocardial perfusion. J Nucl Med 1991;32:2037-42.
27. Nitzsche E, Choi Y, Czernin J, Hoh C, Huang SC, Schelbert HR. Comparison of O-15 water and N-13 ammonia PET measurement of myocardial blood flow in humans. Circulation 1993;88:I-274 (Abstract).
28. Camici PG, Cecchi F, Gistri R et al. Dipyridamole-induced subendocardial underperfusion in hypertrophic cardiomyopathy assessed by positron emission tomography. Coronary Artery Dis 1991;2:837-41.
29. Austin RE Jr, Aldea GS, Coggins DL, Flynn AE, Hoffman JIE. Profound spatial heterogeneity of coronary reserve. Discordance between patterns of resting and maximal myocardial blood flow. Circ Res 1990;67:319-31.
30. Iida H, Rhodes CG, De Silva R et al. Myocardial tissue fraction: Correction for partial volume effects and measure of tissue viability. J Nucl Med 1991;32:2169-75.
31. Yamamoto Y, De Silva R, Rhodes CG et al. A new strategy for the assessment of viable and regional myocardial blood flow using ^{15}O-water and dynamic positron emission tomography. Circulation 1992;86:167-78.
32. de Silva, Yamamoto Y, Rhodes CG et al. Preoperative prediction of the outcome of coronary revascularisation using positron emission tomography. Circulation 1992;86:1738-42.

18   ALTERED AUTONOMIC CONTROL OF THE CARDIOVASCULAR SYSTEM IN SYNDROME X

Joan G. Meeder

Introduction

"Syndrome X" is used to denote the uncertain etiology of chest pain in patients with typical exertional angina pectoris and positive exercise testing (exercise-induced ST-segment depression) despite angiographically normal coronary arteries.[1] If patients with left bundle branch block, diabetes mellitus, arterial hypertension, valve disease (including mitral valve prolapse), epicardial arterial spasm and cardiomyopathy are excluded, then the incidence is probably of the order of 1%-3% of all patients undergoing coronary angiography for a chest pain syndrome.[2] Myocardial ischemia appears to be the underlying mechanism in only 25%-30% of syndrome X patients.[3,4] It is now recognized that syndrome X is a heterogeneous syndrome that encompasses different pathophysiological entities.[5,6] A number of cardiac-related causative factors have been found to play a role in the syndrome: a) restricted coronary vasodilator capacity,[7-9] b) autonomic dysregulation,[11-12] and c) abnormal endothelial function.[13-15] Nevertheless, patchily distributed increased tone of the prearteriolar coronary vessel, interposed between the conductance arteries and the arterioles, and compensatory augmented release of adenosine has been postulated to be the fundamental abnormality in syndrome X.[5,7,16] This chapter reviews the evidence for the altered autonomic control of the cardiovascular system, i.e. the prearteriolar tone in the pathogenesis of angina pectoris in patients with syndrome X.

Prearteriolar coronary vasoconstriction

Traditionally, two compartments of the coronary circulation have been distinguished: 1) *conductive vessels*, constituted by large conduit arteries with a diameter > 1 mm, that can be visualized at coronary angiography; and 2) smaller *resistive vessels*, that are responsible for most of the coronary resistance and

E. E. van der Wall et al. (eds.), Cardiac Positron Emission Tomography, 221–230.

regulation of myocardial perfusion.[17] Resistive vessels can be divided into two functionally distinct compartments.[18,19] The proximal compartment of resistive vessels is constituted by the *prearterioles*, and the distal compartment by the *arterioles*. The function of the prearterioles is to maintain an optimal perfusion pressure at the origin of the arterioles, and this is achieved by constriction when aortic pressure increases, and dilatation when aortic pressure decreases. The function of arterioles is to regulate flow to allow an optimal equilibrium between the supply of nutrients and the washout of metabolites.

In 1986 Epstein and Cannon[20] hypothesized that an increased vasoconstrictor tone of the prearteriolar vessels might be the fundamental abnormality in syndrome X. Recently, Maseri et al.[5] have elaborated this hypothesis. Besides a patchy distribution of prearteriolar constriction, they also proposed that a compensatory release of adenosine may be responsible for chest pain, even in the absence of myocardial ischaemia. An increased release of adenosine, to guarantee an adequate blood flow in myocardial areas with increased prearteriolar tone, also has significant algogenic effects.[21] In the presence of a patchily distributed prearteriolar constriction, local accumulation of adenosine may become sufficient to stimulate cardiac afferent nerves. This may result in an enhanced perception of potentially painful stimuli. This hypothesis explains the wide spectrum of clinical presentations of patients with syndrome X. At one end of the spectrum, the involvement of a large number of prearteriolar vessels would explain the reduced coronary flow reserve and the presence of myocardial ischemia observed in some patients. At the other end, the involvement of a very limited number of prearterioles could explain the occurrence of pain in the absence of detectable signs of ischemia.

Myocardial perfusion heterogeneity

The consequence of the patchily distributed increased vasoconstrictor tone of the prearteriolar vessels to heterogeneity of myocardial perfusion has been recently investigated in patients with syndrome X and healthy control subjects by our group.[22-25] The only non-invasive method for measuring regional myocardial blood perfusion is positron emission tomography (PET). Its quantitative capabilities permit not only an impression of regional perfusion differences, but also absolute measurements.[26] To enhance this technique, we recently developed a method for quantitative mapping, using parametric polar map displays, of myocardial perfusion.[27,28] This method quantifies perfusion in 480 separate segments of the human left ventricle, providing insight in the heterogeneity of myocardial perfusion. As a measure of heterogeneity of myocardial perfusion,[29] the coefficient of variation of perfusion in 480 segments (SD/mean x 100) was calculated.

Visual inspection of the parametric polar maps of syndrome X patients revealed heterogeneous myocardial perfusion (Figure 1). In accordance with these observations, the coefficient of variation of myocardial perfusion calculated from data of 480 separate segments was significantly higher in syndrome X subjects compared to the volunteers (17.0 ± 3.2 versus 13.6 ± 2.2 %; $p < 0.01$). Although syndrome X patients also showed increased myocardial perfusion (123 ± 35 versus 87 ± 16 ml/min/100g; $p < 0.01$), no association could be detected between perfusion

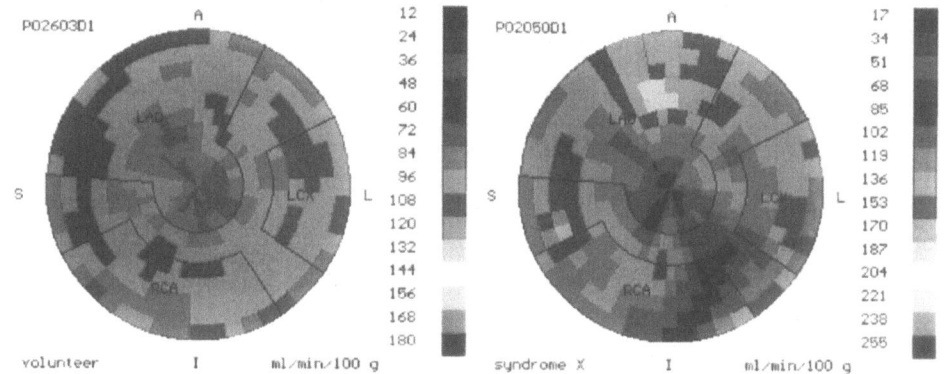

Figure 1. Examples of dynamic parametric polar maps of myocardial perfusion of a healthy volunteer (left) and a syndrome X patient (right). Abbreviations: A (anterior), S (septal), I (inferior), L (lateral). Approximate vascular territories of the three major coronary arteries (LAD: left anterior descending; LCX: left circumflex artery; RCA: right coronary artery) are superimposed upon the polar map. To the right of each graph a quantitative color bar of myocardial perfusion (ml/min/100g). These maps illustrate the much larger heterogeneity of perfusion in the syndrome X patient compared to the healthy volunteer. (see for colourplate of this figure page 247).

heterogeneity and perfusion. Both in syndrome X patients and in healthy volunteers low and non-significant Spearman rank order correlation coefficients were found between coefficient of variation of perfusion and myocardial perfusion. Consequently, the perfusion heterogeneity seems not to be a direct reflection of increased demand. Our study shows that myocardial perfusion in syndrome X patients is heterogeneous on a segmental level despite an overall increased perfusion.

Increased myocardial perfusion at rest has been described previously by Geltman et al.[30] and Galassi et al.[29] The latter group also reported that patients with syndrome X had an abnormal heterogeneity of myocardial perfusion in a total of 25 to 32 tissue regions of interest of the left ventricle. They suggested that this heterogeneity may be due to alterations of vasomotion in even smaller myocardial regions. Our study, which uses for the first time the dynamic parametric polar map method to compare perfusion in 480 separate segments of the left ventricle in syndrome X patients and healthy volunteers, seems to confirm this suggestion. The presence in our patients of small regions with abnormal myocardial perfusion patchily distributed in the myocardium may explain why myocardial perfusion, metabolism and function are frequently found within normal limits when assessed using conventional diagnostics techniques that can only detect abnormalities occurring in large myocardial regions. Our results are in line with the hypothesis that the primary abnormality in syndrome X might be a patchily distributed increased constriction of the prearteriolar coronary vessels with compensatory enlarged release of adenosine. This abnormal constriction impairs local arteriolar blood flow and consequently lowers local myocardial perfusion. Obviously, the patchy distribution of the vascular dysfunction causes heterogeneous perfusion, expressed by the high coefficient of variation of segmental myocardial perfusion in syndrome X patients. Considering the above, the increased coefficient of variation might be the result of regional differences in coronary microvascular diameter causing a segmental reduction of flow in some areas and augmentation in others. An increased release of adenosine to guarantee an adequate blood flow in myocardial areas with increased prearteriolar tone, could explain the augmentation of myocardial perfusion in areas with normal prearteriolar tone. Diffusion of high quantities of adenosine released in the interstitial space could induce vasodilation also, in adjacent arterioles supplied by prearteriolar vessels with normal function. Consequently, this may cause a general increase of myocardial perfusion.

Abnormal autonomic control and perfusion heterogeneity

It is accepted that the autonomic nervous system modulates coronary artery tone and that abnormalities of autonomic control may result in a reduction of coronary blood flow.[31-34] Patients with syndrome X may have an increased sympathetic drive.[11,35-37] Altered autonomic nervous control of the coronary microcirculation has been suggested to be responsible for the increased prearteriolar vasomotor tone in syndrome X.[16,38,39] Analysis of heart rate variability (HRV) is a valuable tool to investigate the sympathetic and parasympathetic function of the autonomic nervous system.[40]

Recently, we assessed segmental myocardial perfusion and heart rate variability during 24 hour Holter ECG monitoring in 16 syndrome X patients and 16 sex- and age-matched healthy controls[22,24,25]. The aim of this study was to investigate the relationship between perfusion heterogeneity and autonomic function. Heart rate variability analysis was performed using commercially available software (Marquette HRV 2A). This system defines six different non-spectral measures of heart rate variability: meanNN (mean of all coupling intervals between normal beats), sdNN (the standard deviation about the mean), SDANN (standard deviation of 5-minute mean R-R intervals), SD (mean of all 5-minute standard deviation of R-R intervals), pNN50 (proportion of adjacent R-R intervals with difference of more than 50 msec), and rMSSD ($\sqrt{}$ mean square of difference of successive R-R intervals). Also the cvNN, the coefficient of variation of heart rate (sdNN adjusted for the meanNN), was calculated. The variables computed from the differences between adjacent cycles such as rMSSD and pNN50 reflects vagal tone. The remaining, more broadly based time domain variables are influenced by diurnal trends, sympathetic influences, and vagal tone.

Only in part, our studies[22,24,25] show clinical evidence to support the hypothesis that an increase in sympathetic tone might be responsible for the increased prearteriolar vasomotor tone In syndrome X. There were no differences In heart rate variability between syndrome X patients and healthy volunteers (Table 1).

However, Spearman rank order correlation coefficients between PET and HRV parameters showed only in syndrome X patients a negative rank order association between coefficient of variation of myocardial perfusion and heart rate variability parameters (Table 2).

Table 1. Heart Rate Variability

	Syndrome X	Volunteers	p
meanNN (ms)	811 (614-1125)	786 (658-1017)	n.s.
sdNN (ms)	144 (52-286)	141 (88-180)	n.s.
cvNN	18 (7.8-33.8)	17 (11.2-25.2)	n.s.
SDANN (ms)	128 (45-220)	123 (69-167)	n.s.
SD (ms)	56 (24-177)	58 (41- 76)	n.s.
rMSSD (ms)	33 (12-210)	33 (18- 46)	n.s.
pNN50 (%)	8.5 (0.2-38.4)	6.2 (1.2-16.1)	n.s.

Median (range) per 24 hours. Abbreviations, see text.

Table 2. Correlation between Perfusion Heterogeneity and Autonomic Function

	Syndrome X		Volunteers	
	r	(p)	r	(p)
meanNN	-0.61	(0.014)	-0.14	(n.s.)
sdNN	-0.54	(0.029)	0.09	(n.s.)
cvNN	-0.50	(0.048)	0.12	(n.s.)
SDANN	-0.53	(0.035)	0.07	(n.s.)
SD	-0.62	(0.011)	0.11	(n.s.)
rMSSD	-0.51	(0.042)	0.11	(n.s.)
pNN50	-0.57	(0.020)	-0.07	(n.s.)

Spearman rank correlation coefficients (p-value). Abbreviations see text.

Also, a significant negative correlation was present between the coefficient of variation of perfusion and the coefficient of variation of heart rate (cvNN). This implies that the observed negative association between heterogeneity of perfusion and sdNN is not a direct result from the negative correlation with the mean NN, i.e the heart rate. These findings indicate that the higher the sympathetic tone or the lower the parasympathetic tone, the more heterogeneous myocardial perfusion is (Figure 2).

Since the heart rate variability parameters did not differ between both groups, it is tempting to speculate that an exaggerated response of coronary vessels to autonomic tone rather than an enhanced tone plays a crucial role in perfusion abnormalities in syndrome X.

Borghi et al.[41] suggested that syndrome X patients may have periods when symptoms are active and periods when there is a resolution of the symptoms. These periods are associated with variations in the ischemic threshold and with changes in sympathetic activity. The syndrome X patients in our study were rather symptomless during 24 hour Holter monitoring. Seven patients (44%) experienced

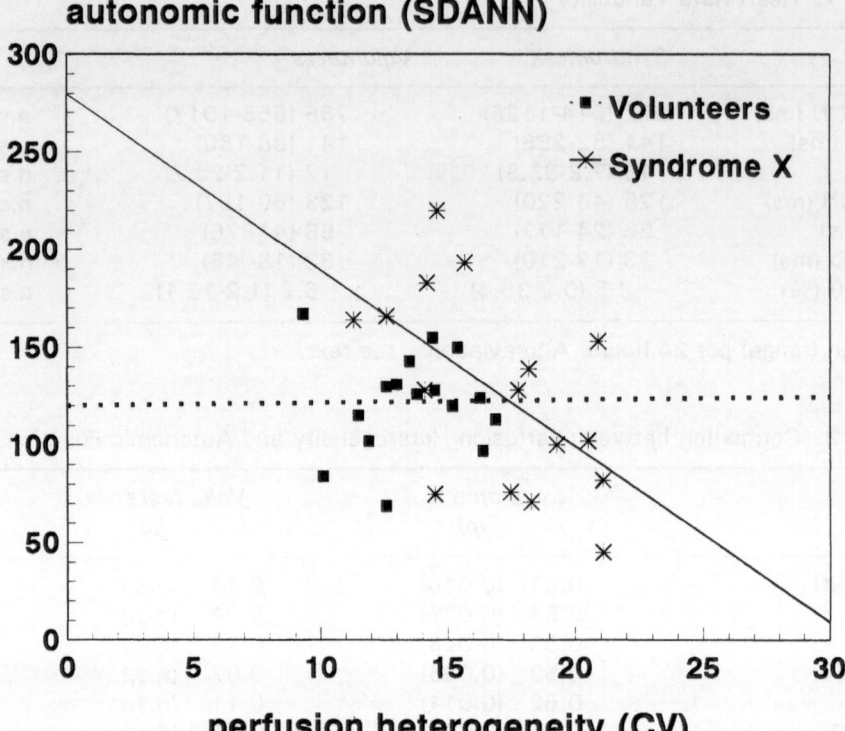

Figure 2.   Example of association between perfusion heterogeneity and autonomic function. Associations of coefficient of variation of segmental myocardial perfusion (CV of MP) with standard deviation of 5-minute mean R-R intervals (SDANN) in syndrome X patients (r = -0.53, p = 0.035) and healthy volunteers (r = 0.07, p = NS).

chest pain during Holter-monitoring, and the electrocardiogram showed in 4 of these patients (25%) ischemia-like ST-segment depression. Three other patients (19%) demonstrated signs of silent ischemia. Our patients seems to remain in a rather "inactive" phase of the disease. This might explain that contrary to the findings of Rosano et al.[11], the heart rate variability parameters in the present study did not differ between syndrome X patients and normal volunteers.

Conclusion

The increased perfusion heterogeneity supports the hypothesis that regionally increased prearteriolar tone is the fundamental abnormality in syndrome X (i.e. angina pectoris and positive exercise testing despite angiographically normal coronary arteries). Patchily distributed increased prearteriolar tone causes increased heterogeneity of myocardial perfusion. Augmented release of adenosine as a response to local constriction may play a role in causing an overall higher myocardial perfusion in these patients. Diffusion of high quantities of adenosine released in the interstitial space could induce vasodilation also, in adjacent arterioles supplied by prearteriolar vessels with normal autonomic function.

Since perfusion heterogeneity is inversely related with heart rate variability in syndrome X, it is tempting to speculate that altered autonomic control of the cardiovascular system plays a pathogenetic role. The higher the sympathetic tone or the lower the parasympathetic tone, the more heterogeneous myocardial perfusion is. Since the heart rate variability parameters did not differ between both groups, an exaggerated response of coronary vessels to autonomic tone rather than an enhanced tone seems to play a crucial role in perfusion abnormalities in syndrome X.

Dynamic parametric positron emission tomography can detect and quantify the perfusion abnormalities, thereby allowing identification of the cardiac origin of pain in syndrome X and provides a means to assess the effects of diagnostic and therapeutic interventions. Obviously, this will enhance the further development of diagnostic procedures and treatment strategies.

References

1. Kemp HG. Left ventricular function in patients with the anginal syndrome and normal coronary arteriograms. Am J Cardiol 1973;32:375-6.
2. Camici PG, Marraccini P, Lorenzoni R et al. Coronary hemodyanmics and myocardial metabolism in patients with syndrome X. J Am Coll Cardiol 1991;17:1461-70.
3. Crake T, Canepa-Anson R, Shapiro L, Poole-Wilson PA. Continuous recording of coronary sinus oxygen saturation during atrial pacing in patients with coronary artery disease or with syndrome X. Br Heart J 1988;59:31-8.
4. Cannon RO, Bonow RO, Bacharach SL et al. Left ventricular dysfunction in patients with angina pectoris, normal epicardial coronary arteries, and abnormal vasodilator reserve. Circulation 1985;71:218-26.
5. Maseri A, Crea F, Kaski JC, Crake T. Mechanisms of angina pectoris in syndrome X. J Am Coll Cardiol 1991;17:499-506.
6. Cannon RO 3d, Camici PG, Epstein SE. Pathophysiological dilemma of syndrome X. Circulation 1992;85:883-92.
7. Cannon RO, Epstein SE. "Microvascular angina" as a cause of chest pain with angiographically normal coronary arteries. Am J Cardiol 1988;61:1338-43.
8. Geltman EM, Henes G, Senneff MJ, Sobel BE, Bergmann SR. Increased myocardial perfusion at rest and diminished perfusion reserve in patients with angina and angiographically normal coronary arteries. J Am Coll Cardiol 1990;16:586-95.
9. Camici PG, Gistri R, Lorenzoni R et al. Coronary reserve and exercise electrocardiogram in patients with chest pain and normal coronary angiograms. Circulation 1992;85:179-86.
10. Rosen SD, Guzzetti S, Tonon G, Lombardi F, Camici PG, Malliani A. Autonomic dysregulation in syndrome X assessed by spectral analysis of 24 hour heart rate variability. Eur Heart J 1993;14:2420 (Abstract).
11. Rosano GMC, Ponikowski P, Adamopoulos S et al. Abnormal autonomic control of the cardiovascular system in syndrome X. Am J Cardiol 1994;73:1174-9.
12. Bugiardini R. Epicardial coronary artery reactivity in syndrome X: the role of increased adrenergic tone. Coronary Artery Dis 1992;3:964-72.
13. Motz W, Vogt M. Rabenau O, Scheler S, Lückhoff A, Strauer BE. Evidence of endothelial dysfunction in coronary resistance vessels in patients with angina pectoris and normal coronary angiograms. Am J Cardiol 1991;68:996-1003.
14. Vrints CJM, Bult H, Hitter E, Herman AG, Snoeck JP. Impaired endothelium-dependent cholinergic coronary vasodilation in patients with angina and normal coronary arteroigrams. J Am Coll Cardiol 1991;19:21-31.
15. Quyyumi AA, Cannon RO, Panza JA, Diodati JG, Epstein SA. Endothelial dysfunction in patients with chest pain and normal coronary arteries. Circulation 1992;86:1864-71.
16. Kaski JC, Crea F, Nihoyannopoulos P, Hackett D, Maseri A. Transient myocardial ischemia during daily life in patients with syndrome X. Am J Cardiol 1986;58:1242-7.
17. Lanza GA, Rosano GMC, Maseri A. Prearteriolar coronary constriction in pathogenesis or syndrome X. Role of adenosine. In: Kaski JC, editor. Angina pectoris with normal coronary arteries: syndrome X. Boston: Kluwer Academic Publishers, 1994:193-210.
18. Marcus ML, Chilian WM, Kanatsuka H, Dellsperger KC, Eatham CL, Lamping KG. Understanding the coronary circulation through studies at the microvascular level. Circulation 1990;82:1-7.
19. Maseri A, Crea F, Cianflone D. Myocardial ischemia caused by distal coronary vasoconstriction. Am J Cardiol 1992;70:1602-5.
20. Epstein SE, Cannon RO III. Site of increased resistance to coronary flow in patients

with angina pectoris and normal coronary arteries. J Am Coll Cardiol 1986;8:459-61.

21. Crea F, Pupita G, Galassi AR et al. Role of adenosine in the pathogenesis of angina pain. Circulation 1990;81:164-72.
22. Meeder JG, Blanksma PK, Anthonio RL et al. Myocardial perfusion dynamics and heart rate variability in syndrome X: evidence for autonomic and endothelial dysfunction. J Am Coll Cardiol 1994;161 (Abstract).
23. Blanksma PK, Meeder JG, Anthonio RL et al. Mechanism of angina pectoris in syndrome X: a study with dynamic myocardial perfusion imaging with ^{13}N ammonia PET. Eur Heart J 1994;15:241 (Abstract).
24. Meeder JG, Blanksma PK, Crijns HJGM et al. Myocardial perfusion and heart rate variability in syndrome X: evidence for autonomic dysregulation and endothelial dysfunction. Eur Heart J 1994;15:245 (Abstract).
25. Meeder JG, Blanksma PK, Crijns HJGM et al. Mechanism of angina pectoris in syndrome X assessed by myocardial perfusion dynamics and heart rate variability. Eur Heart J (accepted for publication).
26. Wisenberg G, Schelbert HR, Hoffman EJ et al. In vivo quantification of regional myocardial blood flow by positron emission computed tomography. Circulation 1983;63:1248-58.
27. Blanksma PK, Willemsen ATM, Meeder JG et al. Quantitative myocardial mapping of perfusion and metabolism using parametric polar map displays in cardiac PET. J Nucl Med 1995 (in press).
28. De Jong RM, Blanksma PK, Willemsen ATM et al. The "posterolateral defect" of the normal human heart investigated with nitrogen-13 ammonia and dynamic positron emission tomography. J Nucl Med 1995 (in press).
29. Galassi AR, Crea F, Araujo LI et al. Comparison of regional myocardial blood flow in syndrome X and one-vessel coronary artery disease. Am J Cardiol 1993;72:134-9.
30. Geltman EM, Henes G, Senneff MJ, Sobel BE, Bergman SR. Increased myocardial perfusion at rest and diminished perfusion reserve in patients with angina and angiographically normal coronary arteries. J Am Coll Cardiol 1990;16:586-9.
31. Chilian WM, Ackell PH. Transmural differences in sympathetic coronary constriction during exercise in the presence of coronary stenosis. Circ Res 1988;22:216-25.
32. Gwirtz PA, Stone HL. Coronary blood flow changes following activation of adrenergic receptors in the conscious dog. Am J Physiol 1982;24:H13-9.
33. Heush G. Control of coronary vasomotor tone in ischemic myocardium by local metabolism and neurohumoral mechanisms. Eur Heart J 1991;12:F99-106.
34. Buffington CW, Feigl EO. Adrenergic coronary vasoconstriction in the presence of coronary stenosis in the dog. Circ Res 1981;48:416-23.
35. Galassi AR, Kaski JC, Crea F et al. Heart rate response during exercise testing and ambulatory ECG monitoring in patients with syndrome X. Am Heart J 1991;122:448-56.
36. Montorsi P, Manfredi M, Loaldi A et al. Comparison of coronary vasomotor responses to nifedipine in syndrome X and in Prinzmetal's angina pectoris. Am J Cardiol 1989;63:1198-202.
37. Ishihara T, Seki I, Yamada Y et al. Coronary circulation, myocardial metabolism and cardiac catecholamine flux in patients with syndrome X. J Cardiol 1990;20:267-74.
38. Montorsi P, Fabbiocchi F, Loaldi A et al. Coronary adrenergic hyperreactivity in patients with syndrome X and abnormal electrocardiogram at rest. Am J Cardiol 1991;68:1698-703.
39. Romeo F, Gaspardone A, Ciavolella M, Gioffre P, Reale A. Verapamil versus acebutolol for syndrome X. Am J Cardiol 1988;62:312-3.

40. Kleiger RE, Stein PK, Bosner MS, Rottman JN. Time domain measurements of heart rate variability. In: Kennedy HL, editor. Ambulatory electrocardiography: current clinical concepts. Philadelphia: Saunders Company, 1992:487-98.
41. Borghi A, Trevisani M, Saccone V, Lucarini S, Puddu GM, Bugiardini R. Resolution of symptoms does not necessarily imply remission of the disease in patients with syndrome X. J Am Coll Cardiol 1992;19:59 (Abstract).

19 POSITRON EMISSION TOMOGRAPHY STUDIES OF CARDIAC NEUROSTIMULATION

Raymond W.M. Hautvast

Introduction

Conventional treatment of angina pectoris involves medication and revascularization procedures, alone or in combination. The main goal of therapy is to restore the imbalance of oxygen demand and supply of the myocardium, resulting in a reduction of anginal complaints. Unfortunately, a considerable number of surgically treated patients remains symptomatic[1] and the process of atherosclerosis is not stopped by revascularization, so new lesions may develop. After bypass surgery only about 75% of the patients are still free from ischemic events for 5 years or more, but this number is only 50% after 10 years or more.[2] Surgical re-intervention however, does take place in only a fraction of these patients post surgery, implying that feasibility and need for repeat surgery do not go parallel. Progression to diffuse coronary artery disease, leaving no options for coronary angioplasty, not infrequently accompanied by impaired left ventricular function, may withhold an increasing number of patients from repeat coronary artery bypass grafting,[3] although their response to regular medical therapy is not adequate. The group of patients answering to this description is considered to have refractory angina pectoris.

Neurostimulation, that is electrical stimulation of the spinal cord, has proven to be an effective therapeutic alternative for these patients. The rationale for its use was based on the gate control theory of Melzack and Wall.[4] They described a model in which the nociceptive, slowly conducting, unmyelated C fibers afferents are inhibited by stimulation of non-nociceptive, fast conducting, myelinated A fibers afferents. In animal studies it was electrophysiologically demonstrated that stimulation of segmental cutaneous A-fibers selectively inhibit noxious-evoked activity in dorsal horn neurones of the spinal cord.[5-7] Wall and Sweet[8] were the first to report a beneficial effect of neurostimulation in pain treatment, later followed by Shealy et.[9] In the mid seventies ischemic pain became a pre-eminent indication for spinal cord stimulation.[10,11] It has been reported that stimulation of the spinal cord improves microcirculation in the afflicted limb, indicating that the relief of ischemic pain may be a consequence of an

E. E. van der Wall et al. (eds.), Cardiac Positron Emission Tomography, 231–240.
© 1995 Kluwer Academic Publishers.

anti-ischemic action.[12]

The first report on spinal cord stimulation in a limited number of patients with severe angina, in the early eighties, described this therapy as clinically effective and safe.[13] In addition we have shown, that besides increase of exercise tolerance with concomitant reduction of ischemic signs on the electrocardiogram also demonstrated by others,[14-16] there was also a reduction of anginal attacks and ischemia during daily life in between periods of neurostimulation,[17,18] indicating post-stimulation analgia.[8] About the mechanism of action of neurostimulation only little is revealed up to date. However, the afore mentioned studies again suggest anti-ischemic properties for spinal cord stimulation, with analgesia, i.e. abolishment of anginal pain, probably as a secondary effect. An assumed anti-ischemic action of spinal cord stimulation may be most likely the result of a change in regional myocardial blood flow during stimulation. With Doppler flow velocity measurements a flow increase was indeed demonstrated by Chauhan et al.[19] in healthy coronary arteries, after only five minutes of neurostimulation. Furthermore, no effect was seen in the coronary arteries of transplanted hearts, suggesting a neurally mediated effect of neurostimulation.[19] About the neural pathways, followed by spinal cord stimulation, again little is known. Chandler et al.[20] have demonstrated that firing of spinothalamic tract cells, as a response to noxious pinching and innocuous brushing, decreases when the spinal cord is stimulated electrically. In our study on spinal cord stimulation and induction of expression of the immediate early gene c-fos, a marker of physiological cell response to stimuli,[21,22] we found c-fos in both hind- and midbrain nuclei, of which some are located in descending cortico-spinal tracts.[23] Almost all c-fos expressing sites were previously found to be involved in cardiac innervation in a viral tracing study we performed in the rat heart.[24] These findings suggest, that higher cerebral centers may be involved in cardiac spinal cord stimulation.

Positron emission tomography studies in spinal cord stimulation

Positron emission tomography (PET) is a very useful tool to study changes in blood flow in specific organs. In two different PET studies we investigated possible changes, induced by spinal cord stimulation, in regional myocardial and cerebral blood flow, as an explanation for an anti-ischemic effect and involvement of specific areas of the brain respectively. For PET recordings an ECAT Siemens 951/31 camera (Siemens CTI, Knoxville, Tennessee) was used, which made 31 simultaneous image planes with an axial length of 10.8 cm. Measured resolution of the system is 6 mm FWHM (Full Width at Half Maximum).

After obtaining informed consent, patients were enrolled in PET-substudies on the effect of spinal cord stimulation on myocardial and cerebral flow, which were embedded in a study on the clinical effect of spinal cord stimulation for their otherwise refractory angina pectoris.[17]

All patients had refractory angina, implying that they met the following conditions: 1) angina pectoris class III or IV according to the New York Heart Association, despite optimal medical therapy, i.e. adequate dosage of ß-blocking agents, calcium antagonists, and long-acting nitrates, 2) with myocardial ischemia as established by at least 0.1 mV ST-depression during treadmill exercise, 3) significant coronary artery disease, as documented by recent coronary angiography, and 4) no option for percutaneous transluminal coronary angioplasty or coronary artery bypass grafting. They were all equipped with a Medtronic Itrell° II (Medtronic Inc., Minneapolis, Minnesota) implantable pulse generator. In the group of patients studied for myocardial blood flow changes the stimulator was placed within a period of two weeks after enrollment. The patients in the substudy were already on spinal cord stimulation. The implantation procedure has been described previously,[25,26] but will be reproduced here in brief: with the patient in prone position an electrode was inserted into the epidural space and moved to C7, under local anesthesia. The electrode was cautiously withdrawn whilst stimulating and was positioned adjacent to the dorsal root, usually at T1 level. Correct positioning was achieved when, at the patients directions, the paraesthesias radiated to the dermatome where anginal pain was referred to. Under the left costal arch a subcutaneous pocket was made for the stimulator, which was connected with the electrode by a subcutaneously tunneled extension lead. Patients were able to switch the device on and off themselves by application of a magnet.

PET study on myocardial blood flow
To investigate whether spinal cord stimulation induced changes in myocardial flow as an explanation for its anti-ischemic effect, a PET study using N-13 ammonia ($^{13}NH_3$) was performed. In nine patients, eligible for spinal cord stimulation, myocardial flow was assessed at rest and after a dipyridamole stress test, both at baseline and after six weeks of spinal cord stimulation. The electrocardiogram and the blood pressure were continuously monitored.

First dynamic imaging was started as a control study, simultaneously with the intravenous injection of $^{13}NH_3$. Images were made according to a standard time frame protocol. After that, a dipyridamole stress test was performed and a second injection $^{13}NH_3$ was given. Data were analyzed using parametric polar mapping, which has been described elsewhere[27] and will be summarized here: by subtracting the last frame from the preceding study, the $^{13}NH_3$ provocation study was corrected for remaining activity. Data for each study were reorientated to 8 - 12 short axis images. The short axis slices were divided into 48 segments. After that, time activity curves were made in all segments of these slices, using maximal activity.[28] A blood pool was defined in three slices near the base, the average of which was used to calculate a single blood pool time activity curve. From these data a parametric polar map was calculated using a two-compartment flow model for $^{13}NH_3$ studies.[29] Flow reserve polar maps were calculated from the $^{13}NH_3$ maps after dipyridamole stress and those at rest, by calculating the ratio of the corresponding segments.

The total myocardium was divided into 9 segments. Coefficient of variation was calculated as standard deviation of the 9 segments, corrected for mean blood flow. Changes in the coefficient of variation reflect changes in myocardial flow heterogeneity.[30,31] The myocardium was divided in ischemic regions and non-ischemic regions, based on their flow reserve, which was decreased or normal, respectively. The defined ischemic regions matched with the supply regions of affected vessels at the coronary angiogram.

After six weeks of spinal cord stimulation a dipyridamole stress test gave in less patients anginal complaints as compared to baseline and there was a reduction of ischemic changes on the electrocardiogram. Also after six weeks of spinal cord stimulation a decrease of the coefficient of variation, both at rest and after dipyridamole stress was demonstrated (Figure 1). However, no evident changes in regional myocardial blood flow, corrected for heart rate and blood pressure, was seen.[32] Instead, a decrease of flow reserve was noticed after six weeks of spinal cord stimulation (Figure 2).

The effects of spinal cord stimulation on myocardial blood flow as we have found are in agreement with a previous PET study.[33] De Landsheere et al.[33] also could not demonstrate changes in regional or total myocardial blood flow. However, a decrease of coefficient of variation, implying homogenization of myocardial flow, may account for fewer anginal complaints and increased exercise tolerance. Homogenization of flow may be the long-term effect of spinal cord stimulation, whereas the findings of the study of Chauhan et al.[19] in normal coronary arteries may illustrate a short term effect, for the results were accomplished immediately after only five minutes of stimulation.

A decrease of flow reserve normally implies worsening of coronary stenoses. However, since it is not accompanied by a rise of anginal attacks and an increase of ischemic signs on the exercise electrocardiogram, this may be translated as a decrease of the effect of dipyridamole, induced by spinal cord stimulation. Dipyridamole acts through inhibition of the re-uptake of adenosine in the cell. Adenosine is believed to play an important role in pathogenesis of anginal pain.[34,35] A direct interaction of spinal cord stimulation with the activity of adenosine can explain the decrease of the dipyridamole effect. This may also be part of the anti-anginal mechanism of action of neurostimulation.

PET study on regional cerebral blood flow (rCBF)

For this study we recruited five dextral patients who were on clinically successful spinal cord stimulation. The aim was to detect regional brain activity, related to cerebral nuclei, which may be related to spinal cord stimulation. In advance, stimulation was stopped for at least one entire week, in order to prevent an assumed carry-over effect of the stimulation.[8]

PET studies of the cerebral blood flow were performed before and during spinal cord stimulation using $H_2{}^{15}O$ as a tracer. By darkening and silencing the PET camera room the patients were deprived of as many as possible external stimuli. The patients heads were fixed in the camera using an individually shaped head mould. During each study an injection of radioactively labeled water was followed by a three minutes scanning period according to a standardized time frame protocol. Recordings of all patients were analyzed in a cumulative evaluation. Image analysis on regional flow differences of the brain was calculated with t-map statistics using Statistical Parametric Mapping (SPM, MRC Cyclotron Unit, London, UK) in an omnibus sense.[36-38] Regional change in cerebral blood flow was interpreted as a sign of activation of that region, implying response to spinal cord stimulation. Regions with change of blood flow are localized using co-ordinates according to the stereotactic space defined by the atlas of Talaraich and Tournoux.[39]

Although only a small number of patients was studied, it was possible to detect flow changes with Z-values ranging from 3.1 to 3.8, which were considered significant. The regions with significant changes in rCBF are listed in Table 1. Increase of flow was seen in Brodman's areas 6, 21, and 44 of the right hemisphere. Flow decrease was noticed in the left hemisphere in Brodman's area 22 and in the right hemisphere in area

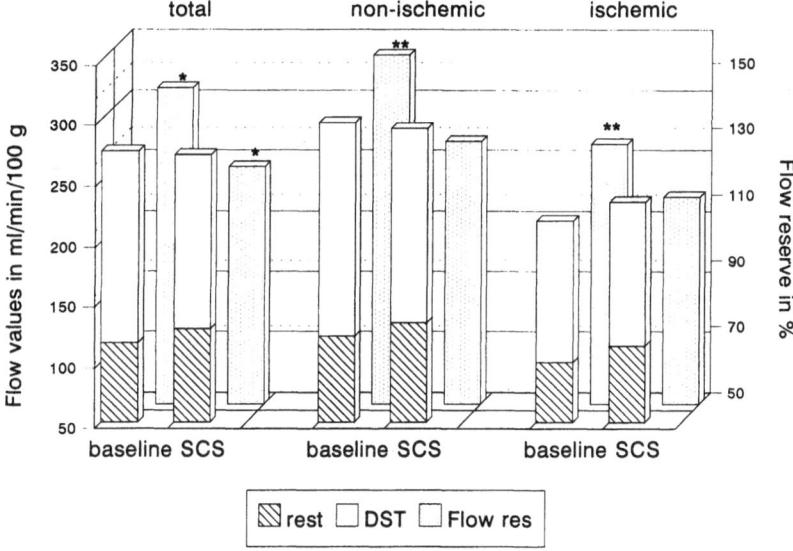

Figure 1. Mean flow values corrected for heart rate and blood pressure (left Y-axis) and corrected flow reserve (right Y-axis) for the total myocardium and for ischemic and non-ischemic regions. DST = dipyridamole stress testing; SCS = spinal cord stimulation. *P = 0.04; **P < 0.01.

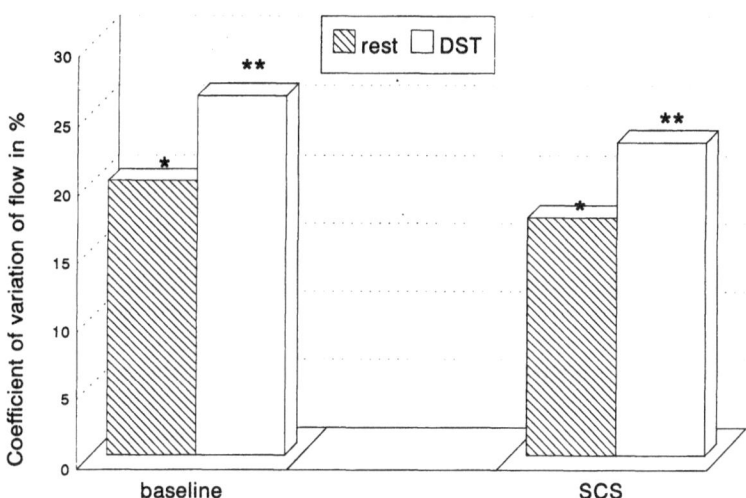

Figure 2. Coefficient of variation of myocardial blood flow, defined as the standard deviation of total myocardial flow corrected for the mean flow, represented as percentages. DST = dipyridamole stress testing; SCS = spinal cord stimulation. *P = 0.04; **P = 0.02.

236 *R. W. M. Hautvast*

Table 1. Areas and co-ordinates of changes in rCBF

Brodman area	x	y	z	Z-value
RIGHT				
21	-44	2	-20	3.3
28	-12	-18	-12	-3.5
Fornix	-8	-14	-8	-3.6
Hyp./C. Mam.	-6	-8	-8	-3.8
Putamen	-14	2	-4	-3.1
Hyp.	-12	0	-4	-3.3
6	-54	2	16	3.1
6/44	-50	4	20	3.7
LEFT				
22	38	-56	16	-3.2

Negative Z-values represent decreased rCBF. Hyp. = hypothalamus; C. Mam. = corpus mammillare.

28, corpus mammillary and hypothalamic region, the fornix and a small part of the putamen.

Recently Rosen et al.[40] have demonstrated rCBF changes during and after induction of angina pectoris by means of dobutamine, in a $H_2^{15}O$ PET study according to the same technique of analyzation as described here. The described areas with changes in rCBF of our study partly match with areas described to be activated during induction of angina pectoris. In contrast with their findings, we could not detect any activity in the thalamus, an important center in pain mediation, which was activated in the afore mentioned study of Rosen et al.[40] during and after angina pectoris. This is probably due to the small sample size, in combination with the nature of the stimulus given, which is not noxious and therefore not severe enough to arouse thalamic activity.[41] A very important finding however, is changed rCBF in the hypothalamic region, which is also believed to play an important role in mediation of pain and which has direct spinal input.[42] It is of interest to notice, that an increase in rCBF is described by Rosen et al.[40] during angina, whereas we found a decrease in rCBF following spinal cord stimulation. Both effects seem opposite to each other and it may be, that this finding indicates a resetting by spinal cord stimulation at hypothalamic level and in some way results in reduction of anginal pain.

Conclusions

PET imaging enables us to reveal some details of the effect of spinal cord stimulation on the myocardium and the central nervous system. The studies described in this chapter should be regarded as pilot studies and need to be continued. However, the results we discussed here allow us to conclude that spinal cord stimulation alters distribution of myocardial blood flow: an anti-ischemic action may be caused by homogenization of myocardial flow, although total flow does not change. Futhermore, we were able to detect, only in a small number of patients, changes in rCBF as a response to spinal cord stimulation. This gives us a clue to which cerebral regions may be involved in its action. However, it remains to be investigated which parts of the central nervous system may account for a possible anti-ischemic effect of spinal cord stimulation.

References

1. Silverman KJ, Grossman W. Angina pectoris - natural history and strategies for evaluation and management. N Engl J Med 1984;310:1712-7.
2. Kirklin JW, Naftel DC, Blackstone EH, Pohost GM. Summary of a consensus concerning death and ischemic events after coronary artery bypass grafting. Circulation 1989;79(Suppl I):I-81-I-91.
3. Foster ED. Reoperation for coronary artery disease. Circulation 1985;72(Suppl V):V-57-V-64.
4. Melzack R, Wall PD. Pain mechanisms: a new theory. Science 1965;150:971-9.
5. Wagman IH, Price DD. Responses of dorsal horn cells of M. Mulatta to cutaneous and sural nerve A and C fibre stimulation. J Neurophysiol 1969;32:803-17.
6. Handwerkert HO, Iggo A, Zimmerman M. Segmental and supraspinal actions on dorsal horn neurons responding to noxious and non-noxious skin stimulation. Pain 1975;1:147-65.
7. Woolf CJ, Wall PD. Chronic peripheral nerve section diminishes the primary afferent A-fibre mediated inhibition of rat dorsal horn neurones. Brain Res 1982;242:77-85.
8. Wall PD, Sweet Wh. Temporary abolitoin of pain in man. Science 1967;155:108-9.
9. Shealy CN, Mortimer JT, Reswick JB. Electrical inhibition of pain by stimulation of the dorsal columns. Anesth Analg 1967;46:489-91.
10. Cook AW, Oygar A, Baggenstos P, Pacheco S, Kleriga E. Vascular disease of extremities: electrical stimulation of spinal cord and dorsal roots. New Y State J Med 1976;76:366-8.
11. Dooley D, Kasprak M. Modification of blood flow to the extremities by electrical stimulation of the nervous system. Southern Med J 1976;69:1309-11.
12. Jacobs MJ, Jorning PJ, Joshi SR, Kitslaar PJ, Slaaf DW, Reneman RS. Epidural spinal cord electrial stimulation improves microvascular blood flow in severe limb ischemia. Ann Surg 1988;207:179-83.
13. Murphy DF, Giles KE. Dorsal column stimulation for pain relief from intractable angina pectoris. Pain 1987;28:365-8.
14. Mannheimer C, Augustinsson LE, Carlsson CA, Manhem K, Wilhelmsson C. Epidural spinal electrial stimulation in severe angina pectoris Br Heart J 1988;59:56-61.
15. Gonzáles-Darder JM, Canela P, Gonzáles-Martinez V. High cervical spinal cord stimulation for unstable angina pectoris. Stereotact Funct Neurosurg 1991;56:20-7.
16. Sanderson JE, Brooksby P, Waterhouse D, Palmer RGB, Neubauer K. Epidural spinal electria stimulation for severe angina: a study of its effect on symptoms, exercise tolerance and degree of ischemia. Eur Heart J 1992;13:628-33.
17. DeJongste MJL, Hautvast RWM, Hillege JL, Lie KI on behalf of the working group on neurocardiology. Efficacy of spinal cord stimulation as adjuvant therapy for intractable angina pectoris. J Am Coll Cardiol 1994;23:1592-7.
18. DeJongste MJL, Haaksma J, Hautvast RWM et al. Effects of spinal cord stimulation on myocardial ischemia during daily life in patients with severe coronary artery disease - a prospective ambulatory electrocardiographic study. Br Heart J 1994;71:413-8.
19. Chauhan A, Mullins PA, Thuraisingham SI, Taylor G, Petch MC, Schofield PM. Effect of transcutaneous electrical nerve stimulation on coronary blood flow. Circulation 1994;89:694-702.
20. Chandler MJ, Brennan TJ, Garrison DW, Kim KS, Schwartz P, Foreman RD. A mechanism of cardiac pain suppression by spinal cord stimulation: implications for patients with angina pectoris. Eur Heart J 1993;14:96-105.
21. Morgan JL, Cohen DR, Hempstead JL, Curran T. Mapping of patterns of c-fos expression in the central nervous system after seizure. Science 1987;237:192-7.

22. Sheng M, Greenberg ME. The regulation and function of c-fos and other immediate early genes in the nervous system. Neuron 1990;4:477-85.
23. Hautvast RWM, Homminga SA, DeJongste MJL et al. C-fos expression in the central nervous system of the rat after myocardial infarction and neurostimulation. Eur Heart J 1994;15:284 (Abstract).
24. Ter Horst GJ, Van den Brink, Homminga SA et al. Transneuronal viral labeling of rat heart left ventricle controlling pathways. Neuro Report 1993;4:1307-10.
25. Augustinsson LE. Spinal cord electrical stimulation in severe angina pectoris: surgical technique, interoperative physiology, complications, and side effect. PACE 1989;12:693-5.
26. DeJongste MJL, Staal MJ. Preliminary results of a randomized study on the clinical efficacy of spinal cord stimulation for refractory severe angina pectoris. Acta Neurochir 1993;58:161-4.
27. Blanksma PK, Willemsen ATM, Meeder JG et al. Quantitative myocardial mapping of perfusion and metabolism using parametric polar map displays in cardiac PET. J Nucl Med (In press).
28. Porenta G, Kuhle W, Czernin J et al. Semiquantitative assessment of myocardial blood flow and viability using polar map displays of cardiac PET images. J Nucl Med 1992;33:1628-36.
29. Bellina RC, Parodi O, Camici P et al. Simultaneous in vitro and in vivo validation of nitrogen-13-ammonia for the assessment of regional myocardial blood flow. J Nucl Med 1990;31:1335-43.
30. Galassi AR, Crea F, Araujo LI et al. Comparison of regional myocardial blood flow in syndrome X and one-vessel coronary artery disease. Am J Cardiol 1993;72:134-9.
31. Meeder JG, Blanksma PK, Anthonio RL et al. Myocardial perfusion dynamics and heart rate variability in syndrome X: evidence for anatomic and endothelial dysfunction. J Am Coll Cardiol 1994;special issue:161A (Abstract).
32. Czernin J, Müller P, Chan S et al. Influence of age and hemodynamics on myocardial blood flow and flow reserve. Circulation 1993;88:62-9.
33. De Landsheere C, Mannheimer C, Habets A et al. Effect of spinal cord stimulation on regional myocardial perfusion assessed by positron emission tomography. Am J Cardiol 1992;69:1143-9.
34. Crea F, Pupita G, Galassi AR et al. Role of adenosine in pathogenesis of anginal pain. Circulation 1990;81:164-72.
35. Maseri A, Crea F, Kaski JC, Davies G. Mechanisms and significance of cardiac ischemic pain. Prog Cardiovasc Dis 1992;35:1-18.
36. Friston KJ, Frith CD, Liddle PF, Lammertsma AA, Dolan RD, Frackowiak RSJ. The relationship between local and global changes in PEt scans. J Cereb Blood Flow Metab 1990;10:458-66.
37. Friston KJ, Frith CD, Liddle PF, Frackowiak RSJ. Comparing functional (PET) images: assessment of significant change. J Cereb Blood Flow Metab 1991;11:690-9.
38. Friston KJ, Passingham RE, Nutt JG, Heather JD, Sawle GV, Frackowiak RSJ. Localisation in PET images: direct fitting of the intercommussural (AC-PC) line. J Cereb Blood Flow Metab 1989;9:690-5.
39. Talaraich J, Tournoux P. A co-planar stereotactic atlas of the human brain. Stuttgard, FRG: Thieme, 1988.
40. Rosen SD, Paulesu E, Frith CD et al. Central nervous pathways mediating angina pectoris. Lancet 1994;344:147-50.
41. Coghill RC, Talbot JD, Evans AC et al. Distributed processing of pain and vibration by the human brain. J Neurosci 1994;14:4095-108.

42. Giesler Jr GJ, Katter JT, Dado RJ. Direct spinal pathways to the limbic system for nociceptive information. Trends Neurosci 1994;17:244-50.

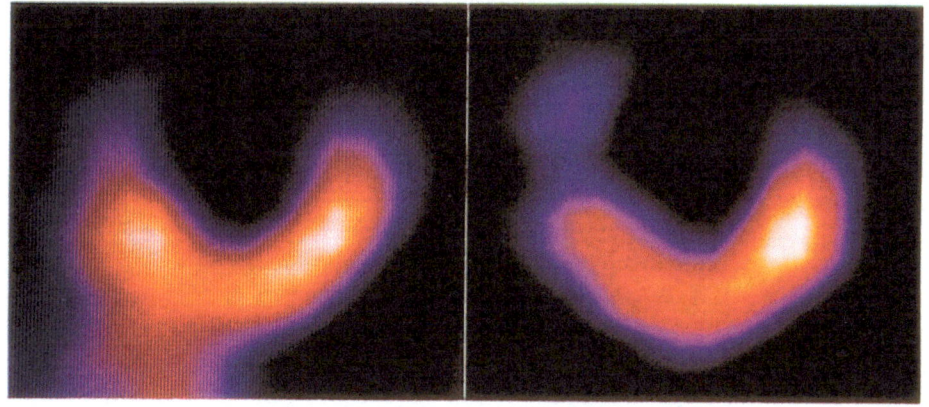

rest perfusion   ml/min/100 g

stress perfusion   ml/min/100 g

glucose uptake   uM/min/100 g

mismatch   S.D.

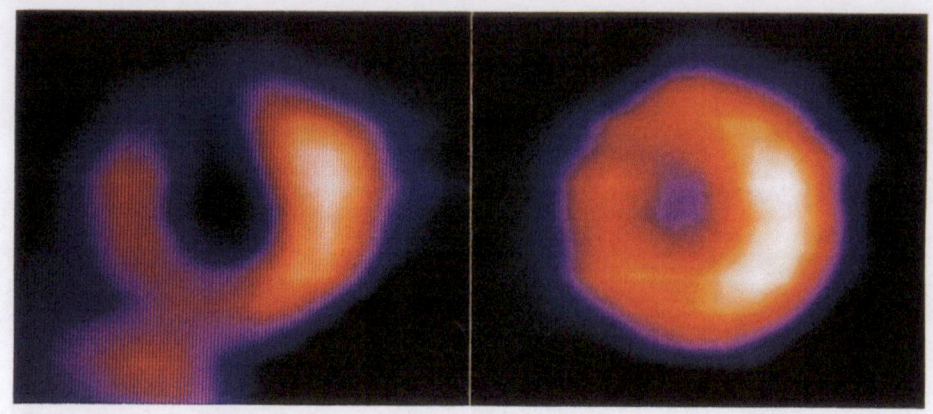

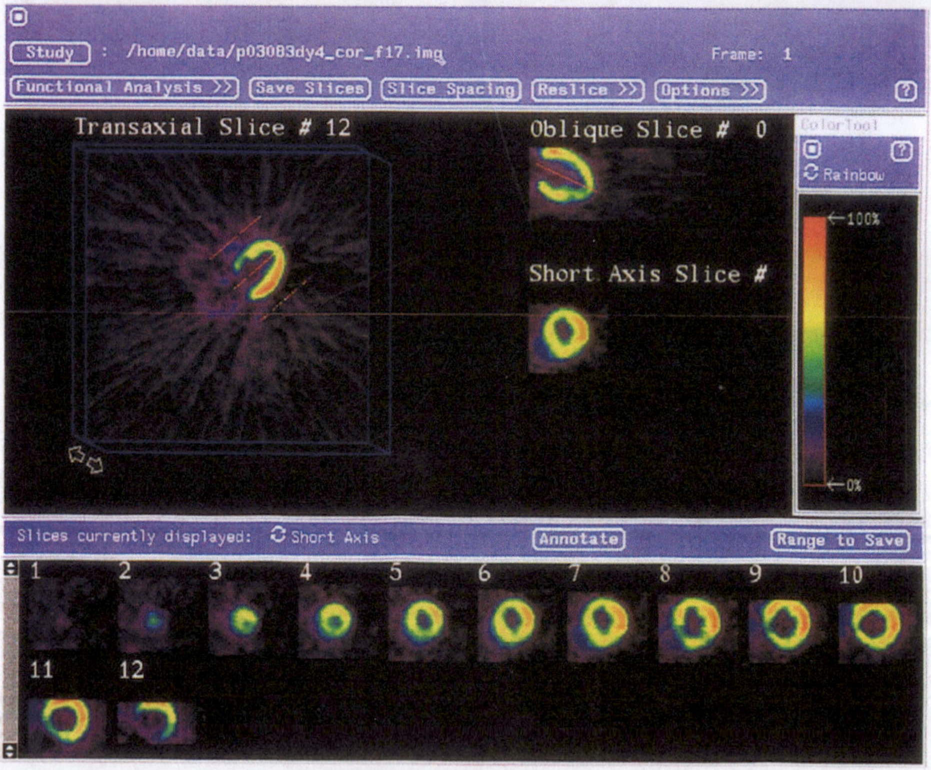

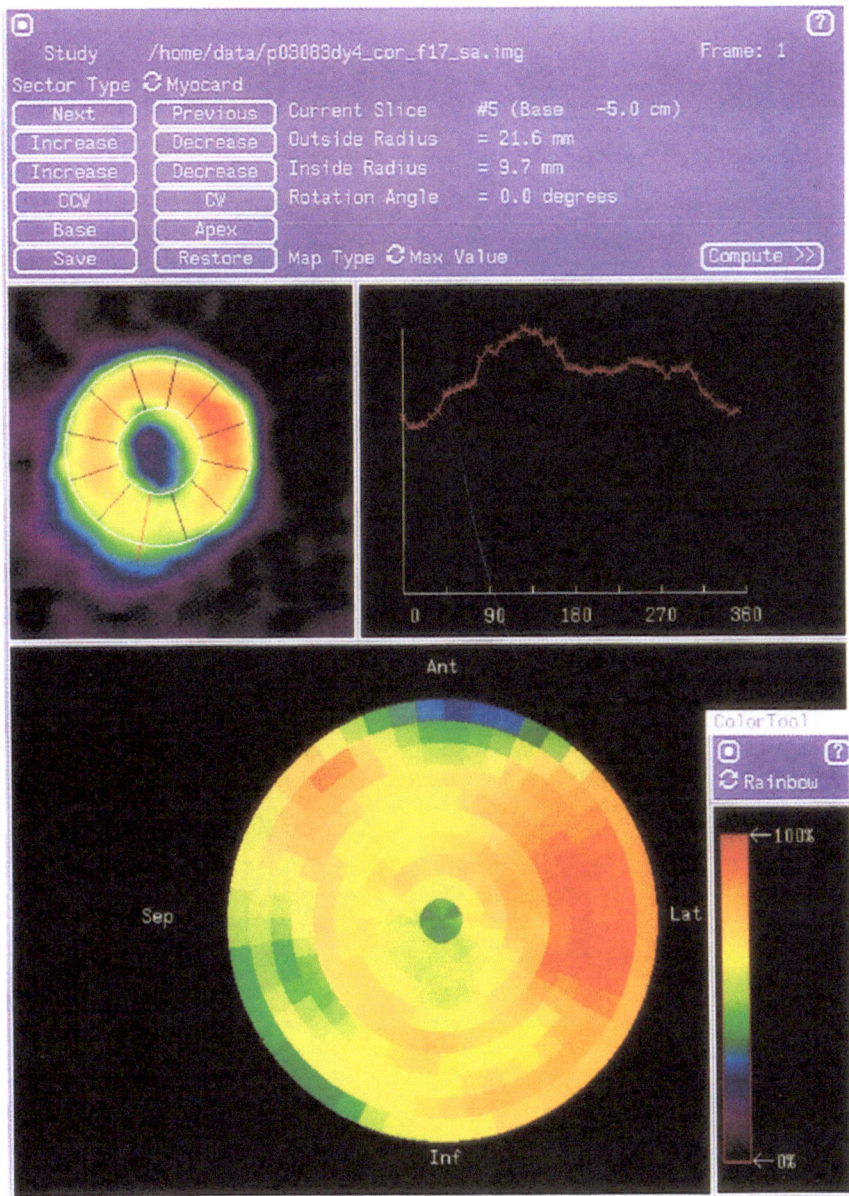

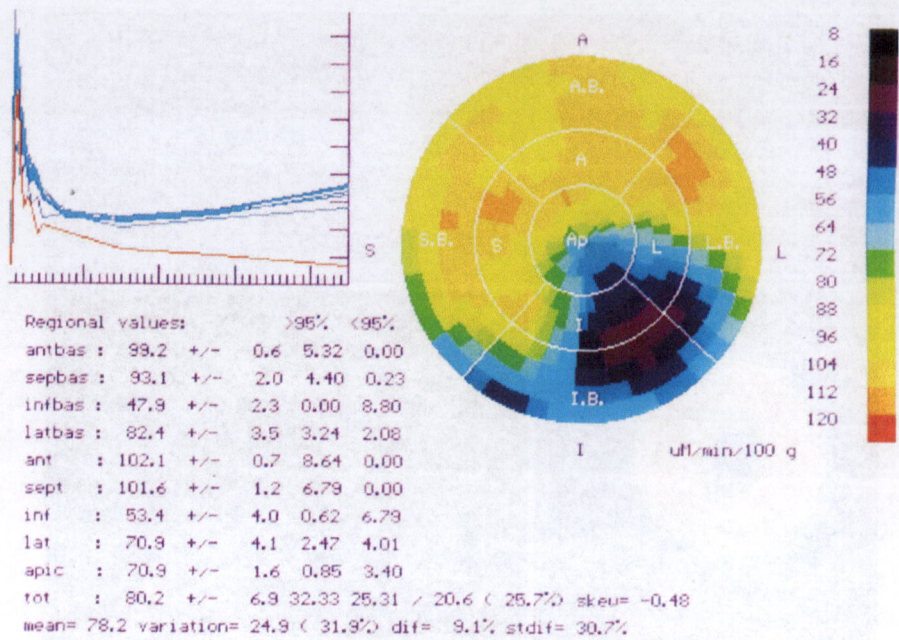

```
Regional values:              >95%  <95%
antbas :  99.2  +/-   0.6  5.32  0.00
sepbas :  93.1  +/-   2.0  4.40  0.23
infbas :  47.9  +/-   2.3  0.00  8.80
latbas :  82.4  +/-   3.5  3.24  2.08
ant    : 102.1  +/-   0.7  8.64  0.00
sept   : 101.6  +/-   1.2  6.79  0.00
inf    :  53.4  +/-   4.0  0.62  6.79
lat    :  70.9  +/-   4.1  2.47  4.01
apic   :  70.9  +/-   1.6  0.85  3.40
tot    :  80.2  +/-   6.9 32.33 25.31 / 20.6 ( 25.7%) skew= -0.48
mean= 78.2 variation= 24.9 ( 31.9%) dif=  9.1% stdif= 30.7%
```

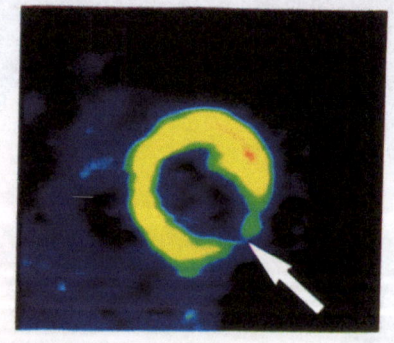

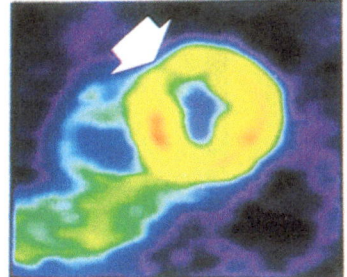

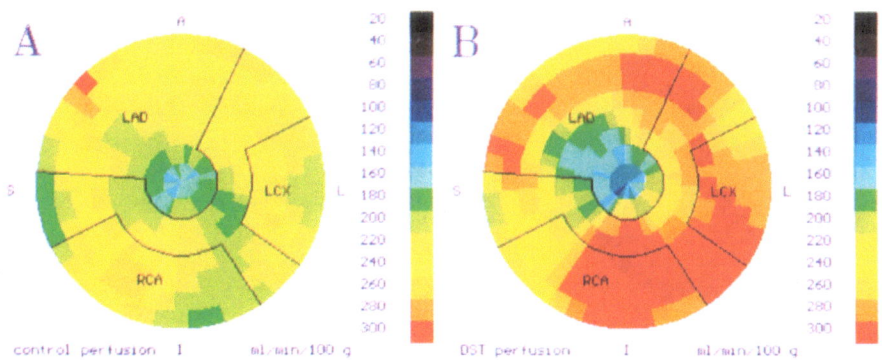

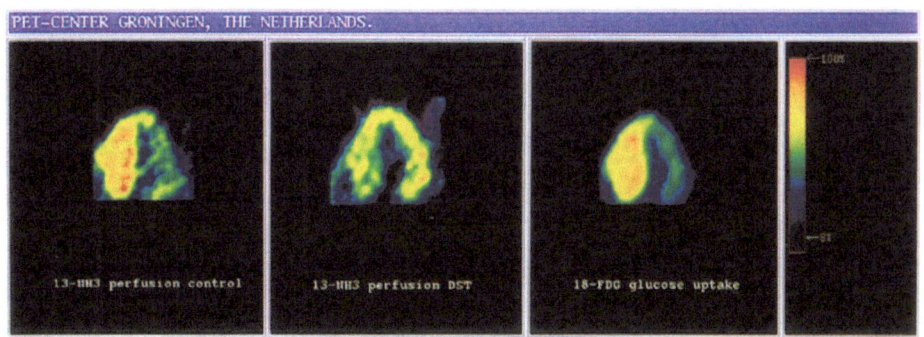

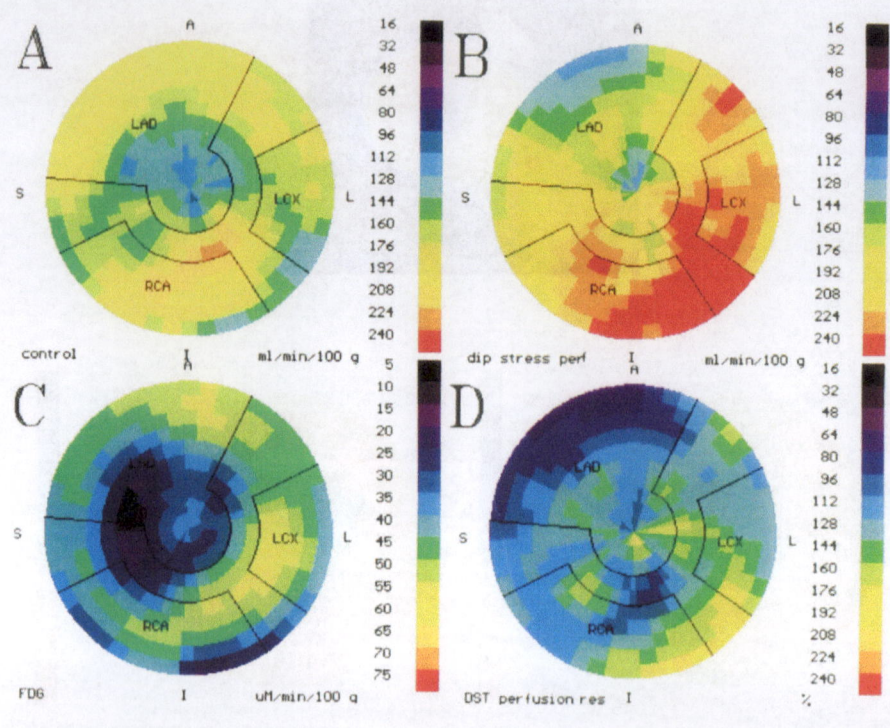

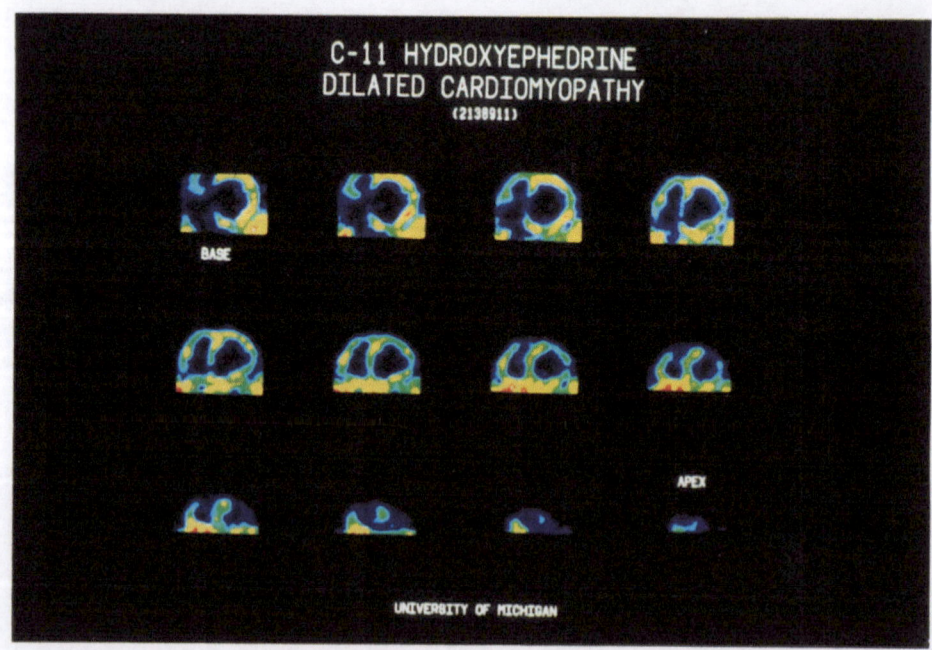

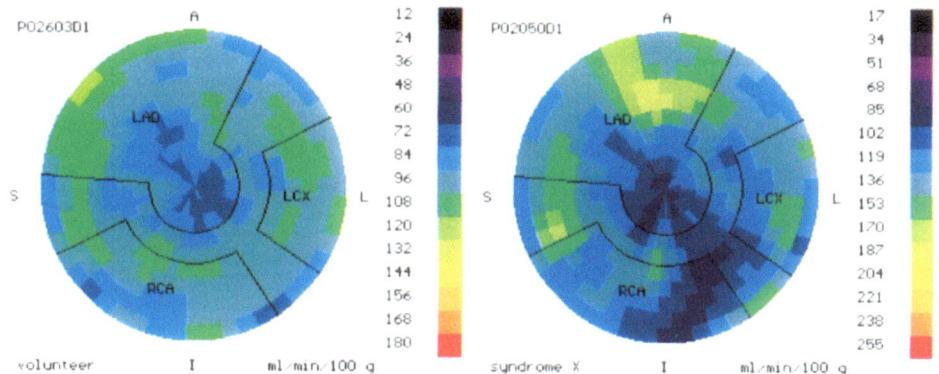

Developments in Cardiovascular Medicine

Developments in Cardiovascular Medicine

121. S. Sideman, R. Beyar and A.G. Kleber (eds.): *Cardiac Electrophysiology, Circulation, and Transport*. Proceedings of the 7th Henry Goldberg Workshop (Berne, Switzerland, 1990). 1991   ISBN 0-7923-1145-0
122. D.M. Bers: *Excitation-Contraction Coupling and Cardiac Contractile Force*. 1991
                                                                    ISBN 0-7923-1186-8
123. A.-M. Salmasi and A.N. Nicolaides (eds.): *Occult Atherosclerotic Disease*. Diagnosis, Assessment and Management. 1991   ISBN 0-7923-1188-4
124. J.A.E. Spaan: *Coronary Blood Flow*. Mechanics, Distribution, and Control. 1991
                                                                    ISBN 0-7923-1210-4
125. R.W. Stout (ed.): *Diabetes and Atherosclerosis*. 1991   ISBN 0-7923-1310-0
126. A.G. Herman (ed.): *Antithrombotics*. Pathophysiological Rationale for Pharmacological Interventions. 1991   ISBN 0-7923-1413-1
127. N.H.J. Pijls: *Maximal Myocardial Perfusion as a Measure of the Functional Significance of Coronary Arteriogram*. From a Pathoanatomic to a Pathophysiologic Interpretation of the Coronary Arteriogram. 1991   ISBN 0-7923-1430-1
128. J.H.C. Reiber and E.E. v.d. Wall (eds.): *Cardiovascular Nuclear Medicine and MRI*. Quantitation and Clinical Applications. 1992   ISBN 0-7923-1467-0
129. E. Andries, P. Brugada and R. Stroobrandt (eds.): *How to Face 'the Faces' of Cardiac Pacing*. 1992   ISBN 0-7923-1528-6
130. M. Nagano, S. Mochizuki and N.S. Dhalla (eds.): *Cardiovascular Disease in Diabetes*. 1992   ISBN 0-7923-1554-5
131. P.W. Serruys, B.H. Strauss and S.B. King III (eds.): *Restenosis after Intervention with New Mechanical Devices*. 1992   ISBN 0-7923-1555-3
132. P.J. Walter (ed.): *Quality of Life after Open Heart Surgery*. 1992
                                                                    ISBN 0-7923-1580-4
133. E.E. van der Wall, H. Sochor, A. Righetti and M.G. Niemeyer (eds.): *What's new in Cardiac Imaging?* SPECT, PET and MRI. 1992   ISBN 0-7923-1615-0
134. P. Hanrath, R. Uebis and W. Krebs (eds.): *Cardiovascular Imaging by Ultrasound*. 1992   ISBN 0-7923-1755-6
135. F.H. Messerli (ed.): *Cardiovascular Disease in the Elderly*. 3rd ed. 1992
                                                                    ISBN 0-7923-1859-5
136. J. Hess and G.R. Sutherland (eds.): *Congenital Heart Disease in Adolescents and Adults*. 1992   ISBN 0-7923-1862-5
137. J.H.C. Reiber and P.W. Serruys (eds.): *Advances in Quantitative Coronary Arteriography*. 1993   ISBN 0-7923-1863-3
138. A.-M. Salmasi and A.S. Iskandrian (eds.): *Cardiac Output and Regional Flow in Health and Disease*. 1993   ISBN 0-7923-1911-7
139. J.H. Kingma, N.M. van Hemel and K.I. Lie (eds.): *Atrial Fibrillation, a Treatable Disease?* 1992   ISBN 0-7923-2008-5
140. B. Ostadel and N.S. Dhalla (eds.): *Heart Function in Health and Disease*. Proceedings of the Cardiovascular Program (Prague, Czechoslovakia, 1991). 1992
                                                                    ISBN 0-7923-2052-2
141. D. Noble and Y.E. Earm (eds.): *Ionic Channels and Effect of Taurine on the Heart*. Proceedings of an International Symposium (Seoul, Korea , 1992). 1993
                                                                    ISBN 0-7923-2199-5
142. H.M. Piper and C.J. Preusse (eds.): *Ischemia-reperfusion in Cardiac Surgery*. 1993
                                                                    ISBN 0-7923-2241-X
143. J. Roelandt, E.J. Gussenhoven and N. Bom (eds.): *Intravascular Ultrasound*. 1993
                                                                    ISBN 0-7923-2301-7
144. M.E. Safar and M.F. O'Rourke (eds.): *The Arterial System in Hypertension*. 1993
                                                                    ISBN 0-7923-2343-2
145. P.W. Serruys, D.P. Foley and P.J. de Feyter (eds.): *Quantitative Coronary Angiography in Clinical Practice*. With a Foreword by Spencer B. King III. 1994
                                                                    ISBN 0-7923-2368-8

Developments in Cardiovascular Medicine

Previous volumes are still available

KLUWER ACADEMIC PUBLISHERS – DORDRECHT / BOSTON / LONDON